WI 529 BAA

DATE DUE

Multidisciplinary Treatment
of Colorectal Cancer

Gunnar Baatrup

Editor

Multidisciplinary Treatment of Colorectal Cancer

Staging – Treatment – Pathology – Palliation

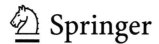 Springer

Editor
Gunnar Baatrup, DMSC
Institute of regional Health Science
University of Southern Denmark
Odense
Denmark

Department of Surgery A
Odense University Hospital
Svendborg
Denmark

Co-Editors
Regina G.H. Beets-Tan, MD, PhD
Department of Radiology
Maastricht University Medical Center
Maastricht
The Nederlands

Hartwig Kørner, MD, PhD
Division of Colorectal Surgery
Department of Gastrointestinal Surgery
Stavanger University Hospital
Stavanger
Norway

Department of Clinical Medicine
University of Bergen
Bergen
Norway

Iris D. Nagtegaal, MD, PhD
Department of Pathology
Radboud University Nijmegen
Medical Center
Nijmegen
The Nederlands

Per Peiffer, MD, PhD
Department of Oncology
Odense University Hospital and
Institute of Clinical Research
University of Southern Denmark
Odense
Denmark

Lars Påhlman, MD, PhD
Department of Surgery
University Hospital of Uppsala
Uppsala
Sweden

ISBN 978-3-319-06141-2   ISBN 978-3-319-06142-9   (eBook)
DOI 10.1007/978-3-319-06142-9
Springer Cham Heidelberg New York Dordrecht London

Library of Congress Control Number: 2014945211

Foreword

During the last 15–20 years, the treatment of colorectal cancer has changed dramatically. From involving almost only surgeons in the treatment, the scientific progress in adjuvant therapy, neoadjuvant therapy, diagnostics and pathology now set the demand for a broader approach when deciding the treatment for the individual patient.

The Calman and Hine report from 1995 [1] first argued for the multidisciplinary approach and has now been implemented in many countries throughout the world and in fact sets the golden standard for modern oncological treatment for all forms of cancer. In the field of rectal cancer, solid documentation exists for the efficacy of this approach in terms of local recurrence rates [2–4]. The reasons for this could be more accurate staging with MRI and ultrasound, the use of neoadjuvant radiochemotherapy – sometimes in selected patients – and, not at least, the evaluations of operative specimens in order to be sure that the correct operative technique has been used [5]. The effect on the improvement in surgical techniques, dissecting in the correct embryological planes, also plays a role for this improvement [6] not only in rectal but also in colonic cancer surgery [7] – although never proven in a proper randomised trial. The use of postoperative adjuvant chemotherapy [8] and the more aggressive approach to salvage surgery and other effective treatments for metastatic disease has become common practise [9]. Apart from these already-achieved improvements, we will, in the future, hear a lot about selective individual therapy based on tumour markers and individual genotypes [10, 11].

In the context of the multidisciplinary approach to colorectal cancer, it seems obvious to have multidisciplinary team conferences – the so-called MDT conference. This has during the last couple of years been introduced in every centre dealing with colorectal cancer treatment with its many different modalities and is in many places a part of the daily practice. Every speciality involved in the handling of these patients is represented – surgery, medical and radiation oncology, pathology, radiology, nuclear medicine, clinical genetics and specialised nurses. The structure on the meetings is locally organised and guidelines for MDT conferences have been launched [12]. In some places a dedicated co-ordinator is nominated and gets special salary for the job [13]. The conferences are ideal forums for discussion and not at least education of younger doctors, and communications between the specialities are thought to be improved [14, 15]. Even though one has to consider the time spent at these conferences and whether it really is cost-effective seen from the patient's point of view [15]. The MDT approach for treatment strategy has been proven to enhance the quality of the operative specimens as regarded from the proportion of circumferential margin (CRM) positivity [16], but whether this is due to the MDT conference itself or just reflects the results of the MDT thinking is unknown. It has been proven that patients which have been objects for a MDT conference have a significant better survival, as compared to patients that did not [17]. These results are to be taken with great reserve due to the historical design of the study, which enhances the risk of bias considerably. During the same period, many new treatment modalities have been introduced such as better anaesthesia, better surgery and fast-track surgery. A proper randomised trial will never be performed due to lack of acceptance and equipoise – not at least among doctors but perhaps also among patients. It is strange that only this study evaluating the efficacy of MDT conference exists, but perhaps others are on their way, now that the MDT approach has gained broad acceptance.

The approach demands training both in organising and in uniforming the language of the different specialities. In this respect national guidelines might be important, although the level of evidences does not seem to improve during the years [18]. National MDT courses and training programmes have been introduced in several countries, and with this book as a backbone for this training, we probably can get even better – although it is difficult to prove. Anyway the MDT conference has probably come to stay.

Copenhagen, NV, Denmark   Peer Wille-Jørgensen, Dr Med Sci

References

1. Calman K, Hine D. A policy framework for commissioning cancer services. London: Department of Health; 1995.
2. Nicholls RJ, Tekkis PP. Multidisciplinary treatment of cancer of the rectum: a European approach. Surg Oncol Clin N Am. 2008;17(3):533–51, viii.
3. Nicholls J. The multidisciplinary management of rectal cancer. Colorectal Dis. 2008;10(4):311–3.
4. Valentini V, Glimelius B, Minsky BD, Van Cutsem E, Bartelink H, Beets-Tan RG, et al. The multidisciplinary rectal cancer treatment: main convergences, controversial aspects and investigational areas which support the need for an European Consensus. Radiother Oncol. 2005;76(3):241–50.
5. Quirke P, Steele R, Monson J, Grieve R, Khanna S, Couture J, et al. Effect of the plane of surgery achieved on local recurrence in patients with operable rectal cancer: a prospective study using data from the MRC CR07 and NCIC-CTG CO16 randomised clinical trial. Lancet. 2009;373(9666):821–8.
6. Daniels IR, Fisher SE, Heald RJ, Moran BJ. Accurate staging, selective preoperative therapy and optimal surgery improves outcome in rectal cancer: a review of the recent evidence. Colorectal Dis. 2007;9(4):290–301.
7. Hohenberger W, Reingruber B, Merkel S. Surgery for colon cancer. Scand J Surg. 2003;92(1):45–52.
8. Gravalos C, Garcia-Escobar I, Garcia-Alfonso P, Cassinello J, Malon D, Carrato A. Adjuvant chemotherapy for stages II, III and IV of colon cancer. Clin Transl Oncol. 2009;11(8):526–33.
9. Segelman J, Singnomklao T, Hellborg H, Martling A. Differences in MDT assessment and treatment between patients with stage IV colon and rectal cancer. Colorectal Dis. 2008;11(7):768–74.

10. Prenen H, Tejpar S, Van Cutsem E. Impact of molecular markers on treatment selection in advanced colorectal cancer. Eur J Cancer. 2009;45(Suppl 1):70–78.
11. Ortega J, Vigil CE, Chodkiewicz C. Current progress in targeted therapy for colorectal cancer. Cancer Control. 2010;17(1):7–15.
12. Ruhstaller T, Roe H, Thurlimann B, Nicoll JJ. The multidisciplinary meeting: an indispensable aid to communication between different specialities. Eur J Cancer. 2006;42(15):2459–62.
13. Soukop M, Robinson A, Soukop D, Ingham-Clark CL, Kelly MJ. Results of a survey of the role of multidisciplinary team coordinators for colorectal cancer in England and Wales. Colorectal Dis. 2007;9(2):146–50.
14. Sharma A, Sharp DM, Walker LG, Monson JR. Colorectal MDTs: the team's perspective. Colorectal Dis. 2008;10(1):63–8.
15. Cheifetz RE, Phang PT. Evaluating learning and knowledge retention after a continuing medical education course on total mesorectal excision for surgeons. Am J Surg. 2006;191(5):687–90.
16. Burton S, Brown G, Daniels IR, Norman AR, Mason B, Cunningham D. MRI directed multidisciplinary team preoperative treatment strategy: the way to eliminate positive circumferential margins? Br J Cancer. 2006;94(3):351–7.
17. Macdermid E, Hooton G, Macdonald M, McKay G, Grose D, Mohammed N, et al. Improving patient survival with the colorectal cancer multi-disciplinary team. Colorectal Dis. 2009;11:291–5.
18. Wille-Jorgensen P. Evidence-based colorectal surgery–facts, fiction or wishful thinking. Colorectal Dis. 2010;12(4):285–6.

Preface

The multidisciplinary team (MDT) approach to rectal or colorectal cancer treatment is becoming the gold standard. It has become mandatory for institutions treating these diseases in more countries and the term is now well established within the involved medical disciplines. The concept has become self-assertive as the number of possible treatments and combinations of treatments have increased. More treatment modalities mean more choices and therefore higher demands to the preoperative staging of the disease and assessment of the patient's physics and preferences.

Multidisciplinarity is defined in the Wikipedia encyclopedia as "a non-integrative mixture of disciplines in that each discipline retains its methodologies and assumptions without change or development from other disciplines within the multidisciplinary relationship". It has been discussed if the correct term should be "interdisciplinary" because "interdisciplinarity blends the practices and assumptions of each discipline involved". The established teams will, with time, have more and more difficulties in defining the interrelationships and their effects on the process leading to decisions at the MDT meetings. No matter what the correct term is, the collaboration is an important means to determine the best treatment, to develop future treatments and to educate the future MDT members.

I was introduced to surgery and colorectal cancer patients by Dr. Carl Zimmermann-Nielsen, DMSc, at Svendborg Hospital in Denmark many years ago. He taught some strange principles of colorectal cancer treatment which seemed quite old fashioned at that time: He emphasised the importance of individualising the treatment. He executed this based on his experience and intuition. At that time, we, youngsters, were learning new words as "evidence based". To our best knowledge it meant that there was only one "best treatment" and this should be offered to all patients without discrimination. We are now beginning to reach the same level of wisdom as that of Carl's, but this time, to some extent, based upon evidence. He also meant that monkeys could be taught the scientific part of patient treatment and that "the art of medicine" was the difficult part. It might have been true then, but our knowledge has grown and even the cleverest monkey will encounter difficulties now. Nevertheless, the art of medicine is still crucial, in particular in the relations with cancer patients and their relatives.

Carl also taught us that whenever you divide a responsibility between two persons, they will be left with approximately five percentages each. This is one of the main dangers of multidisciplinary handling of patients and should be prevented by all means. We will have to prove him wrong on this one in the years to come, and this is actually one of the motivations for this book.

Some of the top European doctors and scientists have agreed to participate in the writing of this book, all of them with experience, dedication and pronounced influence on the development of the MDT concept as well as other aspects of high-quality, individualised treatment of colorectal cancer patients. The book is intended for the MDT members and for those training in the fields of colorectal cancer management. The book presents updated important knowledge but is not intended to be comprehensive within the different disciplines. Focus has been on controversies and on the aspects of common interests amongst the MDT members.

It is the main obligation for any MDT to provide the best possible treatment and care and to implement evidence-based principles whenever possible. It may seem somewhat conflicting that evidence-based principles have to be the foundation of MDT discussions, whereas at the same time we have to admit that the concept of formalised MDT meetings in itself is yet not very strongly evidence based. The near future will provide us with the necessary evidence.

Svendborg, Denmark   Gunnar Baatrup, DMSC

Contents

Part III   Oncology

Part IV   Imaging and Staging

Part V   Pathology

Contributors

Gunnar Baatrup, DMSC Institute of Regional Health Science, University of Southern Denmark, Odense, Denmark

Department of Surgery A, Odense University Hospital, Svendborg, Denmark

Regina G.H. Beets-Tan, MD, PhD Department of Radiology, Maastricht University Medical Center, Maastricht, The Netherlands

Thomas Borschitz, MD Department of Surgery and Coloproctology, Centre of Competence and Reference of Coloproctology, German Clinic for Diagnostic, Wiesbaden, Germany

Gina Brown Department of Radiology, Royal Marsden Hospital, Sutton, Surrey, UK

Christopher Cunningham, MD, FRCSEd Department of Colorectal Surgery, John Radcliffe Hospital, Headington, Oxford, UK

P.G. Doornebosch Department of Surgery, IJsselland Hospital, Capelle a/d IJssel, The Netherlands

Birger Henning Endreseth, MD, PhD Department of Surgery, St. Olavs University Hospital, Trondheim, Norway

Marie-Louise Feddern Department of Surgery P, Aarhus University Hospital, Aarhus, Denmark

Bengt Glimelius, MD, PhD Department of Radiology, Oncology and Radiation Science, Uppsala University, Akademiska Sjukhuset, Uppsala, Sweden

Department of Oncology and Pathology, Karolinska Institutet, Stockholm, Sweden

Robert Glynne-Jones, FRCR Department of Radiotherapy, Centre for Cancer Treatment, Mount Vernon Hospital, Northwood, Middlesex, UK

E.J.R. de Graaf Department of Surgery, IJsselland Hospital, Capelle a/d IJssel, The Netherlands

Dagny Faksvåg Haugen, MD, PhD Regional Centre of Excellence
for Palliative Care, Western Norway, Haukeland University Hospital,
Bergen, Norway
European Palliative Care Research Centre, Department of Cancer Research
and Molecular Medicine, Faculty of Medicine, Norwegian University of
Science and Technology, Trondheim, Norway

K. Havenga Department of Surgery, University Medical Center Groningen,
Groningen, The Netherlands

R.J. Heald Pelican Cancer Foundation, The Ark Conference Centre,
Basingstoke, Hampshire, UK

P.E.A. Hermsen Department of Surgery, IJsselland Hospital,
Capelle a/d IJssel, The Netherlands

Roel Hompes, MD Department of Colorectal Surgery,
John Radcliffe Hospital, Headington, Oxford, UK

Rob Hughes, FRCR Department of Radiotherapy, Centre for Cancer
treatment, Mount Vermon Hospital, Northwood, Middlesex, UK

Chris Hunter Department of Radiology, Royal Marsden Hospital,
Sutton, Surrey, UK

Hartwig Kørner, MD, PhD, Division of Colorectal Surgery,
Department of Gastrointestinal Surgery, Stavanger University Hospital,
Stavanger, Norway
Department of Clinical Medicine, University of Bergen, Bergen, Norway
Regional Centre of Excellence for Palliative Care Western Norway,
Haukeland University Hospital, Bergen, Norway

Cord Langner Institute of Pathology, Medical University of Graz, Graz,
Austria

Søren Laurberg Department of Surgery P, Aarhus University Hospital,
Aarhus, Denmark

Brendan J. Moran Basingstoke and North Hampshire NHS Foundation
Trust, Pelican Cancer Foundation, Basingstoke, Hampshire, UK

Iris D. Nagtegaal, MD, PhD Department of Pathology, Radboud
University Nijmegen Medical Center, Nijmegen, The Netherlands

J. Nonner Department of Surgery, IJsselland Hospital, Capelle a/d Ijssel,
The Netherlands

Per Pfeiffer, MD, PhD Department of Oncology,
Odense University Hospital, Odense, Denmark

Lars Påhlmann, MD, PhD Department of Surgery,
University Hospital of Uppsala, Uppsala, Sweden

Philip Quirke Section of Pathology and Tumour Biology,
Leeds Institute of Cancer and Pathology, University of Leeds, Leeds, UK

Niels Qvist, DMSci Department of Surgery, Odense University Hospital,
Odense, Denmark

Camilla Qvortrup Department of Oncology, Odense University Hospital,
Odense, Denmark

Rune Sjödahl Department of Surgery, Linköping University, Linköping,
Sweden

Rune Svensen Department of Gastroenterological and Acute Surgery,
Haukeland University Hospital, Bergen, Norway

Jon Arne Søreide, MD, PhD, FACS Department of Clinical Medicine,
University of Bergen, Bergen, Norway

Division of HPB Surgery, Department of Gastrointestinal Surgery,
Stavanger University Hospital, Stavanger, Norway

Josep Tabernero Department of Medical Oncology, Vall d'Hebron
University Hospital, Vall d'Hebron Institute of Oncology, Barselona, Spain

Ion Vasile, PhD The 7th Department (Surgical Specialities),
University of Medicine and Pharmacy of Craiova, Craiova, Romania

Michael Vieth Klinikum Bayreuth, Institute of Pathology,
Bayreuth, Germany

Ionica Daniel Vilcea, PhD The 7th Department (Surgical Specialities),
University of Medicine and Pharmacy of Craiova, Craiova, Romania

J.E.R. Waage Department of Surgery, Haukeland University Hospital,
Bergen, Norway

Nicholas P. West Section of Pathology and Tumour Biology,
Leeds Institute of Cancer and Pathology, University of Leeds, Leeds, UK

Arne Wibe Department of Surgery, Sct. Olav University Hospital,
Norwegian University of Science and Technology, Trondheim, Norway

T. Wiggers Department of Surgery, University Medical Center Groningen,
Groningen, The Netherlands

P. Wille-Jørgensen Department of Surgery K, Bispebjerg Hospital,
Copenhagen, Denmark

Part I

Multidisciplinary Treatment of Colorectal Cancer

Organizing the Multidisciplinary Team

Gunnar Baatrup

Abstract

The multidisciplinary colorectal cancer team (CRC MDT) decides the treatment strategy after the disease has been diagnosed, classified, and staged by the team members. It also executes quality control after the treatment has been completed. The core MDT team consists of colorectal surgeons, oncologists, radiologists, and pathologists [3]. Some institutions also include patient care representatives and other disciplines in the team as they take on other obligations concerning the patient's way from referral to discharge from the last follow-up visit [3].

The team should ensure that decisions are evidence based whenever possible and the decisions are based upon all necessary preoperative diagnostic and staging modalities. It is further ensured that diagnostics and staging procedures are of high quality and that no unnecessary procedures are delaying the treatment. The team defines guidelines to ensure that the patient flow is efficient, fast, and without dropouts. The team meetings are learning platforms for younger doctors in specialist training.

G. Baatrup, DMSC
Institute of Regional Health Science,
University of Southern Denmark, Svendborg,
Denmark

Department of Surgery A, Odense University Hospital,
Svendborg, Denmark
e-mail: gunnar@baatrup.com

G. Baatrup (ed.), *Multidisciplinary Treatment of Colorectal Cancer*,
DOI 10.1007/978-3-319-06142-9_1, © Springer International Publishing Switzerland 2015

Organizing the Team

In organizing the CRC MDT, there are local matters to consider. The meetings can be organized in many different ways. The team has to define the tasks they want to take responsibility for. Not all teams will take responsibility for all the jobs listed below, but it may serve as a list from which you can choose those necessary to deal with in your hospital. It is a suggestion for those who have not yet found a satisfactory organization and may act as a checklist for those who have. Weekly meetings are to be recommended. Even if the patient number is low, it is not advisable to prolong the patients' way through the system. The very complex diagnostic, staging, and treatment lead the patient through many consultations and periods of waiting before the treatment is completed. A study conducted in the Section of Colorectal Surgery, Haukeland University Hospital, through 2006–2008 revealed that the patient or the patient's papers are transferred from one person to another 15 times before the patient is operated on in the case of rectal cancer and 6 times for colon cancer patients (not published). For psychological and possibly for outcome reasons [1, 2], the team must strive for an efficient and fast handling in every step toward end of treatment. More national guidelines are now indicating maximum times for the preoperative handling of these patients [3–5], and accidental dropouts have recently made headlines in the Norwegian newspapers. The team must consider cost-effectiveness of their algorithm for the preoperative handling of the patients. Unnecessary procedures should be identified and omitted from the routine. The team setting is, on the other hand, ideal for evaluating new procedures and defining research protocols. The team should, after some time, be able to answer questions as: Are we performing acceptably as compared to national results? Is transrectal ultrasonography or MRI of the pelvic region more accurate for T staging in our hands? Could we restrict MRI investigations to the large cancers? By omitting unnecessary procedures, we may be able to find time and resources to conduct investigations and research.

The team shall be responsible for:

1. Tailoring treatment
2. Deciding the general procedures for diagnostics, staging, and treatment
3. Conducting routine quality control
4. Organizing patient flow
5. Conducting research and quality control studies
6. Training younger doctors and nurses

The team consists of one or more dedicated representatives from colorectal surgery, medical oncology, radiotherapy, radiology, and pathology but serves also as an open meeting for training and education of younger colleagues. The team meets to demonstrate the clinical, radiological, and histological data obtained and from these data decide a treatment strategy. Each specialty takes responsibility for the data they obtain and offers a treatment best fitted to the individual patient. The team decision emerges from these facts. It might therefore seem unnecessary for the team members to have any detailed knowledge about the background for suggestions and decisions taken by their colleagues. The practical experience from the daily work clearly reveals that this is not the case. The quality of the discussion and decisions taken is very much dependent on the team member's transdisciplinary knowledge and insight.

The UK guidelines [3] are defining a more extended MDT group to handle further aspects of the patient's disease and treatment. They recommend the participation of a palliative team, dedicated nurses, physiotherapists, medical coordinator, and a team secretary. Further they describe the staff involved in an "extended MDT" from gastroenterology, liver surgery, thoracic surgery, interventional radiologists, GPOs/primary care teams, diarists, liaison psychiatrist, social worker, clinical genetics, and research nurse.

The participation of a geriatric specialist may be useful to many colorectal cancer cases.

The entire staff taking care of the patient throughout his hospital contact consists of many other specialties and professions. Indeed, the patient may remember his hospitalization as mainly managed by professionals who are not members of the CRC MDT. The CRC MDT is not meant to be a forum for all professionals involved in the treatment and care of the CRC patients, and it is critical for the team to focus on well-defined tasks. The team aspect of problem solving may add further complexity to the administration of the patient flow. The aspects handled by the team should therefore primarily be those which benefit from the team approach.

In larger centers also dealing with surgical treatment of liver metastasis, the CRC MDT is often additionally handling these patients at the same meeting. Alternatively the liver MDT may be held immediately before or after the CRC MDT meetings as some of these patients will need discussion between the two teams. This may be even more important as the "liver-first strategy" is becoming more widespread in the case of synchronous liver metastasis[1]. The entire strategy for resection of the primary tumor and resection or destruction of liver metastasis and oncological adjuvant and neoadjuvant treatment will have to be coordinated.

Ad hoc groups may be formed to discuss the rare cases for intended curative treatment of cancers involving other organs.

Tailoring Treatment for the Individual Patient

During the meetings, easy access to all results, photo-documentation, and radiologic demonstration is ensured. In high-volume centers, it is important that the demonstration is well organized and all relevant data immediately accessible. One appointed member is responsible for the demonstration and the accessibility of data during the meeting. It should be allowed to include patients for demonstration until shortly before the meeting, and the preparation should be done by all team members immediately before the meeting. The file containing data of the patients of the week should therefore be accessible to all team members. The presentation of each patient is often performed by the surgeon who has been talking with the patient about options and preferences. A decision on the treatment strategy is agreed upon for each patient based upon the patient's physical performance and age, the stage and grade of the disease, and the available facilities for treatment. The motivated decision is documented together with the name of the doctor in charge of the patient. This is the main focus of the weekly meeting regarding the treatment of the patient.

If the team has taken responsibility for individualized care and support as well, nurses and physiotherapists will offer a plan for introducing the patient to the facilities for the course of his postoperative recovery and mobilization and to scrutinize the patient's resources and preferences and prepare him in the case a stoma may be necessary.

Some teams also perform quality control and feedback on a weekly basis at these meetings. The final histology of tumors from patients operated earlier is compared with the results from the preoperative staging. Photos documenting the quality of the operation specimen are shown to adjust the patient's prognosis [6] and decide upon any further oncological treatment. Other centers have monthly or rarer meetings for quality control to allow a higher number of patients to be evaluated at the same time.

Some centers treating patients with colorectal cancer do not have all the necessary specialties present at their own hospital. The demands to centers for modern cancer treatment are to solve this by agreements with outside specialists to join the meetings, to arrange video meeting with outside specialists, or to stop the activity.

Patients for MDT Discussion

All patients with rectal cancer should be discussed at a MDT meeting. Individualization is beneficial not only for the advanced cancers that may be subject to possible combination therapy but also for the very early ones, in which cases local treatment may be an option. Despite the fact that most large T2 and early T3 cancers are obvious candidates for surgery-alone treatment, quality control of the staging procedures is necessary. Quality control of the staging procedures is easiest and most reliable in these medium-sized cancers because there is no chemoradiation-induced downstaging between the periods of preoperative staging to the resection specimen is available for evaluation. It has also been argued that the pathologist rather than the surgeon should assess the quality of the resection specimen.

The CRC MDT is also an obvious forum to discuss the advanced anal cancers or those which have recurred after radiation therapy because a collaborative treatment between the oncologists and the surgeons may be an option.

It is debatable if colon cancer patients should be discussed in the MDT. Most patients with a good physical performance and without locally advanced, primary colon cancers might be dealt with by the surgeon himself. Some advanced colon cancer patients definitely need a multidisciplinary approach from the beginning and should only be treated in institutions with the necessary expertise present. The guidelines from the National Comprehensive Cancer Network in the USA are recommending preoperative chemotherapy and radiation in more and more situations of advanced colon cancer treatment [7].

It is likely that multidisciplinary handling of the rectal cancer patient has contributed to the increasing long-term survival observed in most countries during the last 10 years. At present, the 5-year survival of rectal cancer disease is exceeding that of colon cancers in some countries [8]. It may be time to organize, systematize, and prioritize the treatment of colon cancers as it has been done for breast and rectal cancers.

It may, as a minimum, be advantageous to mention all colon cancer patients at the MDT meeting to alert the department of medical oncology of possible candidates for adjuvant chemotherapy and to enroll them in the patient flow control system.

Organizing and Scrutinizing the Patient Flow

It is the obligation of the team to define the patient's pathway from the time of admission to end of treatment and the acceptable maximum time spent during this.

We conducted a study of the paper and patient flow for colorectal cancer patients in our department. From the time the referring doctor sends our department a letter concerning a patient with suspected rectal cancer, the papers are send to a new instance more than 15 times, and the patient will meet 6 times at 5 different clinics or departments before he is operated on (unpublished). The 30 visits for chemoradiation treatment are not included. It is hopefully much better in most hospitals, but the risk of errors leading to delay in treatment or to the loss of the papers is obvious. The patient may be lost to the system. This has in our institution lead to delays of treatment for up to 9 months in a selected case. Therefore, our conclusion was that the ever-increasing complexity of the patients' way to cure needs a well-organized system of scrutinizing the flow of every single patient, with systems of automatic alarm in case of delay at any point. Any unexpected long waiting times for a patient at any stage should be detectable and immediately acted upon, even though it is not necessarily dealt with at the MDT meetings. A survey system also helps the team to identify departments with problems of capacity and to act upon that quickly. It is further important that the clinicians meeting the patient are informed about the waiting time for the different investigations for preoperative oncological treatment and surgery.

In our hospital, the mere focus and investigation of all the steps in the flow resulted in a significant reduction in the time to surgery for our colon and for our rectal cancer patients. This was achieved without utilization of more resources (unpublished).

Acceptable waiting times have to be defined by the MDT taking the patient's best interest, national recommendations, and the realistic capacity of the hospital into account. Acceptable mean times and extremes have to be defined for all out clinic visits and all types of preoperative investigation [3, 4]. This should be systematized to follow all patients entering the department for diagnosis and further handling of colorectal cancers. The system needed, whether it is manual or electronic, depends on local matters such as caseload and the presence of a dedicated secretary. Deviations from the defined standards should be presented at the MDT meeting.

Feedback: Quality Control and Procedure Adjustments

The team needs feedback in order to execute quality control of their decisions and on preoperative diagnostic procedures to find the best possible combination of investigations. This cannot be adapted exclusively from the literature as the accessibility of procedures differs and the accuracy of most of the procedures is highly dependent upon local matters. Accuracy of T and N staging varies between 50 and 95 % even for MRI and perhaps even more for ultrasonography [9].

Results from the preoperative investigations have to be compared with the results from the pathological examination of the resection specimen. Photos of the transanal endoscopic microsurgery (TEM) or the total mesorectal excision (TME) specimens can illustrate the quality of the surgical performance and possibly the advancement of the cancer. The photos are important in the discussion of possible postoperative oncological, adjuvant treatment. The patient's postoperative course and complications should also be discussed. Is the local frequency of neoadjuvant treatment acceptable? The frequency of perineal wound dehiscence in patients having radiation therapy may lead to a discussion on routine plastic surgical reconstruction after abdominoperineal resection. A high frequency of postoperative infections may lead to a discussion on the routine of antibiotics used for prophylaxis. Sudden changes in routines in the clinical departments, the anesthetic department, the ICU, or other places may lead to unexpected changes in outcome. These matters may be difficult to discover in low-volume diseases as rectal cancer. A systematic continuous quality control system may be of great help. It took us almost 6 months to discover a doubling of the frequency of postoperative infections after rectal resections in our department, and it took a further 3 months to identify the cause because we lacked the systematic scrutinizing of postoperative results [10].

The clinical nurse specialist and others may need meetings to discuss and develop services for the nonclinical needs of the patient such as information and support [3].

Quality control cannot be discussed on a weekly basis. It takes several months to obtain a number of procedures high enough to justify any discussion. For some parameters as frequency of local recurrence and T- and N-specific accuracy of staging procedures, it may, in most institutions, take years before the discussion can be meaningful. It is, nevertheless, necessary to collect all these data and to analyze and discuss them in order to improve.

Most MDTs will meet monthly or every third month to discuss these matters. It may be useful to have regular meetings to discuss patient flow, waiting times, and matters such as suggestions for new research protocols, presentations of news from the literature, having guest lecturers, etc.

Research and Teaching

The introduction of TME surgery some 15 years ago reduced the local recurrence rate with more than 50 % in many institutions. It is, however, difficult to demonstrate a significant increase in long-term survival related to the TME technique. This illustrates that the days of single procedure-related significant achievements in terms of increased long-term survival of colorectal cancer patients are over. Improvements of survival will, in the future, come from multidisciplinary collaborations, and the MDT is therefore an obvious forum for discussing and developing new research protocols. This may also be an argument for systematic inclusion of colon cancer patients into the MDT discussions.

The weekly meetings are well suited for education of young doctors seeking training in the treatment for CRC.

One Example of How to Organize the MDT

One example of formalized and systematic presentation of information concerning evaluation and treatment of CRC patient is described below.

Access to Data

Communication on a common electronic meeting platform is very useful for all involved members of the team. Members of the staff at the surgical, medical oncology, radio-physical, pathological, and radiology departments can have access to add information or to create links to the MDT platform. They also have access to all information on the presentation platform in order to prepare themselves before the MDT meeting. All patients to be discussed are present on this platform. This allows for discussing patients a few hours after the needed information has been collected. Once they have been discussed and a decision has been made, the team decision is noted and accessible to all participants.

Preoperative Presentation

Each MDT has to define a set of necessary information and to determine the minimum information accepted for deciding which treatment the patient should be offered. To collect this amount of information within a few days and have them evaluated and discussed in the MDT, the team must organize a very efficient and secure system for patient flow and handling during the preoperative phase.

Information from the Surgeon

The surgeon presents information on the patient's preference, his physical performance, and the operative morbidity and mortality risk. The stage of the disease according to the clinical investigation with photography from the endoscopic examination and video sequences from the transanal ultrasonography is also presented to the team. A drawing of the rectum indicating the position and size of the tumor may be helpful. Complex cases with T4 cancers or metastasis may need additional information.

Information from the Radiologist

The minimum set of radiological investigations for T, N, and M staging is presented, and the radiologist states a radiologic TNM stage for the case in question. For patients undergoing neoadjuvant treatment, a radiologic stage before and after is noted together with the response upon the treatment.

Information from the Pathologist

Benign or malignant biopsy. If any grading features can be deducted from the biopsy, it is also discussed.

Information from the Oncologists

Course of any neoadjuvant treatment.

Preoperative Decision

The conclusion for further investigation or treatment is noted. The file holds clear information on who is in charge of the patient's further handling.

Postoperative Data

Data obtained for decision on further treatment or follow-up and for long-term quality control:

From the Surgeon

1. Type of operation
2. Photography of the resection specimen (mesorectal fascia intact?). Three pictures: left lateral, right lateral, and posterior
3. Completeness of resection
4. Distance to oral and anal margins
5. Special pictures and text for locally resected cancers
6. Morbidity and mortality

From the Pathologist

1. Pictures of the macro preparation
2. Microscopic pictures of the tumor
3. T and N stage

4. Tumor grading and other risk factors
5. Distance to lateral margin
6. Completeness of resection
7. Special pictures and text for locally resected cancers

Advanced Cases

Advanced cases may need the collection of more information and may need discussion with other surgical specialties such as liver surgeons, vascular surgeons, gynecologists, or urologists or may need another regimen for neoadjuvant treatment. Often these cases are handled individually. Only few departments are engaged in the treatment of all types of advanced cases.

Additional Information Needed in Advanced Disease

Locally advanced cases (T4) and recurrences: The surgical options must be evaluated by relevant specialties. The need for special neoadjuvant treatment with chemotherapy and or radiation must be discussed with the oncologists. Participation of vascular surgeons, urologists, gynecologists, etc., must be arranged.

Distant metastasis: The potential for curability must be discussed between the oncologists and the colorectal and liver surgeons. Determination on operability of distant metastasis must be clarified. Timing of medical, radio-physical, and surgical treatment of primary and secondary tumors should be discussed between all parts.

References

1. Gonzales-Hermoso F, Perez-Palma J, Marchena-Gomez J, Lorenzo-Rocha N, Medina-Arana V. Can early diagnosis of symptomatic colorectal cancer improve the prognosis? World J Surg. 2004;28(7): 716–20.
2. Goodman D, Irvin TT. Delay in the diagnosis of carcinoma of the right colon. Br J Surg. 1993;80(10):1327–9.
3. The Association of Coloproctology of Great Britain and Ireland. Guidelines for the management of colorectal cancer. 3rd ed. 2007. http://www.acpgbi.org.uk/assets/documents/COLO_guides.pdf.
4. Danish Colorectal Cancer Group. Guidelines for diagnostics and treatment of colorectal cancer. 4th ed. 2009 in Danish. http://www.dccg.dk/03_Publikation/01_ret_pdf/Retningslinier2009p.pdf.
5. National action plan with guidelines for diagnosis, treatment and follow up of cancer in the large bowel and rectum. In: Norwegian. Helsedirektoratet. 2nd ed. 2010. http://www.helsedirektoratet.no/vp/multimedia/archive/00287/Nasjonalt_handlings_287789a.pdf.
6. Nagtegaal ID, van de Velde CJ, van der Worp E, Kapiteijn E, Querke P, van Krieken JHJM. Macroscopic evaluation of rectal cancer resection specimen: clinical significance of the pathologist in the quality control. J Clin Oncol. 2002;20(7):1714–5.
7. National Comprehensive Cancer Network. Clinical practice guidelines in oncology. Colon Cancer. http://www.nccn.org/professionals/physician_gls/f_guidelines.asp.
8. Paahlman L, Bohe M, Cedermark B, Dahlberg M, Lindmark G, Sjodahl R, Ojerskog B, Damber L, Johansson R. The Swedish rectal cancer registry. Br J Surg. 2007;94(10):1285–92.
9. Baatrup G, Endreseth B, Isaksen V, Kjellmo AA, Tveit KM, Nesbakken A. Preoperative staging and treatment options in T1 rectal adenocarcinoma. Acta Oncol. 2009;48:328–42.
10. Baatrup G, Nielsen RM, Svensen R, Akselsen PE. Increased incidence of postoperative infections during prophylaxis with cephalothin compared to doxycycline in intestinal surgery. BMC Surg. 2009;9:17.

Multidisciplinary Treatment: Influence on Outcomes

Arne Wibe

Abstract

Background. Colorectal cancer is the most common cancer in the western world. Although different treatment modalities are available, many patients suffer from poor functional outcomes, recurrent disease and/or death.

Methods. In 1993 the first national educational programme was launched in Norway in order to improve standards of treatment for rectal cancer and, thus, the prognosis of this disease. Several multidisciplinary workshops were arranged. Simultaneously a national rectal cancer registry was established. In 1995 a similar programme started in Sweden, later several countries have followed. The aim of this chapter is to describe how these projects were developed, how they were run, what were the problems and what were the results and the consequences.

Results. A few years after starting the projects, the prognosis of rectal cancer improved at national levels. There was a considerable variation of results between hospitals. Patients treated by health-care professionals having attended multidisciplinary workshops had better prognosis than other patients. Multidisciplinary teams have been developed in order to secure work-up, decision making and treatment. During the last years, colon cancer has been included into the same projects. The treatment of colorectal cancer has been increasingly multimodal and tailored according to stage of the disease and the status of the patient.

Conclusions. The lesson to learn is that colorectal cancer treatment is no more a matter of a single surgeon working alone in a small hospital. Modern colorectal cancer treatment is advanced medicine that has to be performed by multidisciplinary teams (MDTs). Multimodal tailored treatment has been developed and should be offered to every patient with colorectal cancer. Standards of care can only be evaluated within national audits. Quality assurance of cancer care should be mandatory.

A. Wibe
Department of Surgery, St. Olavs University Hospital,
Norwegian University of Science and Technology,
Trondheim 7006, Norway
e-mail: arne.wibe@ntnu.no

G. Baatrup (ed.), *Multidisciplinary Treatment of Colorectal Cancer*,
DOI 10.1007/978-3-319-06142-9_2, © Springer International Publishing Switzerland 2015

Background

The prognosis of rectal cancer has been generally poor, even for patients undergoing radical surgery. In a review in 1995 including more than 10,000 rectal cancer patients radically treated by surgery alone, the mean local recurrence rate was 18.5 % [1]. The poor outcome after radical surgery for rectal cancer, mainly caused by the detrimental effect of LR, has been regarded as an irrefutable fact even in contemporary literature [2]. Professional bodies had consequently advocated adjuvant chemoradiotherapy as standard treatment [3], as recommended by the National Cancer Institute in the USA in 1990 [4]. This treatment was based on the staging system by Dukes and/or TNM, and according to these guidelines, patients with a tumour growing through the muscularis propria (Dukes B/TNM stage II) and/or with malignant infiltration of any lymph node (Dukes C/TNM stage III) should be offered adjuvant therapy.

However, during the 1980s most opinion leaders of rectal cancer treatment appeared to miss the important message of the work of Richard J. Heald, published in 1982 and 1986 [5, 6]. He named this procedure total mesorectal excision, TME, thus describing a complete removal of the fatty tissue surrounding the rectum, i.e. containing vascular, lymphatic and nervous tissue supplying the rectum. For many years, these milestone reports were not appreciated by the professional international colorectal community. The problem appeared to be the exceptional good results that he presented from his own cohort [7], and he was met with arguments that his low local recurrence rates were consequences of referral or other selection bias [8], although a review suggested otherwise [9]. Another controversy was the alleged technical complexity of the procedure; it was thought impractical to perform this technique outside specialist centres.

At that time, data from some Norwegian university hospitals showed that 21–34 % of radically treated rectal cancer patients developed local recurrence (LR) [10, 11], with a 5-year survival of 55 % [12]. For patients who developed local recurrence, the 5-year survival was 8 %.

Interestingly, there were reported very good results from rectal cancer treatment at one Norwegian hospital, actually similar to Dr. Heald's local recurrence rate of 4 % [13]. Thus, the Norwegian surgical community realised that there was a huge variation of results from hospital to hospital and that the standard of surgery had to play the major role for this variation. At that time in Norway, radiotherapy was only used for fixed tumours, and patients treated with a curative intent neither received radiotherapy nor chemotherapy.

Another support to Dr. Heald's work was the macroscopic and microscopic studies of rectal cancer specimens by the pathologist Philip Quirke. He reported that the major cause of local recurrence was the malignant infiltration of the circumferential resection margins, implying that a high rate of local recurrence is caused by inadequate surgical resections [14].

Although radiotherapy had been used in rectal cancer treatment for decades, and with a significant benefit for reducing local recurrence, still in the early 1990s there had been no effect on overall survival. Despite the fact that postoperative chemotherapy was established as routine treatment for colon cancer in TNM stage III, there was no scientific support for survival benefit of chemotherapy for rectal cancer.

Norwegian Experience

In 1993 the Norwegian surgical community invited Dr. Heald and Dr. Quirke and launched the national Norwegian Rectal Cancer Project. Surgeons and pathologists from all over the country were invited to participate in this first "multidisciplinary" workshop for rectal cancer at the National Hospital in Oslo. During a live video procedure Dr. Heald demonstrated the meticulous TME dissection, and afterwards Dr. Quirke performed detailed examination of the specimen with specific focus on mesorectal spread and the relation between the tumour and the circumferential resection margin according to his recommendations described in his reports. Altogether, there were 16 similar courses in Norway during the

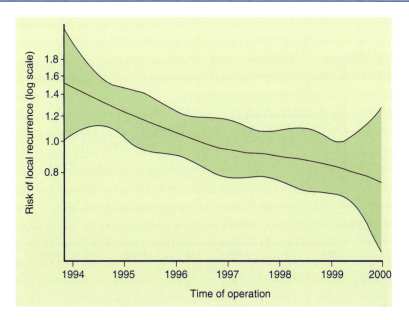

Fig. 2.1 Risk of local recurrence for radically treated rectal cancer patients in Norway during the first years of the project (log scale) (© (2006) Blackwell Publishing Ltd. on behalf of the Association of Coloproctology of Great Britain and Ireland)

next 3 years. The day after the first course, the Norwegian Rectal Cancer Registry started to include rectal cancer patients. This registry contained demographic, clinical, pathological and follow-up data from different sources, thus giving the opportunity to crosscheck the accuracy and the completeness of the data [15]. This rectal cancer registry was the first to include every case of rectal cancer at a national level and to report the results of each hospital, each region and for the whole nation.

At the beginning, the intention was to run this national project through 1999. Financial support was given by the Norwegian Medical Association and by the Norwegian Cancer Society (a non-profit organisation). Assembling data was made possible through a close collaboration with the Cancer Registry of Norway. This registry has collected demographic and clinical data from every case of cancer in Norway since 1952. Due to a compulsory reporting system, both clinicians and pathologists are obliged to report data on cancer patients. In the first years of the project, also the experienced epidemiologists and statisticians at the national cancer registry made an important contribution to secure correct data handling. Together with a clinician as daily manager, a complete research group was established. The project was led by a board consisting of surgeons, oncologists, pathologists and radiologists from all the five health regions of the country, thus securing full geographic participation, necessary for the project in order to be trusted at a national level.

The board established their own regulations on how to handle the database. Thus, every planned study had to be approved by the board. The first results showed that this national initiative had taken a huge step forward in order to improve standards of treatment. Compared to national results prior to the project, the rate of local recurrence had dropped substantially, from 28 to 13 %, and furthermore, there was a considerable ongoing reduction of local recurrence during the project, from 17 % in 1994 to 8 % in 1999 (Fig. 2.1) [16].

At the same time, the overall survival for radically treated rectal cancer patients had increased from 55 % prior to the project to 71 % in the period 1993–1999 (for patients younger than 75 years) (Fig. 2.2) [16, 17].

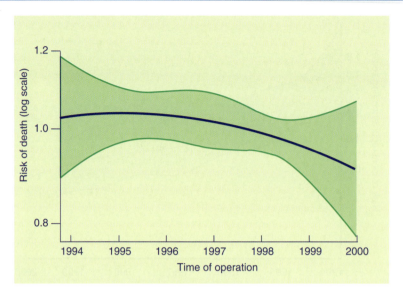

Fig. 2.2 Risk of death of any cause for radically treated rectal cancer patients in Norway during the first years of the project (log scale) (© (2006) Blackwell Publishing Ltd. on behalf of the Association of Coloproctology of Great Britain and Ireland)

What could explain such immediate response? As only 9 % of the patients had radiotherapy and 2 % had chemotherapy, it was obvious that improved surgery had to be the major contributor to the better results. But, there was a huge variation of results between hospitals and also between types of hospitals (Fig. 2.3). The smallest hospitals had doubled the rate of local recurrence and a significant lower survival compared to the largest hospitals. The 5-year local recurrence rates were 17.5 and 9.2 % ($p=0.003$), and the 5-year overall survival rates were 57.8 and 64.4 % ($p=0.105$), respectively, in hospitals with annual caseload less than ten compared to more than 30 [18]. These analyses even strengthened the message that surgery had to be the single most important part of the treatment, as half of the hospitals had to perform better than the mean within each group. What did they do different than the hospitals not performing that well?

Despite the comprehensive educational programme going on from 1993 to 1996, where gastrointestinal surgeons were taught the principles of TME, it was clear that there was a need to continue the project as a continuous quality assurance programme for rectal cancer. Again regular

national workshops were started, including not only live TME surgery but also detailed education in comprehensive preoperative work-up radiology, oncological therapy and pathology. The strategy of the project included systematic training and accreditation of surgeons, ending up with specialised dedicated teams responsible for rectal cancer treatment. The national programme stated that multidiscipline preoperative and postoperative evaluations were mandatory for quality assurance of rectal cancer treatment.

Turning the second millennium, it was obvious that the Norwegian Rectal Cancer Registry contained data that were most important also for the international community. Several study groups were established, and both surgeons and oncologists started as research fellows. The study groups were recruited from every health region, each analysing different topics of rectal cancer treatment. Thus, no competition developed, and the board of the project gained even more support from all over the country. At that time, the project had changed, from a time set developing project, moving on to permanent quality assurance for one of the most common cancer diseases. From 2000 the project has been funded by the Ministry of Health.

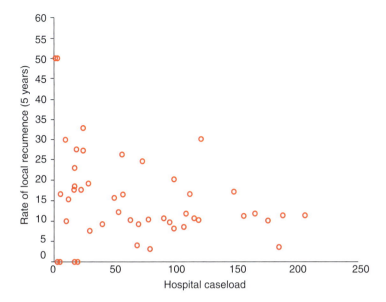

Fig. 2.3 Local recurrence at each hospital in Norway related to hospital caseload in the period November 1993– December 1999 [16] (© (2006) Blackwell Publishing Ltd. on behalf of the Association of Coloproctology of Great Britain and Ireland)

Why had the project succeeded? There may be many reasons for that. First of all, the project was initiated by the clinicians themselves, those doing the work, treating the patients and delivering the data. If this project had been pushed onto the clinicians by the health-care authorities, it may have failed. Secondly, all the clinicians received their own results, i.e. the result of their hospital, and the national means for comparison. That had never happened before in their professional life. In addition, every hospital receives all their data back for their own scientific purpose, thus stimulating to publish their own results, which often happens, especially during the annual national surgical week. Although the results of single hospitals so far have been anonymously reported from the national registry, many hospitals prefer to publish their own data. This feedback of data is a true win-win situation, supporting both the national project and the standard of treatment at each hospital. Another benefit of feedback of results is that underperforming departments make every possible effort in order to catch up with the best performing hospitals. Detailed analyses for single hospitals enable them to identify what may cause inferior results and/or violation of national guidelines.

Thirdly, the board of the project includes experts from different specialities working together towards a common goal. That has increased the competence of the group, securing the development of the project heading in a direction based on international science.

During national workshops the multidisciplinary collaboration of the board has been transferred to each hospital. The clinicians have picked up knowledge and competence from different specialities, showing the necessity of clinicians working together across different specialities. The future of the patient is their common goal.

Another main issue for the success was that the decision of taking part in the national rectal cancer registry was left to the discretion of each hospital. Apart from the compulsory reporting of the standard dataset to the main cancer registry, every hospital was invited to report their detailed data of treatment and follow-up of their rectal cancer patients.

During the first years of the project, although every hospital wanted to take part in the project, a few of the 55 hospitals treating rectal cancer did not report their own data, and the central staff of the project visited these hospitals and collected missing data. However, following the first feedback of results to each hospital, reporting of data has been smooth.

The board has no formal responsibility for the treatment given at each hospital, neither have the members of the board any knowledge of the results of single hospitals. Such results are only known by the office staff. Thus, the board has always voiced that the head of the department is responsible for the quality of care.

One main policy of the project has been that no directives are to be sent to the hospitals, neither from the staff nor from the board. But, based on international and national data, nationwide guidelines have been regularly revised [19].

During the first years of the project, it became obvious that surgery for rectal cancer should be performed by fewer surgeons specially trained in the TME technique. Thus, it was necessary to change the educational programme for general surgery and to remove rectal cancer surgery from the programme. The professional community recommended that rectal cancer procedures only should be performed by specialists in gastrointestinal surgery. A few years later, following the report showing a wide variation of results between hospitals, the regional health-care authorities decided that rectal cancer patients only should be treated by multidisciplinary teams at central hospitals and university hospitals. Although most general surgeons at local hospitals already had ceased rectal cancer surgery due to their very bad results during the first years of the project, some surgeons at small hospitals had to be convinced that without a team of dedicated specially trained experts, many rectal cancer patients would not be cured. Thus, the results of single hospitals changed clinical practice all over the country, and most of this change was initiated by the process itself. Ten years after the project started, rectal cancer treatment had been centralised to less than half of Norwegian hospitals. That solved the problem of missing competence related to low caseload, but what about larger hospitals with bad results?

Reorganising of the whole treatment line was performed at several large hospitals. One example of that was the development of modern treatment principles at Haugesund Central Hospital. In the first 5 years of the project, the rate of local recurrence was 31.5 % at this hospital. The staff was reorganised, and they made several initiatives to improve their standards of care. They attended the national workshops; they got some new retractors for the procedure; they followed the national guidelines for neoadjuvant therapy; CT, rectal ultrasound and MRI became routine for preoperative work-up; a multidisciplinary team was established; and a small dedicated group of specialists in gastrointestinal surgery performed the procedures. In the next 3-year period, their local recurrence was 11 %, later 6 %, and since 2005 none of their patients have developed local recurrence [20]. Similarly, at Levanger Hospital, they had 19 % local recurrence during the 1990s, but, after receiving their results from the national project, the staff came aware of their inferior standards, and in the following period, 2000–2004, they managed to reduce their local recurrence rate to 2 % ($p=0.006$) [21]. In other words, due to the national project, every hospital has got a tool to discover missing standards and to develop their competence and skills through close collaboration with staff members of the project.

The project resulted in much focus on cancer surgery. Newspapers and television companies got interested in the results, especially the wide variation in standards of care between hospitals. That became a political issue which seemed to ease project funding from the Ministry of Health. Similarly, the health-care bureaucracy at the hospital, regional and national level regularly receives results from the project, which seems to have been important in order to keep focus on standards of cancer care in general, and specific regulations for treatment of all gastrointestinal cancers have been implemented all over the country.

European Experience

The Swedish Rectal Cancer Registry was established in 1995. The collection of data is based on regional cancer registries, but complete national rectal cancer analyses are performed on similar data sets as in Norway. The Swedish project is based on similar workshops as in Norway, with live video demonstrations of TME surgery by Dr. Heald. Although the surgical communities in Norway and Sweden have had close collaboration for decades, their treatment policies for rectal cancer have been different. Since the randomised Swedish studies [21, 22], their philosophy for treating rectal cancer has been based on short-course preoperative radiotherapy of 5×5 Gy to most patients and long course with 54 Gy for advanced cases, in contrast to Norway with a tailored treatment policy, with long-course radiotherapy only for advanced cases and no radiotherapy for >90 % of the patients. How could these different guidelines be implemented? May be the explanation is that the literature was interpreted differently. In Norway a nationwide audit of rectal cancer treatment for the period 1986–1988 told us that the prognosis was bad in general, but single-hospital studies showed a huge variation of results between hospitals. Furthermore, rectal cancer surgery was performed by 245 surgeons with an annual median number of one procedure per year [12]. Then, in Norway we trusted the reports from Heald [6] and Bjerkeset [13], both with 4 % local recurrence and almost without any use of radiotherapy. When no other therapy was given and the results were different, there was no other explanation but the standard of surgery had to play the major role for local recurrence and survival. Another reason for not using radiotherapy as routine treatment for rectal cancer was the well-known acute and late toxicity.

That information made the basis of the Norwegian strategy implementing the principle of tailored treatment of the tumour and the patient. The Norwegian surgical and oncological community agreed that routine radiotherapy for all or most rectal cancer patients would imply overtreatment and severe complications resulting in reduced functional outcomes and unnecessary loss of lives. A meta-analysis from the UK of more than 8,500 patients confirmed this view. Radiotherapy increased the risk of death from nonrectal cancer by 15 %, mainly due to vascular and infective complications [23]. For patients over 75 years, there were more side effects than beneficial effects of radiotherapy.

In Sweden the professional surgical and oncological community had experienced a considerable effect of radiotherapy in reducing local recurrence, from 27 to 11 % [22]. It was also thought that preoperative short-course radiotherapy for 1 week and surgery the next week would result in less toxicity and postoperative complications, but with the same positive effect on reducing local recurrence as the long-course schedule.

Although Norway and Sweden established national rectal cancer projects almost simultaneously, in 1993 and 1995, respectively, and with the same professional support, their treatment policies were different. Interestingly, in Norway in 1997, 12 % of the patients had radiotherapy, compared to 55 % in Sweden. But the national mean rates of local recurrence and overall survival were similar in the two countries (10 % and 9 %, and males 62 % and females 58 % and males 56 % and females 56 %, in Norway and Sweden, respectively) [24].

In Denmark a national rectal cancer registry was developed in 1994 [25], and Belgium started a comprehensive registration in 2007 [26]. Since 2006 the Spanish Association of Surgeons has arranged similar workshops as in Norway and Sweden, and a registry is now covering 1/3 of the Spanish rectal cancer patients [27]. Seventy of the largest hospitals in Spain are now included in this initiative. For some years a German-Polish collaboration are collecting data on rectal cancer patients [28], and in 2008 a Dutch national colorectal cancer registry was launched [29]. In Great Britain a colorectal cancer registry is based on administrative data [30]. Although these registries may not have the exact same type of data, all these registries are established with the same goal. All the work with workshops, collecting data, analyses and reporting are established and run by clinicians in order to improve the prognosis of rectal cancer patients. Have all these efforts had any effect on patients' life expectancy? In Norway and Sweden it has had a considerable effect. Before the projects started, the prognosis of rectal cancer was substantially worse compared to colon cancer; now patients with rectal cancer have better survival than those with colon cancer.

Multidisciplinary Meeting and Treatment

That radiotherapy has beneficial effect on rectal cancer in reducing local recurrence has been known for decades, but in the era of TME this benefit has not been translated into an increased overall survival. In spite of that, in many countries radiotherapy has been used, and still is, for most rectal cancer patients.

After implementing optimised surgery by TME, some opinion leaders became even more sceptical to any survival benefit for radiotherapy. This was tested in the Dutch TME trial where patients were randomised to TME surgery alone or with preoperative short-course RT + TME. The last group had less local recurrence, 11 % vs. 6 %, but there was no significant effect on overall survival [31]. In a Swedish study, before TME was implemented, preoperative RT had increased survival, with a 5-year rate of 58 % vs. 48 % for patients treated by surgery alone [22]. However, in this study the effect on local recurrence was much larger than for overall survival, may be due to some radiation toxicity. This information might imply that the Dutch and the Swedish studies did not include anything about tailoring treatment.

As local recurrence was known to be a main contribution for reducing overall survival (HR = 6.0) [7] and according to Dr. Heald and Dr. Quirke's studies in the 1980s, most focus should be directed towards all the details within the mesorectum. During the 1990s there was a technical and radiological development of the use of MRI for rectal cancer. CT scanning of the thorax and the abdomen became more common, and some surgeons and radiologists had used endorectal ultrasound for preoperative staging for some time. But as for every advanced technical medical development, the individual competence and skills are of major importance in order to reach acceptable accuracy. However, in the early 1990s, surgeons realised that collaboration across specialities was necessary in order to improve prognosis for rectal cancer. Treating rectal cancer was no longer a "one-man show". An increasing amount of information was send to and from different specialists in order to stage and treat every single patient until formal multidisciplinary team (MDT) meetings were established as routine in most hospitals. Of course these meetings may be time consuming, but we have to realise that organising medical treatment is an ongoing development and change of traditions. The main focus is the patient. Nowadays the work-up and the treatment of single patients are the responsibility of a group of different specialists working together. The benefits of such an organisation are obvious. It is a matter of safety in medicine. The more competence and skills inside such groups, the better the prognosis of their patients.

All the knowledge of single participants of the MDT group is shared with the other members, and one or a few missing members do not affect outcomes as long as all necessary specialities are present. In biology, there always will be borderline cases, cases being in between different defined groups. Although most rectal cancer patients do belong to one or another defined stage, in some cases it is difficult to decide because of missing accuracy. Commonly the age and the status of the patient are of major importance in order to decide the best strategy for treatment. Due to development of all specialities and the increased amount of detailed information, well known to be crucial for the single patient, modern medicine has reached a level of complexity that overrules the competence of one doctor. Multidisciplinary teams for colorectal cancer most commonly include dedicated colorectal surgeons, MRI and CT radiologists, gastrointestinal pathologists and medical and radiation oncologists. Some teams also include an administrative and a stoma nurse. Usually the MDTs discuss each case following complete work-up, after neoadjuvant therapy and also after surgery in order to decide if additional therapy of any kind is indicated.

In primary advanced tumours with growth into the ureters, the prostate, the pelvis, etc., urologic or orthopaedic surgeons should be included in the discussion within the MDT meeting. For treatment of metastases, the MDT should be supplied by liver surgeons or thoracic surgeons.

The main focus of the MDT is decision making. It is a matter of safety in advanced medical treatment. It is the sum of all the details that decide the prognosis of the patient. This sum is more likely to be present within an MDT compared to one single surgeon working in a local hospital. Thus, the skills and competence of one single physician are not sufficient. Standards of care are best explained by health-care structures and processes of care. For complex medical treatment, the skills of the team of clinicians and the hospital organisational skills are equally important [32, 33].

MDT meetings are the best arena to convey knowledge and experience to colleagues and young doctors. It has also become a secure platform for the administrative part of the handling of work-up and treatment of the patients. Another benefit is that both the patients and the management of the hospital are more likely to trust the decisions made by a group of dedicated experts compared to single doctors' preferences.

There is a lot of evidence that the new knowledge gained at multidisciplinary workshops has beneficial effects [34]. In a paper from Stockholm including 652 patients treated in 1995–1996, Martling et al. found that surgeons having attended multidisciplinary workshops more commonly performed TME, sphincter-saving surgery and preoperative radiotherapy [35]. Outcome was better for patients treated by high-volume surgeons (>12 operations per year) compared to low-volume surgeons, as local recurrence rates were 4 % vs. 10 % in the two groups and cancer-related deaths were 11 and 18 %, respectively. Norwegian data on 1,794 patients treated in 1993–1997 reported similar results. Patients treated by surgeons using TME had 6 % local recurrence and 73 % 4-year survival compared to 12 % local recurrence and 60 % survival for patients treated by non-TME technique [7]. In Denmark the survival of rectal cancer improved following implementation of TME in 1996 [36].

In a Dutch study the rate of local recurrence was 9 % in the TME group compared to 16 % in the non-TME group [37].

Such evidence support the view that participants of multidisciplinary workshops translate their new knowledge into their daily clinical practice, and national initiatives with the focus on developing competence and skills of all the different specialties working within the same field seem to be very appropriate. Interestingly, none of these projects has ceased, and practical and scientific collaboration between countries with rectal cancer specific registries have became common.

In a UK report on 460 colorectal surgeons and colorectal clinical nurses who responded to a questionnaire about the importance of MDT meetings, 96.5 % answered that they considered these meetings improved the overall quality of care of colorectal cancer. They also considered that the MDT concept improves training and that MDTs are cost-effective [38]. Another UK report concluded that 90 % of the MDT decisions were implemented [39]. Reasons for non-implementation were co-morbidity, patient choice and new clinical information not available at the meeting. The changed decisions were more conservative than the original treatment plan. A third UK study of 310 patients reported that undergoing MDT discussion improves survival in Dukes C from 58 to 66 % [40]. The interpretation of their data suggested that this improvement was due to more adjuvant chemotherapy in the MDT group. A Swedish study of 1,449 patients with colorectal cancer stage IV disease analysed the impact of MDT meetings [41]. It was found that MDT increased the proportion of patients who had surgery for metastases, and it concluded that MDT assessment opens up the opportunity for more aggressive treatment with better outcomes. Another UK study confirmed their conclusion and reported improved overall survival if patients with metastatic disease from colorectal cancer was discussed in MDT meetings including a liver surgeon [42]. In one study it was found that the rate of CRM involvement was reduced in rectal cancer patients when MRI was discussed in MDT meetings [43].

What Next?

The first national rectal cancer programme to be developed, the Norwegian project, was planned to run only for 6 years. However, due to the considerable improved outcomes for patients treated at some hospitals and the variation between hospitals, it was thought unmoral to stop developing standards of treatment for all patients. Major differences in the given treatment, the rates of local recurrence, overall survival, 30-day mortality and postoperative complications made a solid platform in order to apply for funding for the Ministry of Health to change the temporary project into permanent quality assurance at a national level, not only for rectal cancer but also for colon cancer, like what happened in Sweden and the Netherlands. Interestingly, although overall survival has been better for colon than for rectal cancer, because of the national projects, now rectal cancer has better prognosis than colon cancer, in both Norway and Sweden [44]. Later it has been decided to establish similar comprehensive educational programmes and registries for all gastrointestinal cancer in Norway. This decision was based on the view that quality assurance at different health-care levels can only be evaluated within audits. Both the professional community treating the patients and the health-care bureaucracy have realised that the rapid development of knowledge and technology makes a demand for continuous quality control. Due to the national project, a close collaboration between the health-care authorities and the professionals has developed, most likely to be very fruitful for the treatment of future cancer patients.

References

1. McCall JL, Cox MR, Wattchow DA. Analysis of local recurrence rates after surgery alone for rectal cancer. Int J Colorectal Dis. 1995;10:126–32.
2. Abulafi AM, Williams NS. Local recurrence of colorectal cancer: the problem, mechanisms, management and adjuvant therapy. Br J Surg. 1994;81:7–19.
3. Cohen AM, Winawer SJ, Friedman MA, Gunderson LL, editors. Cancer of the colon, rectum and anus. New York: McGraw-Hill; 1995.
4. Adjuvant therapy for patients with colon and rectal cancer. JAMA. 1990;264:1444–50.
5. Heald RJ, Husband EM, Ryall RDH. The mesorectum in rectal cancer surgery-the clue to pelvic recurrence? Br J Surg. 1982;69:613–6.
6. Heald RJ, Ryall RDH. Recurrence and survival after total mesorectal excision for rectal cancer. Lancet. 1986;1(8496):1479–82.
7. Wibe A, Møller B, Norstein J, Carlsen E, Wiig JN, Heald RJ, Langmark F, Myrvold HE, Søreide O, on behalf of The Norwegian Rectal Cancer Group. A national strategic change in treatment policy for rectal cancer – implementation of total mesorectal excision (TME) as routine treatment in Norway. A national audit. Dis Colon Rectum. 2002;45:857–66.
8. Isbister WH. Basingstoke revisited. Aust N Z J Surg. 1990;60:243–6.
9. McCall JL, Wattchow DA. Failure after curative surgery alone. In: Søreide O, Norstein J, editors. Rectal cancer surgery: optimisation, standardisation, documentation. Berlin: Springer; 1997. p. 29–45.
10. Dahl O, Horn A, Morild I, Halvorsen JF, Odland G, Reinertsen S, Reisaeter A, Kavli H, Thunold J. Low-dose preoperative radiation postpones recurrences in operable rectal cancer. Results of a randomized multicenter trial in western Norway. Cancer. 1990;66:2286–94.
11. Rein KA, Wiig JN, Sæther OD, Myrvold HE. Local recurrence in patients with rectal cancer. Tidsskr Nor Laegeforen. 1987;107:2318–20. In Norwegian.
12. Norstein J, Langmark F. Results of rectal cancer treatment: a national experience. In: Søreide O, Norstein J, editors. Rectal cancer surgery: optimisation, standardisation, documentation. Berlin: Springer; 1997. p. 17–28.
13. Bjerkeset T, Edna TH. Rectal cancer: the influence of type of operation on local recurrence and survival. Eur J Surg. 1996;162:643–8.
14. Quirke P, Dixon MF, Durdey P, Williams NS. Local recurrence of rectal adenocarcinoma due to inadequate surgical resection. Histopathological Study of Lateral Tumour Spread and Surgical Excision. Lancet. 1986;2:996–9.
15. Wibe A. Rectal cancer treatment in Norway. Standardisation of surgery and quality assurance. Publication from the Norwegian University of Science and Technology (NTNU) 2003. ISSN no. 1503 3465. Thesis no. 234.
16. Wibe A, Carlsen E, Dahl O, Tveit KM, Weedon-Fekjaer H, Hestvik UE, Wiig JN, Norwegian Rectal Cancer Group. Nationwide quality assurance of rectal cancer treatment. Colorectal Dis. 2006;8(3):224–9.
17. Wibe A, Eriksen MT, Syse A, Myrvold HE, Søreide O, Norwegian Rectal Cancer Group. Total mesorectal excision for rectal cancer–what can be achieved by a national audit? Colorectal Dis. 2003;5(5):471–7.
18. Wibe A, Eriksen MT, Syse A, Tretli S, Myrvold HE, Søreide O, Norwegian Rectal Cancer Group. Effect of hospital caseload on long-term outcome after standardization of rectal cancer surgery at a national level. Br J Surg. 2005;92(2):217–24.

19. National guidelines for work-up, treatment and follow-up of colorectal cancer. www.helsedirektoratet.no/kreft/publikasjoner (in Norwegian).

20. Moen A-C, Hansen PEH, Ott M. Rectal cancer surgery in Haugesund. Norwegian Association of Surgeons 2008:Abstract no. 116. (In Norwegian).

21. Holm T, Rutqvist LE, Johansson H, Cedermark B. Abdominoperineal resection and anterior resection in the treatment of rectal cancer: results in relation to adjuvant preoperative radiotherapy. Br J Surg. 1995;82:1213–6.

22. Improved survival with preoperative radiotherapy in resectable rectal cancer. Swedish Rectal Cancer Trial. N Engl J Med. 1997;336:980–7.

23. Colorectal Cancer Collaborative Group. Adjuvant radiotherapy for rectal cancer: a systematic overview of 8,507 patients from 22 randomised trials. Lancet. 2001;358:1291–304.

24. Folkesson J, Engholm G, Ehrnrooth E, Kejs AM, Påhlman L, Harling H, Wibe A, Gaard M, Thornorvaldur J, Tryggvadottir L, Brewster DH, Hakulinen T, Storm HH. Rectal cancer survival in the Nordic countries and Scotland. Int J Cancer. 2009;125(10):2406–12.

25. Bülow S, Harling H, Iversen LH, Ladelund S, Danish Colorectal Cancer Group. Improved survival after rectal cancer in Denmark. Colorectal Dis. 2010;12(7 Online):e37–42. Epub 2009 Jul 15; doi:10.1111/j.1463-1318.2009.02012.

26. Penninckx F, Van Eycken L, Michiels G, Mertens R, Bertrand C, De Coninck D, Haustermans K, Jouret A, Kartheuser A, Tinton N, PROCARE Working Group. Survival of rectal cancer patients in Belgium 1997-98 and the potential benefit of a national project. Acta Chir Belg. 2006;106(2):149–57.

27. Ortiz H. Total mesorectal excision: a teaching and audited initiative of the Spanish Association of Surgeons. Cir Esp. 2007;82(4):193–4 (In Spanish).

28. Mroczkowski P, Kube R, Schmidt U, Gastinger I, Lippert H. Quality assessment of colorectal cancer care – an international online model. Colorectal Dis. 2011;13(8):890–5.

29. van Gijn W, Wouters MW, Peeters KC, van de Velde CJ. Nationwide outcome registrations to improve quality of care in rectal surgery. An initiative of the European Society of Surgical Oncology. J Surg Oncol. 2009;99(8):491–6.

30. Tilney H, Lovegrove RE, Smith JJ, Thompson MR, Tekkis PP, Association of Coloproctology of Great Britain and Ireland. The National Bowel Cancer Project: social deprivation is an independent predictor of nonrestorative rectal cancer surgery. Dis Colon Rectum. 2009;52(6):1046–53.

31. Peeters KC, Marijnen CA, Nagtegaal ID, Kranenbarg EK, Putter H, Wiggers T, Rutten H, Pahlman L, Glimelius B, Leer JW, van de Velde CJ, Dutch Colorectal Cancer Group. The TME trial after a median follow-up of 6 years: increased local control but no survival benefit in irradiated patients with resectable rectal carcinoma. Ann Surg. 2007;246(5):693–701.

32. Porter GA, Soskolne CL, Yakimetz WW, Newman SC. Surgeon-related factors and outcome in rectal cancer. Ann Surg. 1998;227(2):157–67.

33. Penninckx F. Surgeon-related aspects of the treatment and outcome after radical resection for rectal cancer. Acta Gastroenterol Belg. 2001;64:258–62.

34. Daniels IR, Fisher SE, Heald RJ, Moran BJ. Accurate staging, selective preoperative therapy and optimal surgery improves outcome in rectal cancer: a review of the recent evidence. Colorectal Dis. 2007;9:290–301.

35. Martling A, Cedermark B, Johansson H, Rutqvist LE, Holm T. The surgeon as a prognostic factor after the introduction of total mesorectal excision in the treatment of rectal cancer. Br J Surg. 2002;89(8):1008–13.

36. Harling H, Bülow S, Kronborg O et al. Survival of rectal cancer patients in Denmark during 1994–99. Colorectal Dis. 2004;6(3):153–7.

37. Kapiteijn E, Putter H, van de Velde CJ; Cooperative investigators of the Dutch ColoRectal Cancer Group. Impact of the introduction and training of total mesorectal excision on recurrence and survival in rectal cancer in The Netherlands. Br J Surg. 2002;89(9):1142–9.

38. Sharma A, Sharp DM, Walker LG, Monson JR. Colorectal MDTs: the team's perspective. Colorectal Dis. 2008;10(1):63–8.

39. Wood JJ, Metcalfe C, Paes A et al. An evaluation of treatment decisions at a colorectal cancer multi–disciplinary team. Colorectal Dis. 2008;10(8):769–72.

40. MacDermid E, Hooton G, MacDonald M, McKay G, Grose D, Mohammed N, Porteous C. Improving patient survival with the colorectal cancer multi-disciplinary team. Colorectal Dis. 2009;11(3):291–5. doi:10.1111/j.1463–1318.2008.01580.x. Epub 2008 May 9.

41. Segelman J, Singnomklao T, Hellborg H et al. Differences in multidisciplinary team assessment and treatment between patients with stage IV colon and rectal cancer. Colorectal Dis. 2009;11(7):768–74.

42. Lordan JT, Karanjia ND, Quiney N et al. A 10–year study of outcome following hepatic resection for colorectal liver metastases - The effect of evaluation in a multidisciplinary team setting. Eur J Surg Oncol. 2009;35(3):302–6. doi:10.1016/j.ejso.2008.01.028. Epub 2008 Mar 6.

43. Burton S, Brown G, Daniels IR et al. MRI directed multidisciplinary team preoperative treatment strategy: the way to eliminate positive circumferential margins? Br J Cancer. 2006;94(3):351–7.

44. Cancer in Norway 2008; www.kreftregisteret.no (In Norwegian).

Part II
Surgery

Introduction to Surgery

3

Lars Påhlman

Abstract

This chapter describes the evolution in colorectal cancer surgery since the end of the nineteenth century to the beginning of the twenty-first century. The most dramatic changes came in the 1950s when antibiotic and thromboembolic prophylaxis was introduced. Later the knowledge of the negative side effects of bowel preparation was obvious. However, the most important change was when the whole idea to operate in the embryological plane became evident. It was first demonstrated in rectal cancer surgery and later in colonic cancer surgery. During the last three decades, laparoscopic surgery for bowel cancer has been tested, and so far the evidence indicates that a colonic cancer can be treated equally good with a laparoscopic approach as an open one. For rectal cancer the results from randomised trials are still awaited. During the last two decades, reports on the importance of auditing the outcome have become very evident.

From Miles to Heald and Further

With more than one million new cases yearly in the world, colorectal cancer (CRC) is one of the most frequent cancers and approximately one half of the patients will die from the disease [1]. The individual lifetime risk to achieve a CRC is 5 % in developed and industrialised countries [2]. In Europe it is the third most prevalent cancer and the second most important regarding cancer-

L. Påhlman, MD, PhD
Department of Surgery, University Hospital of Uppsala,
Uppsala 751 85, Sweden
e-mail: lars.pahlman@surgsci.uu.se

specific mortality [3, 4]. Surgery has been and is still the only option to be cured for colorectal cancer, and the first report of a successful resection of a colonic cancer including an anastomosis was from Reybard of Lyon in 1833 [5]. However, the majority of patients had a palliative defunctioning colostomy only due to severe complications, but later a resection and double-barrel colostomy were used to achieve intestinal continuity. Successively more surgeons obtained experience with intestinal suture leading to an increasing number of colonic resections being performed but still the mortality for intra-abdominal resection, and anastomosis was approximately 40 % at the end of the nineteenth century due to problems with intra-abdominal leakage and sepsis [6].

The Danish surgeon, Bloch in 1894, presented an idea of preventing intra-abdominal complications by introducing the concept of extraperitoneal resection and anastomosis, based upon two cases in which the loop of colon containing the carcinoma had been mobilised and brought out through the abdominal wall. Later the same manoeuvre was also independently described by von Mikulicz of Breslau [7]. Paul of Liverpool also described a very similar manoeuvre (Paul 1895), but in his operation the protruding loop was excised at the time of exteriorisation and special large, right-angled glass tubes were tied into the lumina of the distal and proximal ends of the colon [8], a procedure which became known as the Paul–Mikulicz procedure (although Bloch's name should have been added) and was popular throughout the world.

In rectal cancer the limitation of radical surgery was more a matter of possibilities to survive why the earliest surgical approaches to carcinoma of the rectum were via the perineum by Faget (1739), Lisfranc (1826) and Verneuil (1873). Subsequently the technique was entirely extraperitoneal, but despite this approach, patients rarely survived the operation due to perineal sepsis locally or a locally non-radical procedure [9–11]. Not until Ernest Miles realised that cancer surgery is more a matter of resecting the lymph node than the bowel, the outcome started to change. Although his initial results was devastation due to postoperative mortality, his philosophy gain acceptance worldwide [12]. Another technique to achieve cure but reduce mortality was an abdominal resection without an anastomosis proposed by Hartmann [13].

However, in the early days, limitations to radical surgery were more a matter of good anaesthesiology and postoperative pain control than surgery by itself. Not until appropriate anaesthesiology was available, surgery could become more radical. Also with the new anastomotic technique, developed in the late nineteenth century, surgery became more reliable to all patients. Doing the first pass of the twentieth century, a major change in the treatment was seen and

surgery was rather standardised with limited segmental resection in colon cancer patients, and for rectal cancer patients an abdominal perineal excision became the standard of care after Earnest Miles' data were presented as well as data from Henry Hartmann. After that it ended up with stomas. The postoperative mortality was very high as well as the postoperative infection rates. During the last century, however, several things slowly changed making surgery more secure.

Mechanical Bowel Preparation

It was a non-disputed knowledge since the late nineteenth century that a better outcome was received if faeces were removed from the bowel. Several sophisticated techniques with mechanical preoperative bowel preparation have been used like salted water enema to per oral bowel preparation with polyethylene glycol or sodium phosphate. However, based upon experience in surgery for emergency cases, where resection has been more common, data from the 1980s and 1990s have proven that the outcome might be worse after mechanical bowel preparation for elective surgery. Two large randomised trials have now shown that bowel prep should not be used in colonic surgery [14, 15]. The evidence is not that strong in rectal cancer surgery, but a lot of data support that surgery can be done safely without major bowel prep even for rectal cancer surgery [16].

Antibiotic Prophylaxis

Before the era of antibiotics, more than 30 % of the patients experienced wound infections. Once antibiotics were introduced, several methods of using antibiotics have been tested. In the beginning both per oral and intravenous antibiotics were given to the patients postoperatively. During the 1960s and 1970s, randomised trials clearly showed that preoperative given antibiotics are better than administrated postoperatively. Moreover, the number of doses has been reduced to one dose preoperatively covering both aerobic and non-aerobic microbes. This is now the standard of care, and only in emergency surgery with extremely contaminated wounds one could consider postoperative antibiotics too.

Thromboembolic Prophylaxis

It is well known that the risk of having a thromboembolic event is increased after major abdominal surgery for cancer. It increases even more if surgery is performed in the pelvis. Based upon the knowledge from randomised trials in hip and knee surgery, new trials have been run showing that there is an increased risk of having deep vein thrombosis but also pulmonary embolism after colorectal cancer surgery if no prophylaxis is used. Subsequently the recommendation is to give some type of prophylaxis and the most commonly used is un-fractionated heparins or equivalent treatment, and this should be ongoing at least 1 week and probably 1 month postoperatively. In cancer surgery of the large bowel, the dose has to be doubled [17].

Anastomotic Techniques

The classic anastomotic technique has for many years been a double- or triple-layer anastomosis with an inner row of adapting the mucosa and an outer row of adapting the serosa. In the late nineteenth century, there was an academic fight between Mikulicz and Billroth whether the mucosa in the anastomosis should be invaginated or not. It was not an evidence-based discussion but merely a matter of who was the strongest surgeon at that time. Billroth won and since his time an invagination of the anastomosis by knitting serosa to serosa became the standard of care. Until the last 25 years of the twentieth century, the most common sewed material was catgut and silk. At that time staplers were introduced, both circular staplers for low rectal anastomoses and also staplers for colonic anastomoses. During the same time period, modern suture material like polyglycolic acid entered the market and handsewn anastomoses with a single-layer interrupted

or non-interrupted anastomosis technique were also introduced. Other techniques like compression anastomoses with metal ring (the Murphy button) or by a biodegradable material (Waltrac®) have also been used but not popularised. The latest type of anastomotic techniques is a compression anastomosis with the use of a memory-shaped nitinol, a metal alloy that contains a nearly equal mixture of nickel and titanium. This technique is still under investigation.

The most common technique is either handsewn or stapled anastomosis, and several randomised trials have shown that stapled anastomoses are as good as handsewn anastomoses, and it is nowadays the preference for surgeons to use either technique.

Important Steps in Modern Rectal Cancer Surgery

In the beginning rectal cancer surgery was performed with a posterior approach, mainly due to the problem with anaesthesia. Once anaesthesiologists were able to take care of the patients, more advanced surgery can be done. Earnest Miles observed a very high local recurrence rate and therefore proposed an abdominal approach to be able to take care of the lymph nodes. In his initial experience with an abdominoperineal excision, the mortality was high for the first time patients could be cured [12]. Henry Hartmann, a French surgeon, also introduced an abdominal resection of the rectum, i.e. the tumour-bearing part of the rectum was resected, the distal rectal stump closed and a sigmoidostomy was performed [13]. This became popular since mortality could be kept on an acceptable level. In the 1930s Dixon proposed that low-situated sigmoid cancer and recto-sigmoid tumours could be treated with an anastomosis instead of a stoma [18]. Dixon has been claimed to be the father of anterior resection. However, a very low anterior resection and sphincter-preserving procedure were not introduced until the stapler device appeared on the market in the late 1970s. Once sphincter-preserving surgery became more common, there were a debate about the safety and length of the distal margin, and for many years the distal margin should be at least 5 cm, based upon anatomical and pathological studies.

When the results were analysed, data on unacceptable high local recurrence rates became more obvious, with reports on recurrence rates of 50 % [19]. Moreover, reports indicated the importance of the operating surgeon [20] and more attention to the circumferential resection margin than the distal margin [21]. With the knowledge of the local recurrence and not only the radicality in the distal margin but also in the lateral margin, it was obvious in the early 1980s that the majority of the local recurrences could be prevented with surgery alone. However, already at that time adjuvant and neo-adjuvant radiotherapy had started to be used and in several countries radiotherapy was thought to be the solution (see Chap. 12).

At the same time as radiotherapy was popularised, reports from single centres showed very good results without radiotherapy [22–24]. Professor Bill Heald introduced the whole concept of total mesorectal excision (TME) [25]. In that concept a dissection following the embryological planes with a radical circumferential resection margin was as important as the distal margin. With the knowledge that the distal margin in very low rectal cancer could be as short as 1 cm, the proportion of sphincter-preserving procedure increased, and in devoted centres 80 % will not have a sigmoidostomy [26]. With the introduction of TME, the local recurrence rate continued to decrease and national training programmes were launched resulting in a dramatic change in the local recurrence rates below 10 % with subsequent survival benefits [27–29].

In one group of the patients, i.e. those having an abdominoperineal resection (APR), the local recurrence rate was still very high mainly due to a non-radical excision with a positive circumferential resection margin. With the introduction of a more cylindrical excision of the levator area when an APR is performed, the coning into the tumour area is prevented. With this technique the local recurrence rate after an APR has been reduced [30]. To achieve a specimen with negative resection margins, it is important to stop the abdominal phase at the level of cervix or vesicles

and start to operate from below and follow the pelvic floor laterally and divide the pelvic floor together with the specimen making a good cylindrical excision.

Important Steps in Modern Colon Cancer Surgery

An important consideration in colon cancer surgery is the distance from the tumour to the resection margin. The rational is to excise lymph nodes along the bowel which can be metastatic. Japanese data have shown that 10 cm from the tumour is a safe margin, since tumour deposits rarely are found more laterally from the primary tumour [31, 32]. The same philosophy as for rectal cancer, i.e. following the anatomical and embryological planes, can also be applied on colon cancer surgery too. Very little attention to the colonic anatomy has been paid, but very recent data from the Erlangen group have emphasised the importance and have also presented very good results [33]. Still it is too early to evaluate this philosophy, but based upon the dramatic change in rectal cancer surgery, this will probably also change colon cancer surgery to the same extent.

Training Organisation

Based upon the national quality register, it is obvious that surgery can be improved. The experience from rectal cancer registries from the Scandinavian countries have showed that surgeons can train and learn better [27–29]. Also the experience from the Netherlands, where surgeons was taught to do a proper TME before they included patients in Dutch radiotherapy trial, could demonstrate an improvement. The training programme in rectal cancer surgery run in Stockholm area, Sweden, has also shown that raining is important [34].

Concentration of surgery to fewer centres with more devoted surgeons has also been proposed, although the individual surgeon is more important than the "unit" [35]. To create a good milieu for surgery, most centres with good results propose two consultant surgeons operating together making the rectal cancer procedure quick and easy and possible to learn from each other. This has become the tradition in the Scandinavian countries and by doing so the results have improved steadily. To follow the process auditing the results is essential.

Laparoscopic Surgery

The first laparoscopic bowel procedure was performed in 1991. Very soon afterwards several reports on feasibility of laparoscopic surgery for cancer were presented. However, the whole idea of laparoscopic colonic resection for cancer was stopped due to several reports of port-site recurrences [36]. It was difficult to understand why a recurrence appeared at the site of the ports. Hypothesis like the "chimney effect", contaminated instruments, creating a tumour cells aerosol and adherence of disseminated cancer cells to different materials were tested experimentally. Unfortunately, all data ended up with a rather simple knowledge that most reasons for having port-site metastases were a matter of bad surgical technique traumatising the tumour during instrumentation.

Due to the uncertainty of the rational of laparoscopic bowel resection for cancer, several randomised trials were started, and all of them showed that in selected patients, no difference in cancer-specific or overall survival could be demonstrated [37–40]. A meta-analysis of these for trials could not demonstrate any difference in outcome, stage by stage [41]. However, one has to remember that there were selections to these trials, and several patients are still not suitable to laparoscopic resection, like T4 tumours growing into other organs. The laparoscopic technique has demonstrated several advantages, less complications, shorter length of stay and quicker return to daily living and work. The laparoscopic technique has illustrated the importance of early discharge, and with an enhanced recovery programme to patients having opened surgery, a similar effect can be reached.

For rectal cancer the evidence is not that strong. There are several hospital reports indicating that the results are as good as with open surgery [42, 43]. In one of the randomised trials, rectal cancer was included [40], but the numbers were few and the evidence is not clear regarding laparoscopic surgery for rectal cancer. At least three ongoing trials will answer this question.

Although, laparoscopic surgery for both colon and rectal cancer is growing, not more than 60 % in dedicated centres will have a laparoscopic procedure. On national level in the majority of countries, less than 10 % of all patients will undergo a laparoscopic procedure. Probably this frequency will increase steadily over the years.

Robotic Surgery

The introduction of robotic surgery has given a new dimension in colorectal cancer surgery. It has been tested in the lesser pelvis treating prostate cancer and has later been used for rectal cancer surgery. It is an expensive tool, but those having learned the technique have stated that the precision in dissection is much better than laparoscopy, mainly due to the degree of freedom on how the instruments can be used. Still there are no randomised trials showing any benefit, but those are ongoing. The most important advantage is dissection in an obese patient with a narrow pelvis [44].

Surgery Is Not Just Operation, It Is Academic

During the last two decades, evidence-based medicine has become more and more important. Lots of dogmas in colorectal cancer surgery have slowly been changed, but this change has only been possible due to a good evidence. The best way to challenge dogmas is of course using randomised trials.

Changes we have seen over the years, based upon randomised trials, are that the drainage will increase anastomotic leakage and should therefore be used selectively. We have also learned that the mechanical bowel preparation will increase morbidity postoperatively, is not well tolerated and should only be used when it is necessary, like finding polyps with a preoperative colonoscopy or other very specific reasons. Enhanced recovery programmes have also been evaluated in randomised trials, and based upon those data, the fast-track idea has become the standard of care in most patients with colorectal cancer. The use of prophylactic antibiotics has been changed, based upon randomised trials, from postoperative to preoperative administration and shorter treatment time. Other important changes, studied in large randomised trials, are the use of thromboembolic prophylaxis.

In this way, with randomised trials, surgery has slowly been changed, and by moving forward, step by step, new hypotheses have been tested rejecting some old-fashioned dogmas. This is the way surgery will improve. However, once the evidence is available, it has been shown that it takes up to 10–15 years until the majority (more than 95 %) of the hospitals have adopted the evidence according to literature and implemented in the practice.

References

1. Parkin DM, Bray F, Ferlay J, Pisani P. Global cancer statistics. CA Cancer J Clin. 2005;55:74–108.
2. Jemal A, Siegel R, Ward E, Hao Y, Xu J, Thun MJ. Cancer statistics. CA Cancer J Clin. 2009;58: 225–49.
3. Ferlay J, Autier P, Boniol M, Heanue M, Colombet M, Boyle P. Estimates of the cancer incidence and mortality in Europe 2006. Ann Oncol. 2007;18:581–92.
4. Weitz J, Koch M, Debus J, Höhler T, Galle PR, Büchler MW. Colorectal cancer. Lancet. 2005;365: 153–65.
5. Rankin FW. Surgery of the colon. New York: Appleton; 1926.
6. Morgan CN. The management of carcinoma of the colon. Ann R Coll Surg Engl. 1952;10:305–23.
7. von Mikulicz J. Small contributions to the surgery of the intestinal tract. Boston Med Surg J. 1903;148:608.
8. Paul FT. Colectomy. Br Med J. 1895;1:1136.
9. Faget JL (1739) Quoted in Rankin FW, Bargen JA, Buie LA. The colon, rectum and anus. Philadelphia: WB Saunders; 1932. p. 768.
10. Lisfranc J. Observation sur une affection cancereuse du rectume guérie par l'excision. Rev Med Franc Etrang. 1826;2:380.
11. Vernenil AA (1873) Quoted by Tuttle JP. A treatise on diseases of the anus, rectum and pelvic colon. 2nd ed. New York: Appleton; 1905. p. 963.
12. Miles WE. A method of performing abdominoperineal excision for carcinoma of the rectum and of the terminal portion of the pelvic colon. Lancet. 1908; 2:1812–3.
13. Hartmann H. Congrès francais de Chirurgie. 1923; 30:411.
14. Jung B, Påhlman L, Nyström PO, Nilsson E. Multicenter randomized trial of mechanical bowel preparation in elective colon resection. Br J Surg. 2007;94:689–95.
15. Contant CM, Hop WC, Van't Sant HP, Oostvogel HJ, Smeets HJ, Stassen LP, Neijenhuis PA, Idenburg FJ, Dijkhuis CM, Heres P, van Tets WF, Gerritsen JJ, Weidema WF. Mechanical bowel preparation for elective colorectal surgery: a multicentre randomised trial. Lancet. 2007;370(9605):2112–7.
16. Guenaga KKFG, Matos D, Wille-Jørgensen P. Mechanical bowel preparation for elective colorectal surgery. Cochrane Database Syst Rev. 2009;(1): CD001544. doi:10.1002/14651858.CD001544.pub3.
17. Enoxacan Study Group. The efficacy and safety of enoxaparin vs unfractionated heparin in prevention of deep vein thrombosis in elective cancer surgery. A double blind randomized multicentre trial in 1116 patients with venographic assessment. Br J Surg. 1997;84:1099–103.
18. Dixon CF. Surgical removal of lesions occurring in sigmoid and rectosigmoid. Am J Surg. 1939;46:12–7.
19. Påhlman L, Enblad P, Glimelius B. Clinical characteristics and their relation to surgical curability in adenocarcinoma of the rectum and recto-sigmoid: a population-based study in 279 consecutive patients. Acta Chir Scand. 1985;151:685–93.
20. Hermanek P, Wiebelt H, Staimmer D, et al. Prognostic factors of rectal carcinoma: experience of the German multicentre study. SGCRC Tumori. 1995;81(Suppl): 60–4.
21. Quirke P, Dixon MF, Durdey P, Williams NS. Local recurrence of rectal adenocarcinoma due to inadequate surgical resection. Lancet. 1986;1:996–8.
22. Heald RJ, Husband EM, Ryall RDH. The mesorectum in rectal cancer surgery: the clue to pelvic recurrence. Br J Surg. 1982;69:613–6.
23. Enker WE, Laffer UT, Block GE. Enhanced survival of patients with colon and rectal cancer is based upon wide anatomic resection. Ann Surg. 1979;190:350–8.
24. Moriya Y, Hojo K, Sawada T, Koyama Y. Significance of lateral lymph node dissection for advanced rectal carcinoma at or below the peritoneal reflection. Dis Colon Rectum. 1989;32:307–15.
25. MacFarlane JK, Ryall RDH, Heald RJ. Mesorectal excision of the rectum. Lancer. 1993;341:457–60.
26. Heald RJ. Towards fewer colostomies: the impact of circular stapling devices on the surgery of rectal cancer in a district hospital. Br J Surg. 1980;60:198–200.
27. Påhlman L, Bohe M, Cedermark B, Dahlberg M, Lindmark G, Sjödahl R, Öjerskog B, Damber L,

Johansson R. The Swedish rectal cancer registry. Br J Surg. 2007;94:1285–92.

28. Wibe A, Möller B, Norstein J, Carlsen E, et al. A national strategic change in treatment policy for rectal cancer – implementation of total Mesorectal excision as routine treatment in Norway. A national audit. Dis Colon Rectum. 2002;45:857–66.

29. Bülow S, Harling H, Iversen LH, Ladelund S. Improved survival after rectal cancer in Denmark. Colorectal Dis. 2009;171:2735–8.

30. Holm T, Ljung A, Häggmark T, Lagergren J. Extended abdominoperineal resection with gluteus maximus flap reconstruction of the pelvic floor for rectal cancer. Br J Surg. 2007;94:232–8.

31. Hida J, Yasutomi M, Maruyama T, Fujimoto K, Uchida T, Okuno K. The extent of lymph node dissection for colon carcinoma: the potential impact on laparoscopic surgery. Cancer. 1997;80:188–92.

32. Hida J, Okuno K, Yasutomi M, Yoshifuji T, Uchida T, Tokoro T, Shiozaki H. Optimal ligation level of the primary feeding artery and bowel resection margin in colon cancer surgery: the influence of the site of the primary feeding artery. Dis Colon Rectum. 2005;48:2232–7.

33. Hohenberger W, Weber K, Matzel K, Papadopoulos T, Merkel S. Standardized surgery for colonic cancer: complete mesocolic excision and central ligation – technical notes and outcome. Colorectal Dis. 2009;11:354–64.

34. Martling AL, Holm T, Rutquist LE, et al. Effect of a surgical training programme on the outcome of rectal cancer in the County of Stockholm. Lancet. 2000;356:93–6.

35. Kressner M, Bohe M, Cedermark B, Dahlberg M, Damber L, Lindmark G, Öjerskog B, Sjödahl R, Johansson R, Påhlman L. The impact of hospital volume on surgical outcome in patients with rectal cancer. Dis Colon Rectum. 2009;52:1542–9.

36. Wexner SD, Cohen SM. Port site metastases after laparoscopic colorectal surgery for cure of malignancy. Br J Surg. 1995;82:295–8.

37. Lacy AM, Garcia-Valdecasas JC, Delgado S, et al. Laparoscopy-assisted colectomy versus open colectomy for treatment of non-metastatic colon cancer: a randomised trial. Lancet. 2002;359:2224–9.

38. Clinical Outcomes of Surgical Therapy Study Group. A comparison of laparoscopically assisted and open colectomy for colon cancer. N Engl J Med. 2004;350:2050–9.

39. COLOR Study Group, Veldkamp R, Hop WCJ, Jeekel J, Bonjer HJ, Haglind E, Påhlman L, Cuesta MA, Msika S, Morino M, Lacy AM. Laparoscopic versus open surgery for colonic cancer: short-term results of the COLOR-trial. Lancet Oncol. 2005;6:477–84.

40. Guillou PJ, Quirke P, Thorpe H, et al. Short-term endpoints of conventional versus laparoscopic-assisted surgery in patients with colorectal cancer (MRC CLASICC trial): multicentre, randomised controlled trial. Lancet. 2005;365:1718–26.

41. Bonjer HJ, Hop WCJ, Nelson H, Sargent DJ, Lacy AM, Castells A, Guillou PJ, Thorpe H, Brown J, Deldago S, Kuhry E, Haglind E, Påhlman L. Laparoscopically assisted versus open colectomy for colon cancer – a meta-analysis. Arch Surg. 2007;142:298–303.

42. Morino M, Parini U, Giraudo G, Salval M, Brachet Contul R, Garrone C. Laparoscopic total mesorectal excision: a consecutive series of 100 patients. Ann Surg. 2003;237:335–42.

43. Laurent C, Leblanc F, Wütrich P, Scheffler M, Rullier E. Laparoscopic versus open surgery for rectal cancer: long-term oncologic results. Ann Surg. 2009;250:54–61.

44. Zimmern A, Prasad L, Desouza A, Marecik S, Park J, Abcarian H. Robotic colon and rectal surgery: a series of 131 cases. World J Surg. 2010;34(8):1954–8.

Surgical Anatomy of the Rectum and the TME Specimen (Total Mesorectal Excision)

4

R.J. Heald and Brendan J. Moran

Abstract

Rectal cancer is a disease where surgical mastery of anatomical detail is the principal determinant of outcome. Classical anatomy is based on cadavers which differ from live humans, whilst inaccessibility and bleeding during surgery have limited our understanding of surgical 'TME anatomy' until this generation. MDT management and the use of preoperative staging by MRI not only show clearly who really needs RT but also introduce a whole new anatomy which must be understood by all who contribute to MDT decisions.

In addition, MRI provides unique opportunities for surgeons to grasp the 3D anatomy of the pelvis and the relations of the surgical specimen to the crucial nerves, organs and muscles that surround it. Each MDT should be an anatomy lesson for every surgeon present.

Introduction

Rectal cancer is a disease where surgical mastery of anatomical detail is the principal determinant of outcome. Classical anatomy is based on cadavers which differ from live humans, whilst inaccessibility and bleeding during surgery have limited our understanding of surgical 'TME anatomy' until this generation. MDT management and the use of preoperative staging by MRI not only show clearly who really needs RT but also introduce a whole new anatomy which must be understood by all who contribute to MDT decisions.

In addition, MRI provides unique opportunities for surgeons to grasp the 3D anatomy of the pelvis and the relations of the surgical specimen to the crucial nerves, organs and muscles that surround it. Each MDT should be an anatomy lesson for every surgeon present (Fig. 4.1).

R.J. Heald (✉)
Pelican Cancer Foundation,
The Ark Conference Centre, Dinwoodie Drive,
Basingstoke, Hampshire RG24 9NN, UK
e-mail: e.hayward@pelicancancer.org

B.J. Moran
Basingstoke and North Hampshire NHS Foundation
Trust, Pelican Cancer Foundation, Aldermaston
Road, Basingstoke, Hampshire RG24 9NA, UK

G. Baatrup (ed.), *Multidisciplinary Treatment of Colorectal Cancer*,
DOI 10.1007/978-3-319-06142-9_4, © Springer International Publishing Switzerland 2015

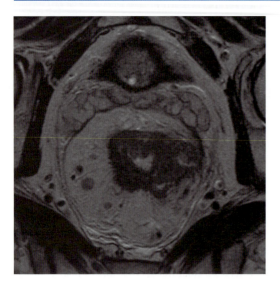

Fig. 4.1 Carcinoma threatening the mesorectal fascia on the left

Total Mesorectal Excision (TME) Current Controversies

TME is the key surgical objective [1–19]—can it however be achieved as well or better by laparoscopy, or by the da Vinci robot? When truly necessary, can the poor results so often obtained by the 'standard' APE be improved upon by superior access—e.g. the Kocher–Holm position face down with excision of the coccyx? All these are controversial issues (Fig. 4.2).

Current priorities include better visualisation and more precise dissection, improved haemostasis and less collateral damage by diathermy (e.g. the use of TriVerse monopolar and LigaSure bipolar electricity). Gradually, surgeons, open, laparoscopic and robotic, are learning to recognise all the components of the autonomic nervous system of the pelvis which surround the TME. Indeed, surgeons are rewriting the anatomy books as surgical technology advances. The preservation of these crucial nerves depends a great part of human happiness and dignity.

There are few branches of surgery where care and effort in the craft of surgery yield so much benefit to our patients or where surgical anatomy is so important and advancing so rapidly.

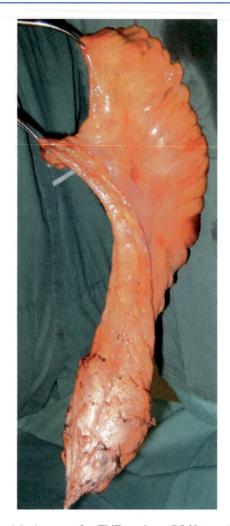

Fig. 4.2 A near perfect TME specimen (PO Nystrom)

Objectives

These are cure of cancer, local control of a disease where local failure causes great misery, keeping permanent stomas to a minimum and avoidance of collateral damage'. As a basic principle of any cancer operation, the block of tissue to be removed should be precisely defined and subjected to scrutiny by an independent pathologist. Thus, surgical anatomy and histopathologic audit should become exact sciences in their own right and surgical practice refined to include meaningful judgement of the oncologic quality of the specimen. It is rewarding to report that naked-eye evaluation of the excised specimen has become mandatory in Germany. Our own teaching workshops always emphasise the importance of 'specimen-orientated surgeons'— i.e. surgeons whose first priority during the procedure is the quality of the fascial-covered untorn envelope of tissue that constitutes an optimal TME specimen.

Definition of the Rectum Itself

Unfortunately, this varies across the world, and all actual definitions are inherently unsatisfactory. For simplicity, we choose arbitrarily to define it as the bowel up to 15 cm above the anal verge (patient conscious). The low rectum is also arbitrarily defined as up to 6 cm, the mid as 6–12 and the upper as 12–15 cm.

Partial Mesorectal Excision (PME)

Height measurement, by general agreement, is from the anal verge in the conscious patient using a rigid sigmoidoscope. In the new world of MRI, the MRI height should also be recorded, and there is an argument for considering as truly 'low' cancers extending below the origins of the levator muscles on the coronal slice. Heights measured under anaesthesia need to be from the dentate line since the external sphincter dilates and retracts (add about 1.5 cm). Care is necessary: any instrument can push a mobile tumour up; flexible ones often give falsely high measurement. With these qualifications, it can be said that, in our view, most cancers with the lower edge at or below 12 cm should have TME as the key component of a radical cancer operation because the mesorectum is the primary field of lymphovascular spread (Fig. 4.3).

The decision as to whether the smaller *partial* mesorectal excision is adequate is finally confirmed after the mobilisation has been completed to the point where the mesorectum must be liberated from the adherent inferior hypogastric plexus—the region is usually referred to as the 'lateral ligament'. It has long been convention

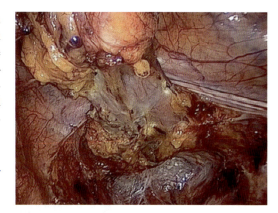

Fig. 4.3 The pelvis after laparoscopic PME

and a very sound rule, borrowed from German surgical practice, that a minimum of 5 cm of mesentery should always be excised both proximal and distal to any colorectal cancer. Whilst lowering of muscle tube margin may safely be reduced to 1 cm in the interest of anal conservation, we have always believed that if less than a total mesorectal excision for a high tumour is contemplated, a minimum of 5 cm of the mesorectum distal to the lower edge of the cancer must be dissected in the perimesorectal (holy) plane. If, therefore, after initial mobilisation there is a clear 5 cm of mesorectum, then tapering into the mesentery, in the interest of making a more minor operation and a higher anastomosis, becomes acceptable.

The operation then becomes perimesorectal mobilisation, mesorectal transection, anterior resection and primary anastomosis for rectal cancers above around 12 cm. Either 5 cm of mesorectum distal to the tumour or the whole mesorectum must be removed intact with the same preoccupation with clear circumferential margins.

Oncologic Envelopes to Be Excised

There is a need for real understanding of where the satellites of cancer commonly occur since the ideal radical cancer operation should encompass only the common fields of spread that do not exact too high a penalty from the patient. The design of the optimal operation that modern surgery can now offer should take into account the field of spread amenable to surgical removal with the primary tumour, the disabilities inflicted by each component of the surgery and the point in time at which cure becomes impossible by local surgery because metastases have already become established. TME is by far the most important oncologic unit of cure in rectal cancer. A perfect surgery is achieved without inflicting lasting morbidity only if the surgical anatomy of TME is fully understood. Preoperative assessment should supplement full clinical and endoscopic appraisal with a computed tomography (CT) scan of the whole body for metastatic spread, and a specialised magnetic resonance imaging (MRI) is necessary for the most precise picture of the primary cancer, its locoregional spread and the anatomical relations of the mesorectum and its contained malignancy.

The Embryologic Basis of Cancer Surgery: Exemplified by Colorectal Cancer: 'The Holy Plane' or 'Holy Space'

Conceptually, TME has a basis in scientific thought which is attractive to all members of the modern multidisciplinary team with background training in basic science. The theory behind it is that all lymphovascular cancer spread will tend, initially at least, to remain within the embryologic hindgut 'envelope'. The gut of the pre-10 mm embryo extruded itself and secondarily became 'plastered' back onto the retroperitoneal structures and into the developing pelvis: it retains its midline lymphovascular integrity, and its artery arises from the front of the aorta. It remains separated from the surrounding paired organs and parietes by a collagenous cobweb of areolar tissue. This allows a degree of movement and is recognisable by the surgeon as a 'surgical dissection plane' and is developed by traction and countertraction into an almost entirely avascular space— 'the holy space'. In a number of publications, the authors have drawn attention to the 'holy plane of rectal surgery' and attempted to point out the value of painstakingly following this perimesorectal avascular plane around the midline hindgut

into the depths of the pelvis as a practical surgical policy. Doing so was eventually shown to improve local recurrence rates in a dramatic way. Straying into the field of cancer spread within the mesorectum was, and still is in conventional practice, an extremely common cause of involved surgical margins and potential residual pelvic disease: straying out can damage the autonomic nerve layers and is a common cause of impotence. Publications from the Karolinska Hospital, Solna, Sweden, demonstrate that more than one-half of all local recurrences are associated with residues of mesorectum left behind by the surgeon. Thus, inadequate TME, i.e. incomplete emptying of the central compartment (within the nerve layer), is a far more important cause of failure than ignoring the internal iliac and other compartments outside the visceral mesorectal 'core'. This is of great practical importance because, although a challenging dissection, TME is a standard reproducible teaching operation. The lateral compartments are surgically much more difficult and much less rewarding—perhaps best left to a few high-volume specialist surgeons along with other extended procedures such as sacrectomy. In summary, TME anatomy describes the precise 'emptying' of the posterial central compartment of the pelvis and the anatomical composition of the relations of each part of the mesorectal surface.

The basic TME hypothesis is essentially that embryology defies the oncologic envelope that encompasses the primary field of all locoregional spread—lymphatic, vascular, perineural and 'random'. Distally, this tapering hindgut 'package', surrounded by the 'holy plane', is inserted into the funnel-shaped sloping levator muscles, which merge and overlap with the skeletal external sphincters distally.

The Anatomy of the Mesorectum for the Surgeon: The Planes of the Pelvis

Surgical Anatomy

The original idea of TME was born from the practice of surgery. The mesorectum only becomes a reality for each individual surgeon from enthusiasm for slow, meticulous, painstaking dissection in difficult but achievable planes. These, once recognised and identified, become the defining objectives of the surgery and the redefined building blocks of the anatomy.

The innermost 'holy plane' is that which surrounds the midline hindgut within its lymphovascular envelope of visceral fascia—the core—whilst the two surrounding lamellae comprise a neural layer and a Wolffian ridge layer, which develop from the paired structures outside the hindgut. This concept has been made easier to comprehend by the Japanese comparison with the layers of an onion—or perhaps the core of the posterior of two onions separated by Denonvilliers' septum.

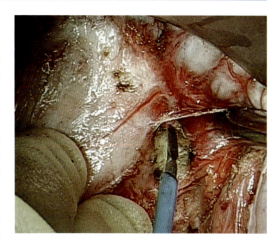

Fig. 4.4 Denonvilliers' septum

Much of the surgery of the whole gastrointestinal tract is a question of pursuing the planes between embryologically distinct lymphovascular entities. The careful and thoughtful surgeon who is mobilising any part of the large intestine by sharp dissection becomes aware of surgically satisfying planes, which assume special value in his or her journey down into the pelvis. The mesorectum is a complete fatty and lymphovascular surround on all aspects of the middle third of the rectum, which constitutes the greater part of the organ and the most common site for cancer. In the upper third, the anterior aspect is covered only by peritoneum with 'mesorectum and mesorectosigmoid' at the back and the sides as the peritoneal reflection tapers forward towards the 'cul-de-sac' or recto-vesical pouch. In the lower third of the rectum, little or no fatty tissue intervenes between the anterior aspect of the rectum and the back of the prostate. Posteriorly, the prostate has an important posterior condensed fascial covering called Denonvilliers' septum. The upper part of the septum is usually adherent to the anterior mesorectal fat of the middle third so that the surgeon must divide this layer from above to enter the plane between the rectum and the prostate in the male. How low this line of division should be may vary according to the position of the cancer—for a very low anterior tumour, it is essential to divide it very low so that the tumour is well cleared anteriorly, preferably with Denonvilliers' fascia as an extra safety layer. In posterior or higher tumours, the surgeon will give greater priority to avoiding damage to the converging nerves lateral to the edges of Denonvilliers' septum. In all cases, a u-shaped incision in the septum must be made so as to clear the tumour safely whilst preserving the converging nerves laterally. In the female, the middle third has only a rather thin and tenuous fatty layer between the rectum and vagina with Denonvilliers' fascia being often scant and difficult to identify; certainly, a recognisable condensed 'septum' is often not found as in the male. Is this perhaps because of its dissolution during childbirth or sexual activity? Denonvilliers' septum is recognised by some embryologists as the downward prolongation of the peritoneum, which has become distally obliterated as a cavity. As we become more fastidious in our dissections, *two layers* of the septum begin to become apparent. It is now clear to surgeons that, in the male at least, this trapezoidal 'bib' with defined lateral margins just medial to the important neurovascular bundles is indeed a reality, and with improving technique, two layers may indeed become apparent (Fig. 4.4).

Posteriorly and posterolaterally, the areolar plane is well defined around the globular expanding bilobed mesorectum. A condensation of the fascia called the rectosacral ligament—or Waldeyer's fascia—often presents a barrier to the surgeon posteriorly below the promontory. It is essential that this be positively divided with either diathermy or scissors. Beyond it, the

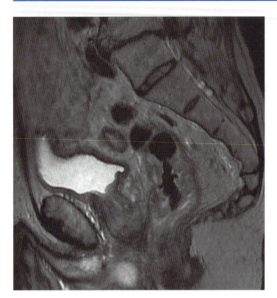

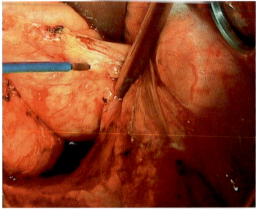

Fig. 4.6 Posterior aspect of a TME, 'the buttocks'

Fig. 4.5 Sagittal MRI cancer at 5 cm posteriorly

forward angulation demands strong anterodistal retraction to facilitate direct visualisation. Understanding the importance of this forward angulation is critical to mastering the traction and countertraction instruments necessary in open, laparoscopic and robotic TME. Confusingly, the middle third of the rectum is often called the horizontal segment because MRIs are typically viewed as if the patient is vertical (Fig. 4.5).

The crucial anatomical reality is that this segment is angled posteriorly relative to the anal canal by almost a right angle. The 'horizontal' segment follows the curve of the sacrum, and the upper third angles backwards to merge with the sigmoid.

Histopathology Audit

For proper independent audit, the surgeon should not cut the specimen except to open the bowel away from the tumour to let in the formalin. Completeness and intactness of the specimen are crucial factors—ideally it should be one recognisable block of tissue with a fascial covering. Its anatomical orientation and former relations should be identifiable. 'Specimen-orientated

surgery' has become an established practice, and recognition of the features of the TME specimen and the freedom of its margins from cancer involvement are the key factors of audit. In most cases, naked-eye inspection provides quality control, with microscopic examination of any suspected areas of margin involvement as a logical primary audit objective for the surgeon.

Visual inspection of the front of a well-performed TME specimen should show three clear landmarks:

- The cut edge of the peritoneal reflection and the whole 'cul-de-sac'
- The smooth shiny anterior surface of the anterior mesorectum of the middle third—Denonvilliers' fascia—or the rectogenital septum (upper half)
- The anterior aspect of the anorectal muscle—in the lowest anterior resections or abdomino-perineal excision (APE) specimens only

Laterally, the fatty mesorectum expands distally beyond an anteroposterior groove made by the nervi erigentes so that an embryologically perfect specimen has a lateral dilatation distally—corresponding with the part related to the inside of the levator muscles beyond their origins from the pelvic sidewall. Posteriorly, a perfect specimen exhibits perfectly curved 'buttocks' with a central midline groove corresponding to the anococcygeal raphe (the pubococcygeus muscle) with distal dilatations from beyond the nerve pillars (Fig. 4.6).

Modern Imaging: Fine-Slice High-Resolution MRI

Brown, Blomqvist and others have shown us that specialised fine-slice high-resolution MRI can visualise this 'holy plane' before the surgery and thus predict the detail of the oncologic specimen that the surgeon endeavours to remove and its relationship to the tentacles of tumour. The recent 'MERCURY' study from the Pelican Centre in Basingstoke has demonstrated reliable equivalence between MRI prediction and histopathologic reality. It also demonstrates that a 1-mm mesorectal 'clearance' does indeed predict a 'safe margin' provided the surgeon is faithfully following the 'holy plane'. Surprisingly, it is not a component of any staging system; extra-mural vascular invasion was an even more important prognostic indicator than nodal involvement at the N1 level. Some may take this as an indication for giving preoperative CRT to all patients with EMVI.

Conversely, 'threats' by proximity of an involved node to the margin did not appear to lead to local recurrence (0/63). This almost certainly reflects the extra care taken by the surgeon to keep clear of such a node by the surgeon who is thus forewarned of the morbid anatomy by the MRI. It thus shows the anatomical value of MRI in relation to surgery.

Similarly, this clearance on MRI between cancer within and mesorectal fascia without can be reliably used to predict a safe margin which does not need neoadjuvant 'downstaging'. It can also warn the surgeon when the mesorectal margin is in danger of being breached during surgery. It can thus provide a 'workshop guide' for anatomical surgery, whether this be performed laparoscopically or open. This may become particularly crucial for laparoscopic surgeons as they increasingly extend their dissections into the challenging depths of the true pelvis where the inability to feel the cancer can be a serious disadvantage. We emphasise the importance of displaying MRIs in the OR during the actual surgery, and surgeons should exercise their ability to correlate MRI anatomy with the surgery.

Critical MRI and Surgical Anatomy in Lower-Third Cancers

One focal area of current controversy centres on the anatomical and embryologic fact that the mesorectal envelope tapers down in this (intralevator) lower third to appear very thin indeed—particularly on the crucial coronal oblique MRI cuts on which decisions in modern multidisciplinary teams (MDTs) are made. On such an MRI, it is extremely tempting to predict that this tapering and narrowing area of the mesorectum will constitute a hazardous margin: thus, a decision may be made to administer preoperative downstaging neoadjuvant therapy or even choose abdominoperineal excision for fear of margin involvement when in fact a carefully orientated axial oblique sequence with the axial cuts precisely at right angles to the tumour segment may demonstrate a potentially safe clearance.

In addition to imaging, it is essential that an experienced surgeon examines the patient himself or herself to establish free mobility of the cancer within the puborectal sling in the conscious patient (with muscle tone). In the authors' opinion, this clinical observation on the sphincter complex and adjacent organs does almost invariably mean that a TME will be an achievable surgical objective. It does not confront the issue of the higher incidence of internal iliac and particularly obturator node involvement in tumours less than 4 cm from the anal margin.

Preoperative MDT 1

This is an exercise in predicting the 'morbid anatomy' in the individual case and cancer in the context of the patient's general health and personal wishes. Thus, the treatment and operation are planned. MRI anatomy provides education for all in the process.

Post-op Review of Patient Recovery, Specimen, and Histology (MDT 2)

- *Review of the Detail of the Surgery*—TME or 'TME plus'. 'TME minus' or 'partial TME' for upper one-third cancers.
- Detailed audit of the specimen after removal with special emphasis on naked-eye assessment of mesorectal integrity and microscopic evaluation of the margins. Postoperative chemotherapy is considered.

Principles of Surgery Based on 'TME Anatomy'

It is impossible to describe TME anatomy without describing the surgery that has defined it. It is truly a set of new pages in the anatomy books from a new source—surgery itself:

- Perimesorectal 'holy plane' sharp dissection by monopolar diathermy and scissors under direct vision. Three-directional traction and countertraction are vital for diathermy dissection as it is essential that the areolar tissue be 'on stretch'—thus creating 'the holy plane'.
- 'Specimen-orientated' surgery and histopathology, of which the object is an intact mesorectum with no tearing of the surface and no circumferential margin involvement (CMI)—naked eye or microscopic.
- Recognition during surgery of, and preservation of, the autonomic plexuses and nerves, on which sexual and bladder functions depend.
- A major increase in anal preservation and reduction in the number of permanent colostomies by skilful extension in the holy plane into the depths of the pelvis.
- Stapled low pelvic reconstruction, usually using the Moran triple stapling technique, plus creation of a short colon pouch or a side-to-end anastomosis to low rectum or anal canal.

Preoperative Assessment of the Morbid Anatomy

CT scans and colonoscopy report should always be at hand in the operating room. Never commence surgery without having examined the patient digitally when awake plus performing bimanual examination under anaesthesia. This is especially true in female patients so as to establish whether the tumour is fully mobile on the posterior vaginal wall.

Laparoscopic Anterior Resection

The authors take a major interest in this area of extending laparoscopic practice but continue themselves to perform open surgery for rectal cancer as detailed. The anatomical principles remain the same, and there is no doubt that excellent clearance of many cancers can be achieved laparoscopically by the increasing skill of specialised surgeons. The elevation of an intact mesorectal package, safely encompassing a large cancer, requires carefully applied but substantial upward traction, which is often difficult to achieve with laparoscopic instruments. Few laparoscopic instruments exist however that bend effectively round a really large cancer to apply upward traction in a safe gentle way.

The Anatomy

Starting Right—the 'pedicle package'—the clue to the top of the 'holy plane' and the anatomical adventure which is TME.

Starting correctly involves three-directional traction on the colon and retroperitoneum to identify the plane between the back of the pedicle package and the gonadal vessels, ureter and preaortic sympathetic nerves—all of which must be carefully preserved. The key to this phase is the recognition of the shiny fascial-covered surface of the back of the pedicle—like a tapering longitudinal 'sausage' with the inferior mesenteric vessels within. The whole sigmoid and its mesentery must be gently lifted forward, usually in open surgery on the left. It is equally satisfactory, as commonly performed in laparoscopic surgery, to start on the right. In either case, the identification of the shiny fascial envelope behind, what we like to call the 'pedicle package', is crucial to proper entry into the pelvis and to the preservation of the nerves.

High Ligation of the Inferior Mesenteric Vessels (IMA and IMV)

These are the principal and often the only major blood vessels supplying the rectum and mesorectum. Small vessels from the pelvic floor and in the area of lateral adherence are present but minor. However, a substantial collateral flow via the rectum itself does maintain viability of the whole organ even when the IMA is ligated.

With the pedicle package lifted gently forward, the dissection behind it can be extended up to its proximal end; separate high ligations of the inferior mesenteric artery and vein can be performed with the pedicle controlled by the left index finger with the surgeon standing on the patient's left side. The artery is taken 1–2 cm anterior to the aorta so as to spare the sympathetic nerve plexuses; the vein is divided above its last tributary close to the pancreas. These two high ligations are an integral part of the otherwise avascular planes, which need to be developed upwards extensively for a full mobilisation of the splenic flexure. The need for this is dictated by the decision to perform a TME and therefore an anastomosis of 3–6 cm from the anal verge. The mobilised colon must lie without tension in the hollow of the sacrum, and the two vessels are the main 'anchors' that prevent this.

The ascending left colic artery and either the accompanying inferior mesenteric vein or its last tributary from the left colon also need to be divided separately to complete the vascular isolation of the specimen with full mobilisation for ultralow pouch anastomosis.

In a minority of cases, a particularly long and healthy sigmoid may obviate the need for this full mobilisation process, which is not entirely without risk (e.g. to the spleen itself). Thus, it is logical, if a decision is made to use such a long healthy sigmoid and thus avoid the splenic flexure, to ligate the inferior mesenteric artery just distal to the ascending left colic, which is essentially a part of its primary blood supply. Particular care over the ligation is necessary as the stump will pulsate vigorously. If there were obvious lymph nodes that would be thus left behind, then so low a division would not be sensible.

The 'Division of Convenience'

The sigmoid mesentery and the sigmoid colon are divided well above the cancer. This is an important step in every cancer dissection as optimal mobility of the top of the specimen facilitates gentle opening of the perimesorectal planes by traction and countertraction in any direction throughout the pelvic dissection. After the division, there is also the best possible visualisation of the pelvis with all of the gut to be retained drawn upwards and to the right. Most laparoscopic surgeons do not find that this division helps them.

Pelvic Dissection: The Anatomy of Pelvic Planes

In both laparoscopic and open surgeries, firm anterior traction lifts the intended specimen forward from the preaortic nerve plexuses. The surgeon is now optimally placed to identify the key planes that must be developed circumferentially around the mesorectum. He or she starts at the back and then follows identifiable areas of the 'holy plane' at various points on the mesorectal circumference in a stepwise manner. If lower down in the pelvis, bleeding in one area is troublesome due to inaccessibility, it is sensible to tackle the opposite circumference so that pressure is applied whilst progress continues.

The Planes Posteriorly

There is no real substitute in open surgery for the St. Mark's retractor or our own reverse concavity version (Heald retractor)—both available from Bolton Surgical of Sheffield or from many instrument manufacturers. Forward traction demonstrates the shiny posterior surface of mesorectum within the bifurcation of the superior hypogastric plexus. This plane is extended downwards towards and eventually beyond the tip of the coccyx, step by step as other sectors of the circumference are developed.

Division of the Rectosacral Ligament or Fascia

This condensation may constitute an apparent barrier to downward progress posteriorly, requiring positive division with scissors or diathermy. Just in front of it, within the mesorectum, the superior rectal vessels can often be seen through the back of the mesorectal fascia, and around them cancerous nodes are likely to occur only millimetres away. An intact shiny visceral fascia over these must be jealously guarded and tearing avoided at all costs. This poses one of the greatest dangers of blunt manual extraction or of any haste or roughness, since the rectosacral ligament may be stronger than the surface fascia over the nodes. Thus, tearing into the lymphatic field by the inserted hand becomes a real risk and must have disrupted the anatomy frequently in the past. Sharp dissection under direct vision is crucial and lighting essential. A further safety factor in identifying positively the 'holy plane' posteriorly in front of the presacral fat pad (when present) is that one avoids the risk of tearing thin-walled presacral veins, which often have no valves and can bleed prodigiously when cut or torn. The key to the 'holy space' anatomy is that the surgeon must remain on the yellow mesorectal inner dissection plane which is opened by traction and countertraction. Sometimes there is a presacral fat pad behind the plane, and it is important to recognise and leave this in situ.

Planes of the Lateral Pelvic Sidewall

Dissection involves forward extension of the plane around to the sides, gently easing the adherent hypogastric nerves laterally off the mesorectal surface under direct vision. Freedom to lift the divided rectosigmoid forward often means that the tangentially running hypogastric nerves are first positively identified at this stage, the superior hypogastric plexus itself only becoming obvious proximal to the nerves after they have been dissected away from the mesorectal surface on each side. The superior hypogastric plexus is sometimes ensheathed by fatty tissue and not immediately recognised as a nerve bifurcation.

These nerves are far more important than hitherto appreciated because they subserve many of the functions of orgasm in both sexes, whilst the inferior, more distal plexus is necessary for the more obvious parasympathetic function of erection—certainly in the male and presumably clitoral function in the female as well.

The Loss of the Plane in the 'Lateral Ligament' Area

The 'holy plane' is followed downwards towards the vesicles with the expanding plexiform band of inferior hypogastric plexus outside it but increasingly adherent to it. In essence, there is no actual ligament, but there is an area of adherence between the mesorectum medially and plexus laterally: small branches of nerves and vessels penetrate through at this point, but none generally reaches more than 1 mm in diameter. The key nerves entering this flattened band from above are largely sympathetic hypogastric nerves curving distally from the superior plexuses and more distally the 'erigent' parasympathetic nerves coming forward to it from behind. These arise from the front of the roots of the sacral plexus (especially S3, out of sight behind the parietal sidewall fascia). This fascia is quite robust laterally, and the surgeon will note that he or she usually cannot even see the internal iliac vessels, which are outside it. Posteriorly, these

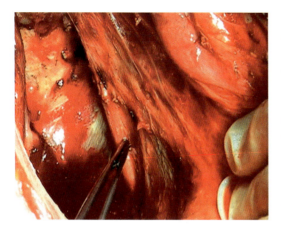

Fig. 4.7 The right erigent pillar and neural plate

'erigent pillars' from the roots around S3 curve forward outside the parietal fascia but medial to the branches of the internal iliac vessels (Fig. 4.7).

A little way behind the vesicles, the erigent pillars pierce the fascia to join the inferior hypogastric plexus and often contribute nerve branches to the mesorectum and rectum. These 'neural T-junctions' are the nearest structures to 'lateral ligaments' that the most careful surgeon will find with precise dissection. Another often described structure that we believe to be found only rarely by the surgeon during this dissection is a true middle rectal artery. We also believe that in the past what the surgeon believed to be a middle rectal artery was most often a lateral intra-mesorectal artery, and the so-called lateral stalk being divided represented a 'coning in' to the mesorectum. The surgeon dissecting perfectly between the mesorectum and the inferior hypogastric plexus discovers nothing more than a tiny vessel that requires no more than a touch of diathermy. Thus, the clamp and cut routine implied a poor quality of the dissection, damaged nerves and left a substantial residue of dangerous tissue—probably all a part of the prodigious 30–40 % local recurrence rate that was once commonplace.

Occasionally, the perivascular plane medial to the internal iliacs is the only way to achieve a clear margin. Rarely it may become necessary to go outside these vessels, but venous bleeding can be a problem.

Anterior: Denonvilliers' Septum

Dissection anterolaterally and anteriorly following the correct plane forward will encompass the peritoneal reflection that remains on the specimen and thus allows positive identification of the backs of the seminal vesicles. Forceful forward retraction on these with a St. Mark's retractor will facilitate the development of the areolar space between the vesicles and the smooth front of the mesorectal specimen. We call this smooth surface that is generally adherent to and clearly a part of the mesorectum Denonvilliers' fascia or the rectogenital septum. As one works distally, there comes a point where this fascia must be divided transversely as it becomes adherent to the posterior capsule of the prostate. The neurovascular bundles (of Walsh) constitute the distal condensation of the inferior hypogastric plexuses and are here joined by numerous veins and small arteries—hence the title neurovascular. More distally, they run posterolateral to the prostate and converge in the bulb of the penis to supply it and subserve erection as the so-called cavernous nerves.

These bundles are impossible to see in open surgery from above because of the forward angulation behind the vesicles, bladder and prostate and are in particular danger from surgeons who somewhat blindly 'take a slice off the back of the prostate'. This is highly likely to cause impotence because of the close relationship of the neurovascular bundles to the back of the prostate.

The pillar-like appearance is in part due to the forcible forward traction on the prostate and bladder to see the structures during an open operation, and this tends to bow the nerves medially and thus make them stand out. This retraction does not occur to the same extent in a laparoscopic operation, which may account for the reported higher incidence of nerve damage recorded from several centres.

Anatomy of the Most Distal Mesorectum from Above

The anatomy of the insertion of the mesorectal 'package' into the pelvic floor also becomes increasingly difficult for the surgeon to grasp from above—again because of inaccessibility behind the vesicles and prostate and behind the vagina in females. The situation is further complicated by the fact that the levators are like a 'flower pot' in continuity with the tube of external sphincter distally.

Careful pursuit of the plane at this level eventually liberates the mesorectal package and takes the operator down to a clean muscle tube. Although crossed by a few small arteries and veins from the puborectal sling and some slips of sphincter muscle, the 'holy plane' here becomes the intersphincteric plane, which is familiar to proctologists from below—a tube of red skeletal muscle outside a tube of whiter smooth muscle within. On the inner aspect, the mucosal lining of the rectum becomes a transitional zone which interdigitates with pectineal skin as the dentate line. This marks the transition from pain-sensitive to insensitive mucosa.

The Anatomy of Abdominoperineal Excision: New TME Anatomy from Behind with the Patient Facedown (The Kocher–Holm Position)

The views into the pelvis from behind are considered by many surgeons to be superior to those in the conventional steep Trendelenburg position (a point originally observed by Theodor Kocher more than 100 years ago). In particular, spectacular access is provided if the coccyx is excised with the cancer. Once the coccyx has been liberated by diathermy and osteotome, the presacral fascia is incised—hopefully onto the gauze swab left on the abdominal side. The levators are divided far out near to their origins from the surface of the obturator internus muscle, working gradually across various levator bundles towards the puborectal sling which must be carefully identified.

Provided all the abdominal operation has been completed, the colon and rectum can be fully delivered below to provide maximum access to the all-important interface between cancer specimen and prostate.

As this dissection progresses, the liberated bowel segment with coccyx attached can be eased downwards to open the recto-prostatic planes (12 o'clock) upwards through the transverse perineal muscles and perineal body (6 o'clock) and then laterally (3 and 9 o'clock). The advantage becomes even greater as the neurovascular bundles are carefully identified coursing towards the bulb of the penis. Random fatty tissue tends to obscure these, and it helps to identify them if a LIGACLIP has been placed on the top of the neurovascular inferior hypogastric plexuses by the abdominal operator.

The key to not damaging these hitherto largely unrecognised nerves is care in dividing the puborectal sling which can be seen just after its division on the right side of the prone male in a white divided muscle bundle in close proximity to the longitudinally running nerve bundle—now called the cavernous nerves.

'Lipo-anatomy' in APE

The authors have a particular preference for the avoidance of surgical removal of the macroglobular ischiorectal fat so well adapted to sitting upon (and also elegant in a swimming costume!). Apart from rare extremely advanced cancers, whose MRI will clearly show invasion through the levator muscle, the inferior haemorrhoidal vessels and lymphatics are not a field of spread for adenocarcinoma. The facedown APE can therefore usually be commenced in a tidy bloodless way following a perfect surgical plane outside the external sphincters but within the macroglobular fat. This reduces the ultimate size of the dead space and hopefully the need for plastic surgeons' assistance to fill it (Fig. 4.8).

The urethra is not far away anteriorly: during operation, it should always have a

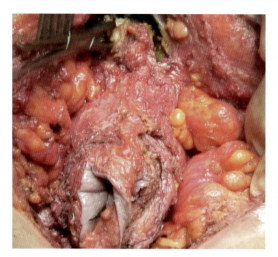

Fig. 4.8 Retention of ischiorectal fat

substantial (easy to feel) catheter in place—
even if this is removed at the end and its function taken over by the suprapubic catheter,
which is our preferred routine for both AR and
APE. A curious muscle called rectourethralis
intervenes and connects the urethra to the pre-
rectal muscle.

Distally, the perineal body is worrying for the
surgeon because it is fibromuscular and dissection through it is not in a recognisable surgical
plane. The rectourethralis remains something of a
practical challenge, but the essence of this part of
the procedure is carefully to find a safe covering
for the urethra on the one hand and for the tumour
specimen on the other.

The Ideal APE Specimen

The surgeons' objective is a perfect TME with its
distal component wrapped in levators and
sphincter muscles with the coccyx attached but
no significant 'waist', i.e. the distal one-third of
the 'holy plane' has not been converted into a
'space' by dissection. The authors' personal
preference is for the MR to be used for planning,
applying similar principles to those outlined
above—but using as the defined margin the plane
outside the anal sphincters and levator muscles,
so that if these are clear low rectal cancers may

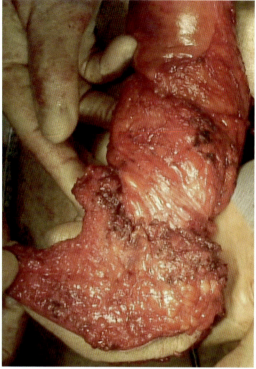

Fig. 4.9 The APE specimen

not need to have radiotherapy with its disastrous
implications for wound healing in this area
(Fig. 4.9).

The Posterior Vaginal Wall

This is very close to the anterior aspect of a TME
specimen. Bimanual examination via the rectum
and the vagina in the anaesthetised patient is
essential. If there is free mobility of the cancer on
the posterior vaginal wall, then it need not be
excised. If tethered over a small area, a disc of
vagina may be taken with the tumour, or in a case
that requires APE because of a margin threatening the sphincters, the whole or most of the posterior wall from the perianal skin upwards may
need to be removed.

During abdominal dissection, the anatomy of
the vaginal fornix and the relation of an anterior
cancer to it and to the uterine fornix are crucial:
these must be determined before the surgery by
EUA and MRI.

Other Organs Occasionally Requiring En Bloc Removal on Account of a Direct Invasion: Anatomical Relation and Adherence to a Cancer

- Seminal vesicles.
- One or both ureters.
- Ileum.
- The folded-over sigmoid.
- One or both hypogastric plexuses.
- Parts of the neural lamella may have to be removed in continuity with the primary or even a node—going laterally until a clear plane can be identified.
- Appendix.
- Uterus, ovaries and adnexal structures.
- Bladder wall.
- Extra-mesorectal lymph nodes.

Conclusion

Rectal cancer surgery is probably the most rewarding of all the challenges to the aspiring gastrointestinal surgeon. Arguably, there is no cancer operation where proper understanding of the complex anatomy, what we may call 'TME anatomy', and surgical skill of the highest order can bring so much benefit to the patient.

References

1. Adam IJ, Mohamdee MO, Martin IG, et al. Role of circumferential margin involvement in the local recurrence of rectal cancer. Lancet. 1994;344:707.
2. Birbeck K, Macklin C, Tiffen N, et al. Rates of circumferential resection margin involvement vary between surgeons and predict outcomes in rectal cancer surgery. Ann Surg. 2002;2354:449.
3. Dukes CE. The classification of cancer of the rectum. J Pathol Bacteriol. 1932;35:323.
4. Heald RJ. The "holy plane" of rectal cancer. J R Soc Med. 1988;81:503.
5. Heald RJ, Moran BJ, Ryall RDH, et al. The Basingstoke experience of total mesorectal excision 1978–1997. Arch Surg. 1998;133:894.
6. Hermanek P, Wiebelt H, Staimmer D, et al. The German Study Group Colorectal Carcinoma (SGCRC). Prognostic factors of rectal carcinoma—experience of the German Multicentre Study. Tumori. 1995;81:60.
7. Jass JR, Atkin WS, Cuzick J, et al. The grading of rectal cancer: histological perspectives and multivariate analysis of 447 cases. Histopathology. 1986;10:437.
8. Karanjia ND, Schache DJ, North WR, et al. "Close shave" in anterior resection. Br J Surg. 1990;77(5):510.
9. MacFarlane JK, Ryall RD, Heald RJ. Mesorectal excision for rectal cancer. Lancet. 1993;341(8843):457.
10. Miles WE. A method of performing abdomino-perineal excision for carcinoma of the rectum and terminal portion of the pelvic colon. Lancet. 1908;35:320.
11. Moran MR, James EC, Rothenberger DA, et al. Prognostic value of positive lymph nodes in rectal cancer. Dis Colon Rectum. 1992;35(6):579.
12. Moriya Y. The "onion rings" of rectal fascia. In: Heald R, editor. 2002.
13. Quirke P, Durdey P, Dixon MF, et al. Local recurrence of rectal adenocarcinoma due to inadequate surgical resection. Histopathological study of lateral tumour spread and surgical excision. Lancet. 1986; 2(8514):996.
14. Quirke P, Scott N. The pathologist's role in the assessment of local recurrence in rectal carcinoma. Surg Oncol Clin North Am. 1992;1:1.
15. Silen W. Mesorectal excision for rectal cancer. Lancet. 1993;341.
16. Wolmark N, Wieand HS, Rockette HE, et al. The prognostic significance of tumor location and bowel obstruction in Dukes B and C colorectal cancer. Findings from the NSABP clinical trials. Ann Surg. 1983;198(6):743.
17. Syk E, Torkzad MR, Blomqvist L, Ljungqvist O, Glimelius B. Radiological findings do not support lateral residual tumour as a major cause of local recurrence of rectal cancer. Br J Surg. 2006;93(1):113–9.
18. Syk E, Torkzad MR, Blomqvist L, Nilsson PJ, Glimelius B. Local recurrence in rectal cancer: anatomic localization and effect on radiation target. Int J Radiat Oncol Biol Phys. 2008;72(3):658–64.
19. Holm T, Ljung A, Haggmark T, et al. Extended abdominoperineal resection with gluteus maximus flap reconstruction of the pelvic floor for rectal cancer. Br J Surg. 2007;94:232–8.

Low-Risk Early Rectal Cancer

5

Roel Hompes and Christopher Cunningham

Abstract

The treatment pathways for rectal cancer are evolving, in particular for patients who present with an early detected rectal cancer. Currently, the golden standard for rectal cancer treatment is radical surgery, i.e. low anterior resection or abdominoperineal resection both with adherence to the total mesorectal excision (TME) principles as advocated by Bill Heald. This type of meticulous surgical technique together with neo-adjuvant (chemo)radiotherapy in selected cases has led to high cure rates. However, the excellent oncological results are offset by significant morbidity, adverse functional outcome (bowel, urinary and sexual function) and even mortality. In patients with early rectal cancer, these 'side effects' of radical surgery become even more significant since in a proportion of these patients, radical surgery is overtreatment and local excision with preservation of the rectum is adequate. It is undisputed that local excision of poorly selected rectal cancers results in an unacceptably high incidence of local recurrence; however, some impressive results have been obtained with the use of local excision for low-risk early stage cancers or when used in combination with neo-adjuvant treatment for less favourable T2 disease.

Here we will describe the application of local excision (predominantly transanal endoscopic microsurgery, TEM) for early rectal cancer (ERC), from pragmatic assessment of patients, operative techniques and most importantly management decisions on the basis of postoperative pathology.

R. Hompes, MD • C. Cunningham, MD, FRCSEd (✉)
Department of Colorectal Surgery,
John Radcliffe Hospitals, Old Road,
Headington, Oxford OX3 9DU, UK
e-mail: roelhompes@gmail.com;
chriscunningham.ogi@gmail.com

G. Baatrup (ed.), *Multidisciplinary Treatment of Colorectal Cancer*,
DOI 10.1007/978-3-319-06142-9_5, © Springer International Publishing Switzerland 2015

Introduction

Over the last few decades, we have been fortunate to witness the dramatic improvement in outcome that can be achieved by meticulous surgical technique of total mesorectal excision (TME). Some surgeons already had an anatomical awareness within the pelvis, intuitively preserving natural planes, but it was the evangelical popularisation of this technique by Bill Heald that translated optimum surgical technique into better outcomes for patients with rectal cancer throughout the world. Rates of local recurrence after TME for rectal cancer have been reduced to less than 10 % in routine practice with appropriately trained surgeons, and this can be further reduced with preoperative short-course radiotherapy [1]. However, this oncological excellence comes at a cost. Mortality rates vary from 1 to 13 % being particularly high in the elderly and co-morbid population. Anastomotic dehiscence can occur in up to 20 % of cases, and the sequelae of pelvic sepsis and stoma formation can have catastrophic effects on quality of life. Even for those who make an uncomplicated recovery, bowel, urinary and sexual dysfunction compromise daily living.

These poor functional and quality of life outcomes are more significant when we consider that for a proportion of patients with early stage cancer, there is evidence that radical surgery is overtreatment and local excision (LE) with preservation of the rectum is adequate. The challenge arises in identifying these early stage cancers and presenting patients with a reasonable estimate of risk of recurrent disease to be balanced against their individual risk of mortality and serious morbidity. This concept of 'trading off' oncological excellence against reduced surgical morbidity and maintenance of quality of life is controversial, and the strongest critics often reflect on the dreadful results of LE following transanal excision of rectal cancer [2–4]. However, for many of these patients, treatment was viewed as a compromise from the outset, follow-up was not rigorous and recourse to radical surgery in the face of unfavourable prognostic factors was not considered after LE. Addressing these weaknesses and providing LE within a carefully managed strategy offer the opportunity to minimise overtreatment in early stage rectal cancer while avoiding the disasters of oncological compromise by inappropriate application of LE. This approach is founded on meticulous pathological assessment and recourse to completion resection in the face of poor histology along with close surveillance of those managed by LE to detect early disease recurrence and offer salvage surgery. For many clinicians this will not be acceptable but many patients devastated with a cancer diagnosis and the prospect of major surgery are willing to explore this option.

Patient Selection

The defining feature of an ERC suitable for local excision is the absence of lymph node disease, and thus, the goal in selection is to identify the risk of lymph node disease in a given patient. Depth of tumour invasion is a potent predictor of this, as T1 cancers with invasion restricted to the submucosa are less likely to metastasise due to the paucity of lymphatics within the colorectal mucosa. Furthermore, small cancers, particularly less than 3 cm, are less likely to have nodal disease, and the absence of poor differentiation, tumour budding and vascular or lymphatic invasion are also associated with reduced incidence of nodal disease [5]. These factors are considered in selecting patients for LE and recommending radical surgery for less favourable cancers. Early cancers deemed 'oncologically' suitable for LE must then be judged if they are technically amenable for a safe excision (i.e. ideally lying in the extraperitoneal rectum and of a size that is amenable to an adequate TEM), coining the phrase 'TEM-able'.

Preoperative Staging

As in any rectal cancer assessment, digital examination, rigid sigmoidoscopy and endoscopic assessment are important in determining suitability for LE. The site, size and height above the anal verge and anorectal junction should be determined and recorded. Position of the lesion can be difficult to establish at flexible endoscopy, and instilling some water into the lumen during endoscopy can help considerably by providing a reference point. Morphology plays an important role; those cancers showing non-exophytic ulcerated characteristics tend to be of a more advanced stage than exophytic tumours [6]. Histological confirmation of cancer is desirable but not essential before undertaking LE; in fact 40 % of cancers in the UK TEM database were only confirmed as such on post-TEM pathology [5]. Controversy exists as to how vigorously preoperative pathology should be sought with some experts advocating a generous biopsy to obtain sufficient tissue to allow realistic assessment of differentiation grade and possible lymphovascular invasion, the presence of which may preclude LE. On the other hand, some avoid repeated biopsies as final histological assessment may be difficult due to post-biopsy artefacts. The architectural disruption resulting from biopsies and fibrosis can mimic malignant infiltration which is interpreted as pseudo-invasion; however, the distinction with true invasion is difficult. A more direct determination of the local extension of tumour growth (T stage) and lymph node involvement (N stage) is provided by imaging. This should include endorectal ultrasound (ERUS), magnetic resonance imaging (MRI) and a multi-detector computed tomography (MDCT). ERUS provides evaluation of the T stage with high discrimination of the rectal wall and its layer configuration with a reported accuracy of 82–93 %. However, for more advanced lesions and those in the upper rectum, the accuracy of ERUS decreases and additional information can be provided by MRI and to a lesser extent by CT. Although the risk of lymph node involvement in ERC is low, positive lymph nodes can still be present in 2–14 % [7], but preoperative identification of nodal disease is challenging, with the conventional imaging modalities all lacking accuracy. These modalities are unable to identify small metastatic deposits in normal-sized lymph nodes, and nodal size alone is a poor predictor if there is no extracapsular extension or lymph node necrosis. Encouraging results to improve

accuracy of MRI for nodal disease have been achieved with the use of lymphotrophic contrast media [8]. However, their use needs to be further investigated in larger clinical trials. It is likely that developments in applying molecular profiling to cancers will be valuable in the next 5 years. This approach has already been used in finer discrimination of prognosis in advanced cancer [9], and a role in selecting early stage cancers suitable for LE is a natural extension of this work. The value of CT is mainly in the exclusion of distant disease, which is an uncommon but important factor in early rectal cancer as the treatment options alter dramatically.

A pragmatic approach suitable for most practice is to assess the primary tumour for 'TEM-ability' by clinical examination and ultrasound and use MRI to identify those with unexpected advanced T stage and more importantly evidence of nodal involvement. So, an ERC most suitable for a local excision needs to be <3 cm, freely mobile, ultrasound stage T1, well or moderately differentiated on biopsy, lack lympho-vascular invasion and mucinous architecture and be free from nodal disease on MRI.

Surgical Procedures for Local Excision

As a general rule, whichever technique is used for LE of an ERC, it must ensure a complete macroscopic excision with safe margins and an intact specimen for accurate histopathological examination [10]. The most common conventional technique for lesions within 6–10 cm from the anal verge is the Parks' per anal resection. The major drawback of this technique is the restricted access and view that can lead to less precise excisions with a higher rate of specimen fragmentation and positive resection margins. This is the likely cause of the reported high local recurrence rates [11]. Alternative local techniques for the resection of larger tumours of the mid or upper rectum are the Kraske (suprasphincteric/trans-sacral) or York-Mason (trans-sphincteric) procedures. These are however technically demanding and associated with high postoperative morbidity rates. Gerhard Buess introduced and popularised transanal endoscopic microsurgery (TEM) which has become the treatment of choice for local excision of tumours throughout the rectum and even the distal sigmoid. It provides a magnified and stable view of the operative field which allows an accurate resection of the lesion with adequate margins and avoiding fragmentation. TEM is furthermore associated with low postoperative morbidity and mortality rates.

Patient Preparation and Set-up for TEM

The patient can be admitted on the day of the procedure and receives a cleansing enema 2 h before surgery. Some surgeons advocate a complete bowel preparation, both mechanical and antibiotic, especially if there is a risk for perforation into the peritoneal cavity with higher lesions. This is however not our practice. The patient is positioned such that the bulk of the tumour lies at the 6 o' clock position: lithotomy for posterior lesions, lateral decubitus for lateral lesions and for anterior lesions the patient is positioned in prone position with the legs spread.

TEM Procedure

Once the patient is positioned, the perianal area is prepped, and an anal local anaesthetic block is injected to improve anal dilatation allowing the rectoscope to be gently inserted. The rectoscope is advanced to the desired position under direct vision and fixed with a supporting arm. The tumour, with a 1-cm margin of clearance of normal mucosa, is outlined with eschar dots. The dissection is started by incising the rectal wall layer by layer until the desired level, which is usually full thickness. A partial-thickness excision is associated with a sixfold increase in risk of a positive resection margin, so a full-thickness excision should be standard for any lesion distal to the peritoneal reflection where TEM is performed with curative intent. The extraperitoneal part of

the rectum runs up to 20 cm from the dentate line posteriorly, 15 cm laterally and 10–12 cm anteriorly, but these heights can vary particularly in female patients. The dissection should always be carried out close to the rectal wall to avoid inadvertent damage to the vaginal wall and urethra or accidental entry into the abdominal cavity. For posteriorly located lesions, the mesorectal fat can be resected by continuing the dissection onto the presacral fascia. This allows for lymph node sampling but can lead to troublesome bleeding, and a subsequent classical resection will encounter a spoiled mesorectal margin and will be technically more difficult. After removal of the specimen, the defect is rinsed with a copious amount of a tumoricidal agent to prevent the theoretical possibility of tumour implantation. The defect is usually closed with a running 2-0 PDS suture, with silver clips to the secure the ends. Some surgeons leave all defects open provided there is no peritoneal breach. The specimen should be handled with care and pinned out on a piece of cork with dressmaker's pins to preserve the orientation and relationship between the normal margin and the tumour. These specimens are best delivered fresh to the pathologist, with all the relevant clinical information.

Complications and Risks of TEM

A possible major complication is perforation into the peritoneal cavity. If the peritoneal cavity is accidentally entered, the defect should be closed to prevent soiling and loss of a stable pneumorectum. For large defects, it may be prudent to perform a laparoscopic exploration at the end of the procedure to test the site of closure and washout of the pelvis. Postoperative morbidity rates after TEM are low (5–10 %), and complications are predominantly minor. The most frequent complication is dysuria or urinary retention which usually resolves spontaneously in the first 24 h after surgery or may need temporary urethral catheterisation. This complication tends to be more common after excision of lesions within 2 cm of the dentate line. Postoperative haemorrhage can be treated conservatively in the majority of cases, but if severe enough, an urgent rectoscopy is required to deal with the focus of bleeding, which is usually the suture line or a mucosal tear. Pelvic sepsis can be controlled by local drainage via the rectum and antibiotics, but if sepsis persists, a diversion colostomy or ileostomy may be necessary. Other less frequently reported complications are fistulas to the perineum or vagina, surgical emphysema and rectal strictures.

Postoperative Follow-up and Treatment Strategies

Subsequent management after LE of early rectal cancer depends predominantly on histological parameters, and, of course, the patient's physiology and wishes are also critical. Further treatment may demand radiotherapy, chemotherapy, radical surgery or a combination of these. The final histology will provide information based on which one can estimate the chance of subsequent development of local recurrence and the likelihood of positive lymph nodes being left behind. The reported incidence for lymph node involvement in T1, T2 and T3 tumours are 0–12 %, 12–28 % and 36–66 %, respectively [11–13], and the risk of local recurrence after LE also correlates directly with the depth of rectal wall invasion: 5–29 % for T1 tumours, 18–62 % for T2 tumours and greater than 40 % for T3 tumours [2, 14, 15].

Therefore, LE can only be accepted as an oncological safe procedure in T1 tumours, but even within this early stage, important subdivisions exist which allow cancers to be divided into 'low' and 'high' risk including Haggitt's classification for pedunculated polyps, Kikuchi submucosal invasion for sessile lesions and several important histological criteria as described in Table 5.1. In the case of completely excised 'low-risk' cancers, local recurrence rates are low and comparable to those after radical surgery for an ERC, so no further surgical treatment is necessary (Table 5.2).

Although recurrence rates following LE in carefully selected cases should be low, it is imper-

Table 5.1 Pathological determinants of risk of local recurrence after local excision for early rectal cancer

	Low-risk ERC	High-risk ERC
Absolute factors		
Morphology	Polypoid	Ulcerated
	Sessile	Flat raised
Tumour grade	G1–G2	G3–G4/signet ring
Depth of invasion	Haggitt 1–3	Haggitt 4
	pT1sm1	pT1sm2–3
Lympho-vascular invasion	No	Yes
Resection margin	R0	Rx or R1
Relative factors		
Tumour budding	–	+
Mucinous histology	–	+
Distal 1/3 rectum	–	+
Tumour size	<3–4 cm	>3–4 cm

Table 5.2 Recurrence rates and survival after local excision for early rectal cancer

	No. of patients	Local recurrence (%)	5-year survival rate (%)
Borschitz et al. [16]	Low risk $n=89$	6	89
	High risk $n=21$	39	93
Heintz et al. [17]	Low risk $n=46$	4.3	79
	High risk $n=12$	33	62
Lee et al. [18]	52	4.1	100
Winde et al. [19]	24	4.2	96
Bretagnol et al. [20]	31	9.6	81

ative that those that fail should be identified at the earliest opportunity. The aim is to provide a safety net for those who choose some degree of oncological 'trade-off' detecting recurrence at a presymptomatic stage. Preliminary evidence suggests that salvage surgery under these circumstances can have more favourable outcomes than traditionally reported and can be managed without recourse to multiviscera resection and offer acceptable rates of margin involvement [21]. There is however no real consensus on follow-up schedule after local excision of an ERC. Recurrences usually occur within the first 2 years after resection, so investigation should be rigorous in this time period. The Oxford protocol consists of follow-up in clinic and flexible endoscopy at 3-monthly intervals for 2 years, thereafter 6-monthly for up to 5 years. Pelvic MRI is performed at 3, 9 and 24 months postoperatively, and a CT of the chest, abdomen and pelvis is performed annually for 3 years. At present PET-CT is not routinely recommended but can be employed to resolve uncertainty if local recurrence is suspected on MRI or CT. Although not part of our protocol, CEA levels can be determined every 3–6 months for 2 years, then every 6 months for a total of 5 years in patients who are potential candidates for resection of isolated metastasis. Many institutions with enthusiasm and expertise for ERUS will use this instead of MRI with impressive results but without the reproducibility and valuable baseline reference images of MRI.

In case of 'high-risk' ERC or unexpected pT2 cancer, the patient should be offered 'completion surgery' or early salvage as it is usually referred to in the literature, if there are no extenuating circumstances. The term 'completion surgery' is preferable to 'salvage' which has a negative connotation, and the patient must understand that the TEM specimen is an excisional biopsy and that further treatment (completion of therapy) may be necessary. Furthermore, data from the literature suggests that completion surgery, i.e. anterior resection or abdominoperineal excision, can offer comparable oncological outcomes after TEM compared to radical surgery performed as a primary treatment [5, 22]. Thus, if adverse pathology is detected following TEM, completion surgery can be undertaken without compromising oncological excellence. However, certain technical issues may make radical surgery after TEM more difficult, and there is perhaps a tendency towards abdominoperineal resection rather than restorative anterior resection in cancer of the lower third. There is no consensus on the timing of completion surgery nor on the use of preoperative radiotherapy. In the authors' practice, patients are usually not given neo-adjuvant radiotherapy, and surgery is performed when the TEM site has completely healed and the inflammation at the site has subsided. In patients with significant co-morbidities that preclude major abdominal surgery, completion surgery is of course not an option for 'high-risk' early rectal cancer or pT2 disease. For these patients, adjuvant radiotherapy is a reasonable option. There is no high-quality data in the literature regarding postoperative adjuvant radiotherapy; however, a report by Duek et al. hints at some benefit [23]. Twelve patients with T2 rectal adenocarcinoma who had undergone radiotherapy after TEM remained disease free after a median follow-up of 3 years, while a 50 % recurrence rate was seen in four patients who refused adjuvant treatment. Patients may also choose close follow-up with regular scanning and sigmoidoscopy as outlined above; however, they must be counselled and made clear that this is an oncological compromise.

Conclusion

LE for ERC is controversial not least because we have invested considerably in improving outcomes from radical surgery since the 1980s. However, the presentation of rectal cancer is changing with a significant proportion of cancers presenting at an early stage as a result of screening. In addition, we are slowly gaining insight into tumour behaviour through molecular analyses and will be able to create a tumour profile that allows us to tailor treatment to fit more precisely with the needs and desires of individual patients. For the vast majority, radical surgery along the principles of total mesorectal excision will continue to be the standard of care, but an important minority may choose to compromise oncological excellence in favour of quality of life. The challenge is to allow this practice to evolve in a safe, carefully managed and audited environment. It is imperative that any move towards avoiding radical surgery is tempered by adherence to a strategy that embraces LE for carefully selected early rectal cancers. It must also provide appropriate guidance should adverse features be identified and a safety net for those who develop recurrent disease in an effort to do no harm.

References

1. Kapiteijn E, Marijnen CA, Nagtegaal ID, et al. Preoperative radiotherapy combined with total mesorectal excision for resectable rectal cancer. N Engl J Med. 2001;345:638–46.

2. Paty PB, Nash GM, Baron P, et al. Long-term results of local excision for rectal cancer. Ann Surg. 2002; 236:522–9.

3. Mellgren A, Sirivongs P, Rothenberger DA, et al. Is local excision adequate therapy for early rectal cancer? Dis Colon Rectum. 2000;43:1064–71.

4. Endreseth BH, Myrvold HE, Romunstad P, et al. Transanal excision vs major surgery for T1 rectal cancer. Dis Colon Rectum. 2005;48:1380–8.

5. Bach SP, Hill J, Monson JRT, et al. A predictive model for local recurrence after transanal endoscopic microsurgery for rectal cancer. Br J Surg. 2009; 96:280–90.

6. Michelassi F, Vanucci L, Montag A, et al. Importance of tumour morphology for the long term prognosis of rectal adenocarcinoma. Am Surg. 1988;54: 376–9.

7. Sitzler PJ, Seow-Choen F, Ho YH, et al. Lymph node involvement and tumor depth in rectal cancers: an analysis of 805 patients. Dis Colon Rectum. 1997;40:1472–6.

8. Thrall JH. Nanotechnology and medicine. Radiology. 2004;230:315–8.

9. Kerr D. Quantitative multigene RT-PCR assay for prediction of recurrence in stage II colon cancer: selection of the genes in four large studies and results of the independent, prospectively designed QUASAR validation study. 2009, ASCO Annual Meeting Proceedings. J Clin Oncol. 2009;27:15S.

10. Langer C, Liersch T, Suss M, et al. Surgical cure for early rectal carcinoma and large adenoma: transanal endoscopic microsurgery (using ultrasound or electrosurgery) compared to conventional local and radical resection. Int J Colorectal Dis. 2003;18:222–9.

11. Gall FP, Hermanek P. Cancer of the rectum-local excision. Surg Clin North Am. 1988;68:1353–65.

12. Hermanek P, Gall FP. Significance of local control of colorectal cancer. Fortschr Med. 1985;103:1041–6.

13. Nascimbeni R, Burgart L, Nivatvongs S, et al. Risk of lymph node metastasis in T1 carcinoma of the colon and rectum. Dis Colon Rectum. 2002;45:200–6.

14. Madbouly KM, Remzi FH, Erkek BA, et al. Recurrence after transanal excision of T1 rectal cancer: should we be concerned? Dis Colon Rectum. 2005;48:711–9.

15. Sengupta S, Tjandra JJ. Local excision of rectal cancer: what is the evidence? Dis Colon Rectum. 2001;44:1345–61.

16. Borschitz T, Heintz A, Junginger T. The influence of histopathologic criteria on the long-term prognosis of locally excised pT1 rectal carcinomas: results of local excision (transanal endoscopic microsurgery) and immediate reoperation. Dis Colon Rectum. 2006;49: 1492–506.

17. Heintz A, Morschel M, Junginger T. Comparison of results after transanal endoscopic microsurgery and radical resection for T1 carcinoma of the rectum. Surg Endosc. 1998;12:1145–8.

18. Lee W, Lee D, Choi S, et al. Transanal endoscopic microsurgery and radical surgery for T1 and T2 rectal cancer. Surg Endosc. 2003;17:1283–7.

19. Winde G, Nottberg H, Keller R. Surgical cure for early rectal carcinomas (T1): transanal endoscopic microsurgery vs anterior resection. Dis Colon Rectum. 1996;39:969–76.

20. Bretagnol F, Merrie A, George B, et al. Local excision of rectal tumours by transanal endoscopic microsurgery. Br J Surg. 2007;94:627–33.

21. Doornebosch PG, Ferenschild FT, de Wilt JH, et al. Dis Colon Rectum. 2010;53:1234–9.

22. Hahnloser D, Wolff BG, Larson DW, et al. Immediate radical resection after local excision of rectal cancer: an oncologic compromise? Dis Colon Rectum. 2005; 48:429–37.

23. Duek SD, Issa N, Hershko DD. Outcome of transanal endoscopic microsurgery and adjuvant radiotherapy in patients with T2 rectal cancer. Dis Colon Rectum. 2008;51:379–84.

'High-Risk' Early Rectal Cancers and (Neo)Adjuvant Therapy for Advanced Carcinomas in Addition to TEM Surgery

Thomas Borschitz

Abstract

Allocation into high- and low-risk cancers is useful when considering local excision of rectal cancers. It is referring to the risk of local recurrence after the transanal procedure as compared with open major surgery.

T1 cancers in the early substages sm1 and sm2 are generally considered low risk, whereas T1sm stage 3 is classified as high risk together with tumours of higher T stages. The risk can be modified by histological features. Patient-related factors determine the acceptable level of risk in individual cases.

The risk of local recurrence may be significantly reduced by combining the transanal surgery with radiation or chemoradiation to a level where previously 'high-risk' cancers become 'low risk'. This is still experimental. The accumulating evidence of the oncological outcome after combined treatment is still not sufficient for a firm conclusion. Early reports suggest that complete responders and good responders to chemoradiation or radiation may have acceptable long-term cancer-free results after local resection.

In case of preoperative under-staging, early, major 'rescue surgery' may produce a late outcome comparable with primary major surgery, whereas late 'salvage surgery' has a high risk of being non-curative.

Introduction

The suggestion to divide early, i.e. pT1, rectal carcinomas into 'low-risk' and 'high-risk' criteria was first published in 1986 by Hermanek and Gall [1]. They defined risk factors for lymph node metastases in pT1 carcinomas and thus criteria for local carcinoma excisions. Hermanek et al. were able to demonstrate that in well- to moderately differentiated (G1–2) tumours, which

T. Borschitz, MD
Department of Surgery and Coloproctology,
Centre of Competence and Reference of
Coloproctology, German Clinic for Diagnostic,
Wiesbaden, Germany
e-mail: thomas@borschitz.de

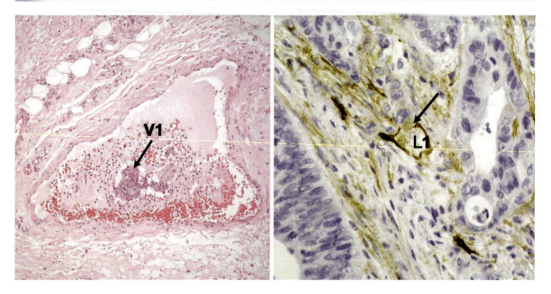

Fig. 6.1 Tumour cell migration within a vein (*V1*) and tumour cell invasion in a lymphatic vessel (*L1*)

did not show invasion of the lymphatic systems (L0) or of blood vessels (V0), lymph node metastases occur in <3 % of cases. In pT1 tumours with tumour-related L1/V1 findings (Fig. 6.1) or with bad differentiation (G3–4), N+ findings were present in >10 % of cases. In a literature analysis, Deinlein et al. further confirmed this observation and calculated a percentage of 1.4 % for 'low-risk' pT1 carcinomas and 14 % lymph node metastases for 'high-risk' pT1 tumours [2]. The aim of this classification was to identify risk factors which speak for a 'low' or 'high' potential of local recurrence development after local treatments. The results suggested that so-called high-risk pT1 rectal cancers are not treated adequately by local surgery, since lymph node metastases are not considered and a high number of local recurrences can be expected.

Independent from this, it was documented that the proportion of 'high-risk' tumours to be expected is ~13 % [3]. Nevertheless, only a few studies about local excisions of rectal carcinomas provide information about these 'high-risk' criteria [3–9].

The relevance of tumour-related blood vessel invasion (V1) was relativized since, in cases with V1 situation, a systemic spread is already present.

However, the impact of the risk potential of V1 findings on the development of local recurrences is unclear but is generally estimated to be low (low evidence level).

Apart from this classification, further definitions for 'high-risk' tumours exist. Some authors do consider tumour differentiation (G3–4) only; others include incomplete (R1) or inadequate resections (Rclose/Rdoubtful) without providing detailed explanations or definitions [5–9].

Results After Local Excision of pT1 'High-Risk' Rectal Carcinoma and the Influence of the Submucosa Level (sm1–3) as well as the Surgical Quality on the Risk for Local Recurrences

The differentiation of pT1 rectal cancers into 'low-risk' and 'high-risk' criteria was already recommended ¼ of a century ago, and a large number of studies about local excision exist. The majority of investigations, however, ignored this classification. One possible reason may be that these so-called high-risk criteria (G34/L1/V1) are difficult to determine preoperatively and that patients decline further therapeutic steps after local excision after receiving these results [3, 10, 11].

From large single mono- or multicentre studies, it became clear that a local recurrence rate of >20 %, and thus unfavourable oncological courses, can be expected in patients with pT1 'high-risk' rectal cancers [3–10, 12–26]. If these results are further split into inadequate local excisions (R1) and tumours that were not excised 'en bloc' or if the minimal distance of the tumour to the resection margin is smaller than 1 mm, the local recurrence rates rose to 50, 38, and 50 %, respectively [3, 4, 12]. Even if other researchers did not consequently separate their results according to these criteria, they indirectly confirmed the above-mentioned results since the median of recurrence rates from these studies was much higher (Table 6.1) [12–26].

The importance of the invasion level of the tumour into the submucosa (sm), for the development of local recurrences, was proven by other studies. Bach et al. and previously Schäfer et al. have demonstrated that the sm level is important for the risk for local recurrences (e.g. ~20 % for sm3 rectal carcinomas) [4, 26]. If only 'low-risk' (G1–2/L0) criteria were considered, similar results of 5 % local recurrences were found, as if

Table 6.1 Local recurrences after local excision of pT1 rectal cancer without excluding prognostic unfavourable histological finding

	Local recurrences		Follow-up
	$n =$	%	(months)
15 studies[a]	126/788	15.4 (9–40)	53 (29–85)
Bentrem, Chakravarti			
Endreseth, Doornebosch			
Helgastrand, Floyd, Garcia-Aguilar			
Gopaul, Lamont, Mellgren			
Nascimbeni, Paty, Stipa			
Taylor, Whitehouse, Wirsing			

[a]11 studies without information about R1/Rdoubtful/ Rclose; 6 studies without information about L1/V1; 5 studies including 0–34 % G3–4, 0–17 % R2, 9–17 % R1, 2–20 % Rdoubtful, 17–32 % R1/Rdoubtful, 5 % Rclose

the sm level (sm1/G1–2/L0) was additionally included. The reason for this is unclear.

One reason for this may be that the division of the submucosa (sm1–3) can vary from one investigator to the next. Further, with increasing depth of tumour invasion into the submucosa, the risk for lymph vessel invasion increases. In this context it is unclear if determination of one parameter (sm2–3 level or L1) is sufficient or if both are needed for consideration.

Novel factors such as tumour buddings at the tumour front and molecular biological markers (factors for angiogenesis, their receptors, pro- and anti-apoptotic markers, regulatory T cells, etc.) have potential as prognostic markers for the development of local recurrences and lymph node metastases [27–30]. However, it needs to be mentioned that these have only been investigated in single studies with small patient collectives so far.

Results of Local Excision of pT2 Rectal Carcinomas

The studies of local excision of pT2 rectal cancers are heterogeneous and reveal a broad range of local recurrences of 0–67 %. The reason is the inclusion of tumours with varying histological features. All studies considered prognostic unfavourable results ('high grade'/'high risk'/R1/ Rdoubtful/Rclose) to different degrees (0–47 %) and included only few patients with short follow-ups [5–9, 31].

Studies which separately described 'low-risk' pT2 tumours and adequate resections (R0 und R >1 mm) demonstrated that local recurrences can be expected in 29 % for these tumours. Thus, local excision in this situation cannot be considered oncologically adequate. The rate of local recurrences rises to >50 % if other high risk factors are added (G3–4/L1/V1 R1/Rdoubtful/ Rclose) [5–9, 31]. This high rate of local recurrences may be influenced by the potential to develop lymph node metastases, which is ~22 % for pT2 rectal cancers [32].

If one wants to accept an increased risk for recurrences after local excision of 'high-risk' pT1 or pT2 carcinomas to avoid functional disturbances (impotence, incontinence) after conventional radical resection, the oncological approach should be in the foreground. But the possibility for using local excision as palliative approach is given. Such a highly individual approach should, however, be discussed with the patient.

Adjuvant Therapy After Local Excision of Rectal Cancers

For pT2 tumours, the option to perform adjuvant radio(chemo)therapy exists as an alternative to local excision alone. Only retrospective heterogeneous results support this concept of adjuvant therapy after local excision, and interpretations should only be considered with caution [33]. The single studies included different adjuvant therapeutic regimens, and even within one study, the patients were treated differently, i.e. with combined radiochemotherapy or with radiation or chemotherapy only. Thus, the results obtained cannot be compared directly (Table 6.2) [33].

The studies also included patients with varying risk factors [33]. Up to 44 % 'high-grade' or 'high-risk' findings, up to 29 % of cases with R1 resections, and 57 % Rdoubtful or Rclose findings were included. The high rates of inadequate resections of pT2 rectal carcinomas do point to the difficulties associated with the surgical procedure if the tumour could not be excised by full-thickness technique. If, against expectation, a T2 carcinoma is detected in a tumour preoperatively staged as adenoma or cT1 tumour, a high frequency of inadequate resections can be expected if only mucosa or submucosa resection was performed [31, 32].

Patients receiving radiochemotherapy after surgery developed local recurrences in 12 % of the cases. If only irradiation was offered, the local recurrence rate increased to 18 % [33].

In comparison to local excision of pT2 rectal cancers alone, the local recurrence rate was halved using adjuvant radio(chemo)therapy. However, compared to results after primary radical surgery, these recurrence rates are still unacceptably high [32, 33].

Immediate Radical vs. Salvage Surgery After Local Excision

After local excision of a pT1 rectal carcinoma with prognostically unfavourable criteria (G3–4/L1/V1 R1/Rdoubtful/Rclose) or a pT2 carcinoma, an immediate radical reoperation can be performed instead of an adjuvant therapy. Investigations have documented that after immediate conventional reoperation, i.e. within 4 weeks after local excision, oncological results comparable to those after primary radical surgery can be obtained [14, 33].

In contrast, after follow-up and later salvage surgery for the recurrence, the developed recurrence is associated with a significant higher risk of positive lymph nodes and systemic metastases [14, 33]. Therefore, if inadequate resections and 'high-risk' pT1 or pT2 carcinomas are detected after the local excision, the procedure should be considered as an extended diagnostic procedure,

Table 6.2 Recurrences after local excision of pT2 rectal cancer and adjuvant therapy

13 studies	$n=$	RT (%)	CT (%)	LR (%)	M	Follow-up (months)
Bleday, Russell, Steele, Lamont	107	100	100	12	11 %	49 (33–73)
Gopaul, Wagmann, Chakravarti, Bouvet	96	100	~50	18	k.A.	45 (37–51)
Benson, Minsky, Le Voyer, Valentini, Fortunato	91	~100	None	18	17 %	48 (37–56)
Total	294	~100	~40	16	11 %	47 (33–73)

R1 14 % (7–21 %), Rdoubtful/Rclose 16 % (8–18 %), G3–4/L1/V1 27 % (20–34 %)

RT radiation, *CT* chemotherapy, *LR* local recurrences, *M* metastases

which requires additional therapeutic actions. In this context, adjuvant radiochemotherapy is clearly inferior to immediate radical reoperation [14, 32, 33].

Local Excision After Neoadjuvant Radio(chemo)therapy

The first results of local excision after neoadjuvant radiochemotherapy of rectal cancers showed consistently favourable results (Table 6.3) [14–39]. The local recurrence rate after neoadjuvant radiochemotherapy of cT2–3 carcinomas was only about 11 %. Prerequisite for this success and thus a decisive prognostic parameter for recurrence freedom was the primary response of the tumour to radiochemotherapy.

In the case of 'complete responders' (ypT0), no local recurrences have been observed so far [34]. But also patients with a good response, i.e. a tumour response up to the submucosa level (ypT1), showed an encouraging low local recurrence rate of 2 % (0–6 %). Less clear-cut were the results of ypT2 findings, since the local recurrences were 6–20 % in this group and they are therefore to be judged as less favourable. In addition, in the case of ypT2 tumours, persisting lymph node metastases is to be expected in more than 19 % of cases [40]. Unfavourable results were observed in nonresponders (ypT3), who in

our analysis developed recurrences in 21 % of cases [34].

The above-mentioned results in combination with the good results observed after radical surgery combined with neoadjuvant radiochemotherapy led to the discussion regarding if this approach does represent an alternative therapy for patients with a distal T2–3 rectal cancer [34]. Even in cases with more advanced (cT3) and primary non-resectable rectal cancers (cT4), complete remission can be achieved in ~20 %. After successful pretreatment of these patients (with a response to ypT0–1 level) followed by local excision, a stoma may be avoidable in a significant number of patients.

However, almost all prior studies about local excision after neoadjuvant radiochemotherapy were retrospective analyses with selected patients. In addition, the follow-up was in the median 35 months. Therefore, more long-term results are needed. An extension of the indication of local excision of rectal cancers can only be discussed after appropriate, controlled studies have been performed.

Table 6.3 Local recurrences after local excision and neoadjuvant chemoradiation of cT2–3 rectal carcinomas

13 studies	cT category	Local recurrences	Follow-up (months)
Bon nen, Borschitz	n = 41 cT1–2 (11.6 %)	40/354 (11 %)	39 (24–64)
Callender, Caricato	n = 113 cT2 (31.9 %)		
Hershman, Kim	n = 11 cT2–3 (3.4 %)		
Lezoche,[a] Meadows	n = 207 cT3 (58.5 %)		
Park, Nair, Ruo	n = 1 cT4 (0.3 %)		
Schell, Stipa	n = 1 cTX (0.3 %)		

[a] 1 prospective study; 12 retrospective studies

References

1. Hermanek P, Gall FP. Early (microinvasive) colorectal carcinoma. Int J Colorectal Dis. 1986;1:79–84.
2. Deinlein P, Reulbach U, Stolte M, Vieth M. Risikofaktoren der lymphogenen Metastasierung von kolorektalen pT1-Karzinomen. Pathologe. 2003;24: 387–93.
3. Borschitz T, Heintz A, Junginger T. The influence of histopathologic criteria on the long-term prognosis of locally excised pT1 rectal carcinomas: results of local excision (transanal endoscopic microsurgery) and immediate reoperation. Dis Colon Rectum. 2006;49: 1492–506.
4. Bach SP, Hill J, Monson JR, Simson JN, Lane L, Merrie A, Warren B, Mortensen NJ, Association of Coloproctology of Great Britain and Ireland Transanal Endoscopic Microsurgery (TEM) Collaboration. A predictive model for local recurrence after transanal endoscopic microsurgery for rectal cancer. Br J Surg. 2009;96:280–90.
5. Borschitz T, Junginger T. Value of local surgical therapy for rectal cancer. A literature analysis. Zentralbl Chir. 2003;128:1066–74.
6. Dias AR, Nahas CS, Marques CF, Nahas SC, Cecconello I. Transanal endoscopic microsurgery: indications, results and controversies. Tech Coloproctol. 2009;13:105–11.

7. Middleton PF, Sutherland LM, Maddern GJ. Transanal endoscopic microsurgery: a systematic review. Dis Colon Rectum. 2005;48:270–84.

8. Sengupta S, Tjandra JJ. Local excision of rectal cancer: what is the evidence? Dis Colon Rectum. 2001;44:1345–61.

9. Sharma A, Hartley J, Monson JRT. Local excision of rectal tumours. Surg Oncol. 2003;12:51–61.

10. Baatrup G, Endreseth BH, Isaksen V, Kjellmo A, Tveit KM, Nesbakken A. Preoperative staging and treatment options in T1 rectal adenocarcinoma. Acta Oncol. 2009;48:328–42.

11. Ueno H, Mochizuki H, Shinto E, et al. Histologic indices in biopsy specimens for estimating the probability of extended local spread in patients with rectal carcinoma. Cancer. 2002;94:2882–91.

12. Bentrem DJ, Okabe S, Wong WD, Guillem JG, Weiser MR, Temple LK, Ben-Porat LS, Minsky BD, Cohen AM, Paty PB. T1 adenocarcinoma of the rectum: transanal excision or radical surgery? Ann Surg. 2005;242:472–9.

13. Chakravarti A, Compton CC, Shellito PC, Wood WC, Landry J, Machuta SR, Kaufman D, Ancukiewicz M, Willett CG. Long-term follow-up of patients with rectal cancer managed by local excision with and without adjuvant irradiation. Ann Surg. 1999;230:49–54.

14. Doornebosch PG, Ferenschild FT, de Wilt JH, Dawson I, Tetteroo GW, de Graaf EJ. Treatment of recurrence after transanal endoscopic microsurgery (TEM) for T1 rectal cancer. Dis Colon Rectum. 2010;53:1234–9. Garcia-Aguilar J, Mellgren A, Sirivongs P, Buie D, Madoff RD, Rothenberger DA. Local excision of rectal cancer without adjuvant therapy: a word of caution. Ann Surg. 2000;231:345–51.

15. Endreseth BH, Myrvold HE, Romundstad P, Hestvik UE, Bjerkeset T, Wibe A, Norwegian Rectal Cancer Group. Transanal excision vs. major surgery for T1 rectal cancer. Dis Colon Rectum. 2005;48:1380–8.

16. Gopaul D, Belliveau P, Vuong T, Trudel J, Vasilevsky CA, Corns R, Gordon PH. Outcome of local excision of rectal carcinoma. Dis Colon Rectum. 2004;47:1780–8.

17. Helgstrand F, Iversen E, Bech K. Transanal endoscopic microsurgery. The latest 5 years' experience in Roskilde County. Ugeskr Laeger. 2007;169:1784–8.

18. Lamont JP, McCarty TM, Digan RD, et al. Should locally excised T1 rectal cancer receive adjuvant chemoradiation? Am J Surg. 2000;180:402–6.

19. Mellgren A, Sirivongs P, Rothenberger DA, Madoff RD, García-Aguilar J. Is local excision adequate therapy for rectal cancer? Dis Colon Rectum. 2000;43:1064–74.

20. Nascimbeni R, Burgart LJ, Nivatvongs S, Larson DR. Risk of lymph node metastasis in T1 carcinoma of the colon and rectum. Dis Colon Rectum. 2002;45:200–6.

21. Paty PB, Nash GM, Baron P, Zakowski M, Minsky BD, Blumberg D, Nathanson DR, Guillem JG, Enker WE, Cohen AM, Wong WD. Long-term results of local excision for rectal cancer. Ann Surg. 2002;236:522–9.

22. Stipa F, Burza A, Lucandri G, Ferri M, Pigazzi A, Ziparo V, Casula G, Stipa S. Outcomes for early rectal cancer managed with transanal endoscopic microsurgery: a 5-year follow-up study. Surg Endosc. 2006;20:541–5.

23. Taylor RH, Hay JH, Larsson SN. Transanal local excision of selected low rectal cancer. Am J Surg. 1998;175:360–3.

24. Wirsing K, Lorenzo-Rivero S, Luchtefeld M, Kim D, Monroe T, Attal H, Hoedema R. Local excision of stratified T1 rectal cancer. Am J Surg. 2006;191:410–2.

25. Whitehouse PA, Armitage JN, Tilney HS, Simson JN. Transanal endoscopic microsurgery: local recurrence rate following resection of rectal cancer. Colorectal Dis. 2008;10:187–93.

26. Schäfer H, Baldus SE, Gasper F, Hölscher AH. Submucosal infiltration and local recurrence in pT1 low-risk rectal cancer treated by transanal endoscopic microsurgery. Chirurg. 2005;76:379–84.

27. Homma Y, Hamano T, Otsuki Y, Shimizu S, Kobayashi H, Kobayashi Y. Severe tumor budding is a risk factor for lateral lymph node metastasis in early rectal cancers. J Surg Oncol. 2010;102:230–4.

28. Ljuslinder I, Melin B, Henriksson ML, Oberg A, Palmqvist R. Increased epidermal growth factor receptor expression at the invasive margin is a negative prognostic factor in colorectal cancer. Int J Cancer. 2011;128(9):2031–7.

29. Schulze-Bergkamen H, Weinmann A, Moehler M, Siebler J, Galle PR. Novel ways to sensitize gastrointestinal cancer to apoptosis. Gut. 2009;58:1010–24.

30. Nosho K, Baba Y, Tanaka N, Shima K, Hayashi M, Meyerhardt JA, Giovannucci E, Dranoff G, Fuchs CS, Ogino S. Tumour-infiltrating T-cell subsets, molecular changes in colorectal cancer, and prognosis: cohort study and literature review. J Pathol. 2010;222:350–66.

31. Borschitz T, Heintz A, Junginger T. Transanal endoscopic microsurgical excision of pT2 rectal cancer: results and possible indications. Dis Colon Rectum. 2007;50:292–301.

32. Borschitz T, Gockel I, Kiesslich R, Junginger T. Oncological outcome after local excision of rectal carcinomas. Ann Surg Oncol. 2008;15:3101–8.

33. Borschitz T, Kneist W, Gockel I, Junginger T. Local excision for more advanced rectal tumors. Acta Oncol. 2008;47:1140–7.

34. Borschitz T, Wachtlin D, Möhler M, Schmidberger H, Junginger T. Neoadjuvant chemoradiation and local excision for T2-3 rectal cancer. Ann Surg Oncol. 2008;15:712–20.

35. Callender GG, Das P, Rodriguez-Bigas MA, Skibber JM, Crane CH, Krishnan S, Delclos ME, Feig BW. Local excision after preoperative chemoradiation results in an equivalent outcome to total mesorectal excision in selected patients with T3 rectal cancer. Ann Surg Oncol. 2010;17:441–7.

36. Caricato M, Borzomati D, Ausania F, Tonini G, Rabitti C, Valeri S, Trodella L, Ripetti V, Coppola R. Complementary use of local excision and transanal

endoscopic microsurgery for rectal cancer after neoadjuvant chemoradiation. Surg Endosc. 2006;20: 1203–7.

37. Meadows K, Morris CG, Rout WR, Zlotecki RA, Hochwald SN, Marsh RD, Copeland EM, Mendenhall WM. Preoperative radiotherapy alone or combined with chemotherapy followed by transanal excision for rectal adenocarcinoma. Am J Clin Oncol. 2006; 29(5):430–4.

38. Nair RM, Siegel EM, Chen DT, Fulp WJ, Yeatman TJ, Malafa MP, Marcet J, Shibata D. Long-term results of transanal excision after neoadjuvant chemoradiation for T2 and T3 adenocarcinomas of the rectum. J Gastrointest Surg. 2008;12:1797–806.

39. Park C, Lee W, Han S, Yun S, Chun HK. Transanal local excision for preoperative concurrent chemoradiation therapy for distal rectal cancer in selected patients. Surg Today. 2007;37:1068–72.

40. Perez RO, Habr-Gama A, Proscurshim I, Campos FG, Kiss D, Gama-Rodrigues J, Cecconello I. Local excision for ypT2 rectal cancer—much ado about something. J Gastrointest Surg. 2007;11:1431–40.

Hartmann's Resection

7

Ionica Daniel Vilcea and Ion Vasile

Abstract

The resection of the rectosigmoid followed by intraperitoneal closure of the rectal stump and a terminal colostomy in a rectosigmoid junction cancer was first described by Henri Albert Hartmann, as having the advantage of removal of the tumor and the avoidance of an anastomosis on an unprepared and severely affected colorectum.

Nowadays, indications for Hartmann's resection are related especially to complicated rectal cancer: tumoral perforation with peritonitis or abscess formation, obstructive rectal cancer with severely affected colonic wall, and postoperative peritonitis following an anastomotic dehiscence after an anterior rectal resection. A patient's severely altered general status, difficulties in performing a very low anastomosis, or important dysfunctions of the anal sphincter may also represent a formal indication for Hartmann's resection.

From a technical point of view, there are two major options: In a clearly palliative procedure (residual tumor, distant inoperable metastasis), the resection may be limited, without high ligation of the inferior mesenteric pedicle, but in cases with chance for cure, the principles of curative anterior resection must be observed. The stoma formation has no peculiarities, but the surgeon must keep in mind that colostomy will be definite in many of these cases.

Although postoperative results of Hartmann's resections have considerably improved over time, an important number of cases will continue to develop postoperative general complications and some specific morbidity: stoma-related complications, pelvic abscesses, and rectal stump fistula formation.

Regardless of its high morbidity and mortality, Hartmann's resection remains a life-saving surgical procedure in the aforementioned conditions.

I.D. Vilcea, PhD (✉) • I. Vasile, PhD
The 7th Department (Surgical Specialities),
University of Medicine and Pharmacy of Craiova,
Craiova, Romania
e-mail: danielvldoc@rdslink.ro; vasileion52@yahoo.com

G. Baatrup (ed.), *Multidisciplinary Treatment of Colorectal Cancer*,
DOI 10.1007/978-3-319-06142-9_7, © Springer International Publishing Switzerland 2015

Definition: Indications

The resection of the rectosigmoid followed by intraperitoneal closure of the rectal stump and a terminal colostomy in an obstructive colorectal cancer was first described by Henri Albert Hartmann in 1921 at the 30th Congress Françoise de Chirurgie [9]; his idea was extended later for lower rectal tumors (extended Hartmann's procedure) and even for colon tumors in cases in which an anastomosis cannot be performed (á la Hartmann's or Hartmann's-like procedure) [8]. The main advantage of this approach is represented by the removal of the tumor at the time of primary surgery and also by the avoidance of an anastomosis on an unprepared and severely affected colorectum.

In the long run, indications for Hartmann's resection suffered several modifications; considered initially for obstructive carcinomas, nowadays the main indications for Hartmann's procedure are represented by emergency rectal cancer surgery. The incidence of Hartmann's resection varies between 11.5 and 31.9 % in acutely complicated colorectal cancer, being related to surgeon preferences and patient status [2, 5, 22].

The most definite indication of Hartmann's procedure in rectal carcinoma remains tumoral perforation with peritonitis or abscess formation, although several studies brought even this indication ton debate [3, 18]. It is highly recognized that, in such cases, performing an anastomosis is highly contraindicated, while tumor resection is imperative in order to remove the primary source of contamination [11, 12, 21, 22]. Also, in postoperative peritonitis following an anastomotic dehiscence after an anterior rectal resection, the Hartmann's procedure represents the best possible solution, especially for high anterior resections, and also for low colorectal anastomosis, in case of a large dehiscence or colic necrosis [16, 21].

In obstructive rectal or left-sided colonic cancer, Hartmann's resection remains an important option, even though a series of modern procedures (intraoperative colic lavage, self-expanding metallic stents, bowel manual decompression and lavage with antiseptics, and protective ileostomies) have decreased its incidence [13, 15, 17, 21]. Still, the procedure of bowel decompression requires a longer operative time, a disadvantage for these patients; it also appears that not bowel cleansing itself contributes to a lower dehiscence risk, but especially the quality of the bowel wall (bowel wall thinned or thickened by important edema, colonic vascularization affected by ateromatosis, colonic diverticulitis). The placement of a self-expanding metallic stent may alleviate the quality of the bowel wall after decompression, but this procedure is not always possible or, more often, is not available, Hartmann's resection being a salvatory procedure in these cases.

In patients with severe altered general status (severe comorbidities, low life expectancy, multiple metastases, severe occlusive shock), the resection itself is under question, but, if it is possible, a Hartmann resection may be preferable to a proximal diverting stoma, due to its favorable effects (removal of the primary tumor creates a better quality of life and sometimes an improvement in local control and even survival) [10, 14]. A Hartmann procedure may also be employed during a presumed anterior resection or abdominoperineal resection, when the patient's condition is altered severely, determining a reduction of the operative time [8].

Advanced age of the patients may represent a formal indication for Hartmann's resection, especially due to multiple comorbidities affecting such cases [12].

Another indication for Hartmann's resection in rectal carcinoma is like a palliative type of resection, in advanced cases, in which an anastomosis is difficult to be performed; in these cases, cure cannot be achieved, due to inoperable distant metastasis, or due to local extent of the tumor, in which local recurrence is to be expected very soon after the resection (involved circumferential margins or even macroscopic residual tumor – R_2 resections). In these cases, the purpose of palliation is to alleviate the patient's symptoms, which is better achieved through the Hartmann's procedure than an abdominoperineal resection (persistent perineal pain, sepsis related to perineal wound) [10]. Also, an anastomosis performed under these circumstances will be quickly invaded by cancer, imposing a rapid, unjustified reoperation, or, even worse, will lead to an anastomotic dehiscence and further severe complications. Hartmann's procedure will also be preferable to a low anterior resection, whenever anal sphincter function is poor, leading to a postoperative anal incontinence [7, 22].

Surgical Technique

When discussing the Hartmann's surgical technique, many authors consider it as an anterior rectal resection without an anastomosis; still, there are several differences in the technical approach over the Hartmann's resection.

The surgical approach is routinely made by a median pubo-umbilical incision, prolonged above the umbilicus; a complete abdominal exploration is mandatory before considering a Hartmann's resection: Synchronous colonic tumors, colonic diverticulitis, severe altered colorectal wall, and multiple metastases may influence the type of surgery. When the decision for resection without anastomosis is made, the resection is usually commenced with lateral mobilization of the sigmoid and, sometimes, descending colon (short, retracted sigmoid).

When the resection has a clearly palliative intention (short life expectancy, advanced cases, too frail patients with severe comorbidities), the mobilization may be more limited, specimen resection including the distal part of the sigmoid and the tumor-bearing rectum, along with at least 4–5 cm of the distal rectum, in order to ensure a good cleaning of both the mesorectum and distal margin. In case of a middle rectal cancer, in order to preserve enough length of the distal rectum, the sectioning may be performed 2 cm below the tumor, but this recommendation makes sense when a future reversal procedure is foreseen [4].

In these cases, lateral mobilization is followed by sigmoid mesentery sectioning at the level of presumed upper resection; the ligation and sectioning of the inferior mesenteric artery and vein at the origin has no sense, due to the obvious character of palliation, so the vascular time will

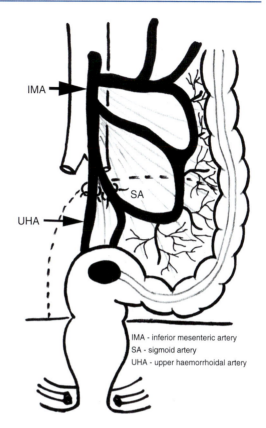

Fig. 7.1 Low ligation of the distal sigmoid artery in a clearly palliative Hartmann's resection

IMA - inferior mesenteric artery
SA - sigmoid artery
UHA - upper haemorrhoidal artery

include only one or two of the sigmoid arteries and superior hemorrhoidal artery, which are distributed to the virtually removed colorectal segment (Figs. 7.1 and 7.2). Obviously, below the tumor, the rectal supplying arteries and veins will be divided until the distal limit of resection is reached. This technique has the advantage of a shorter operative time, which has a paramount importance in the postoperative evolution of a very frail patient, in spite of modern techniques in anesthesia and intensive care. Obviously, as I have already mentioned, this is recommended to be done only in clearly "no-chance for cure" patients, with a median of 11–12 months of survival after the operation.

When Hartmann's procedure is employed only because of the local condition (too altered colonic wall, peritonitis), otherwise in a patient with good condition and apparently localized rectal cancer, the resection type must be as

Fig. 7.2 Final aspect after a clearly palliative Hartmann's procedure; the rectal stump is closed with sutures and two drains are placed around it

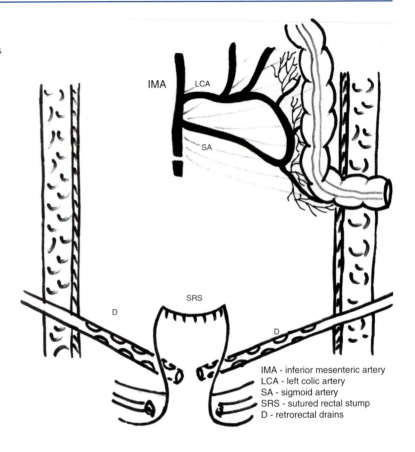

IMA
LCA
SA
SRS
D
D

IMA - inferior mesenteric artery
LCA - left colic artery
SA - sigmoid artery
SRS - sutured rectal stump
D - retrorectal drains

similar as possible to the anterior resection. In these cases, ligation of the inferior mesenteric artery and vein must be done as close as possible to their origin, with or without preserving the left colic artery, but with the removal of the lymph node at this level (Figs. 7.3 and 7.4). The dilated bowel may induce difficulty at this moment, but the exteriorization of the small bowel loops from the abdomen (covered with soft, moistened drapes) and a good lateral mobilization of the sigmoid and descending colon make the individualization and sectioning of these vessels possible. Except for a very short and retracted sigmoid or its mesentery, or a previously affected sigmoid by diverticular disease, which recommend the removal of the entire sigmoid, the mobilization of the splenic flexure is not usually necessary for future stoma creation.

From this moment, the resection of the sigmoid and rectum may be performed in the same manner as in the curative anterior resection: The colic mesentery will be divided, preserving the vascular marginal arcade along the segment which will be preserved. Different from rectal resection, dividing the sigmoid, at the level chosen for resection, is not recommended in obstructive rectal cancer due to the increased risk of stercoral spillage in the peritoneal cavity, so the rectal resection will be made with sigmoid "in situ," which may create some difficulties in mesorectal dissection. Similar to the anterior resection, much attention must be given to preserving the upper hypogastric plexus and hypogastric nerves and especially to not entering the mesorectal fascia, with subsequent risk of residual microscopic cancer, which may compromise the oncologic result. Obviously, this is easier in upper rectal cancers, while in middle rectal cancers, dilated upper rectum will create many difficulties in doing a correct mesorectal excision. This is also an explanation for some failures after Hartmann's resection (or extended Hartmann's resection) in

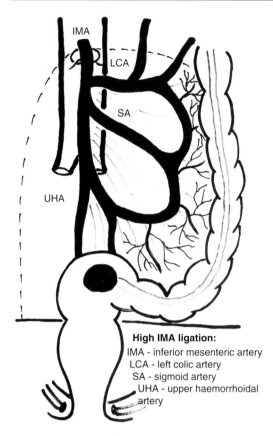

High IMA ligation:
IMA - inferior mesenteric artery
LCA - left colic artery
SA - sigmoid artery
UHA - upper haemorrhoidal artery

Fig. 7.3 The high ligation in Hartmann's resection: inferior mesenteric artery and vein ligated and divided just below the pancreatic border

patients otherwise suitable for cure (local disease leading only to intestinal obstruction, without perforation or metastasis). Nevertheless, it has been proven that circumferential margin involvement is significantly higher after Hartmann's resection (31.7 % of cases) than after anterior resection or Miles' procedure; this was explained partially by the palliative and emergency character of resection [19].

When the distal point of resection is achieved, the rectum will be transected, directly or using a stapling device. Usually, conditions claiming a Hartmann's resection do not allow a total mesorectal excision to be performed, but if cancer cure may be considered an endpoint, the total mesorectal excision must be performed in spite of all mentioned difficulties. Still, in many cases, the mesorectal dissection will stop at the level of the rectal sectioning.

If a stapling device is not available or cannot be used, the rectal stump may be closed simply with interrupted or continuous sutures or may even be left open with a drain in it (usually, when the closure is very difficult, in case of a very narrow pelvis and a very low resection). In both such cases, due to the risk of pelvic sepsis (abscess formation), pelvic lavage followed by pelvic drainage is mandatory. It is now the moment for the sigmoid sectioning and rectal specimen removal.

Colostomy Formation

There are several possibilities of performing a colostomy, all of them being related to the surgeon's preferences. Regardless of the technical varieties, there is a series of conditions to which a colostomy must submit: good vascularization of the exteriorized bowel, with no tension, and the possibility of being easily and efficiently covered by a colostomy bag that implies a comfortable distance from the midline incision in order to avoid its contamination but also a sufficient distance from the bony structures or cutaneous folds. Every time a colostomy creation is anticipated, the stoma area must be evaluated preoperatively and marked for the ease of intraoperative completion of the above enounced conditions. In Hartmann's resection, the surgeon must also keep in mind that usually colostomy will be a definite in most of the cases.

Usually, the stoma-creation time commences with an incision on the left side of the rectus abdominis projection area, dissection of the subcutaneous layer, and incision of the anterior sheet of the rectus abdominis. After the dissociation of the muscular fiber, an incision is made on the posterior sheet of the rectum abdominis and peritoneal sheet, and the sigmoid (or the mobilized descending colon) is exteriorized. A series of sutures are then placed around the exteriorized bowel to ensure its fixation to the tegument. In the case of good local condition, per primam maturation of the stoma might be possible, but sometimes a secondary opening of the stoma is performed 2 or 3 days later (Fig. 7.5).

Fig. 7.4 Final aspect after a high ligation in Hartmann's resection, also with closing of the rectal stump and pelvic drainage

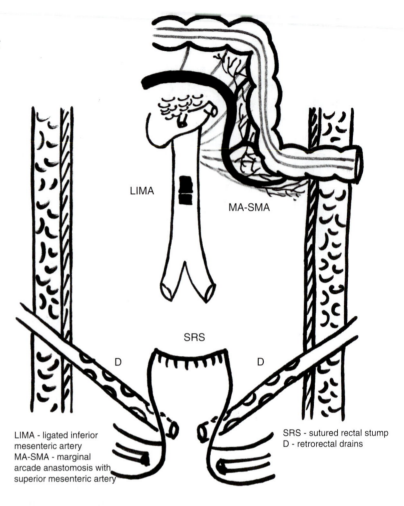

LIMA

MA-SMA

SRS

D   D

LIMA - ligated inferior mesenteric artery
MA-SMA - marginal arcade anastomosis with superior mesenteric artery

SRS - sutured rectal stump
D - retrorectal drains

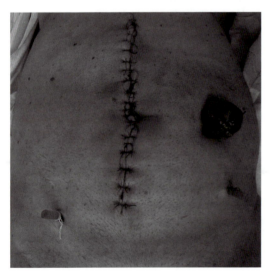

Fig. 7.5 Final aspect after a Hartmann's resection: a midline large incision with left colostomy; the exteriorized bowel will maturated 7 days after the resection

Postoperative Results

Although postoperative results of Hartmann's resections have considerably improved over time, still an important number of cases will continue to develop postoperative complications, leading to an important morbidity and mortality after this procedure. The main cause of this situation is represented by the conditions themselves imposing a Hartmann's resection: severely altered general status and advanced neoplastic disease at the time of surgery, emergency operation for obstructing or perforated rectal cancer, or, even worse, a reoperation for a postoperative peritonitis after failure of an anterior rectal resection.

Excluding general complications, favored especially by the patient's existing comorbidities and stoma-related complications, Hartmann's resection has a particular frequent type of postoperative morbidity, represented by pelvic abscess and rectal stump fistula formation. The latter has relatively little consequences in terms of gravity (except for its contribution in pelvic abscess formation), but the former represents an important cause of death of these patients.

The incidence of pelvic sepsis after a Hartmann's resection decreases from 30 (even 75 % for extended Hartmann's resection) to 18.6 % in the study of Tøttrup et al. The incidence of pelvic sepsis after Hartmann's resection seems to be significantly higher in men (45 %), with low closure of the rectal stump (below 2 cm from the pelvic floor) – 32.9 % [20].

In order to reduce the incidence of pelvic sepsis after Hartmann's resection and especially after extended Hartmann's resection, the best method is to permit a good drainage of the rectal stump and its surroundings; therefore, a policy of non-peritonealization and a good drainage of the pelvis and presacral space are mandatory. Transanal drainage of the rectal stump may be useful in low or very low rectal resections, when the rectal stump suture line is difficult to be performed or even impossible.

Postoperative mortality after Hartmann's resection for rectal cancer decreases significantly; still, it is impossible to disappear completely due to severe conditions imposing such type of resection. The highest mortality after Hartmann's procedure is encountered in the study of Biondo et al., with 56.2 % of patients dying after this type of resection, but explained by the patient selection for the procedure: Only high-risk (ASA IV) patients with fecal peritonitis, renal failure, hemodynamic instability, or advanced cancer were selected for resection without anastomosis [2].

Regardless of its high morbidity and mortality, Hartmann's resection remains a life-saving surgical procedure, which makes it difficult to believe that it will be surpassed by other therapeutic methods, at least for a specific category of rectal cancer patients: perforated tumors, advanced intestinal obstruction, and advanced locoregional or distant disease, otherwise requiring an abdominoperineal resection.

In terms of long-distance results, the proportion of patients with a chance of cure is still low: Only 30–34.1 % of patients with an apparently curative resection survive at 5 years. However, a percentage of patients initially considered in a palliative resection will survive long enough to permit reevaluation of the initial stage and prognosis [8, 19].

Hartmann's Reversal Procedure

Sometimes after a Hartmann's resection for rectal cancer, it is possible to dismantle the initial colostomy and perform a colorectal anastomosis (Hartmann's reversal). The percentage of Hartmann's reversal in rectal cancer is relatively low, only about 24 % of cases; the reasons are represented by the initial conditions claiming a Hartmann's resection, by the technical difficulties (a very low rectal stump, hidden behind important urinary structure), or by the patient's lost to follow-up or their refusal to be submitted again to surgery [22].

The time of reversal also represents an opportunity to explore the peritoneal cavity, seeking metastasis or locoregional recurrences. This is the reason why a Hartmann's reversal procedure after rectal cancer must not be employed before 6 months or even a year after the initial operation and only after a good general preoperative evaluation (CEA dosage, abdominal CT, pelvic MRI, or endorectal ultrasound). Only after the preoperative imaging modalities have excluded a distant or locoregional recurrence can a Hartmann's reversal be taken into consideration.

If the reversal is possible, a good preoperative evaluation of the rectal stump and anal sphincter must be employed: anal manometry to test the quality of the anal sphincter (not mandatory but recommended in cases with weak preoperative anal pressure on rectal digital examination or if a history of preoperative anal incontinence is present, especially in elderly patients) [11]. The length and quality of the rectal stump is needed to assess for the possibility of a low or a very low colorectal anastomosis or for associated pathology (proctitis); additionally, a good evaluation of the large bowel frame is mandatory, seeking for synchronous or metachronous lesion (full-length colonoscopy or barium enema) [11]. After the decision of

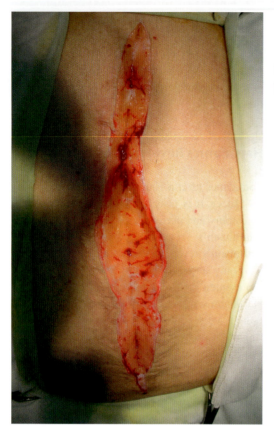

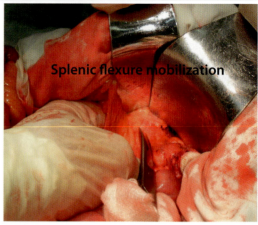

Fig. 7.7 The mobilization of the left colon and splenic angle for Hartmann's reversal.

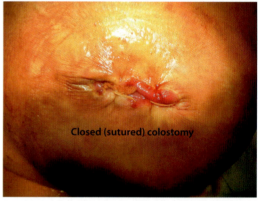

Fig. 7.6 The iterative pubo-umbilical incision for Hartmann's reversal.

the reversal has been made, a good preoperative mechanical preparation of both the rectal stump and large bowel frame should be employed.

The reversal surgery usually commences with an iterative midline laparotomy, followed by a thorough exploration of the entire peritoneal cavity and liver status (intraoperative ultrasound is very useful); only after that, the colostomy will be dismantled usually with a circumferential incision around the exteriorized sigmoid. A large mobilization of the large bowel frame is then necessary to ensure a sufficient length of the colon to perform a low colorectal anastomosis; the exteriorized portion of the sigmoid is recommended to be resected, in order to ensure a good healthy colic partner for the anastomosis. Obviously, the presence of diverticular disease or other colonic pathology will change the good progress of the surgery (Figs. 7.6, 7.7, 7.8, 7.9, 7.10, and 7.11).

Fig. 7.8 The colostomy is closed and protected with povidone-iodine gauze

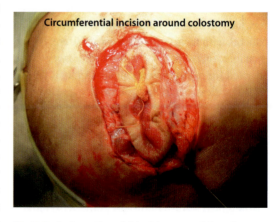

Fig. 7.9 A circumferential incision around the colostomy for Hartmann's reversal

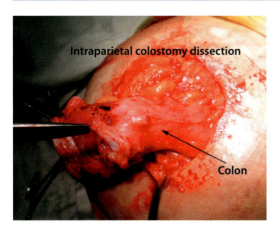

Fig. 7.10 Dissection of the exteriorized large bowel for Hartmann's reversal

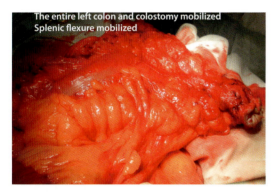

Fig. 7.11 Hartmann's reversal. The colon is mobilized and the terminal end will be resected

The identification of the rectal stump represents a very important time of the reversal procedure (a sigmoidoscope, a Hegar's dilator, an anal tube, or even a circular stapling device may be very useful, but with much attention to avoid rectal wall damage or perforation); unpleasant surprises may still arise, even with a good preoperative exploration (important adhesions between the rectum and urinary bladder in men, with risk of ureteral or bladder lesion, undetected local recurrence). In order to minimize the risk of intraoperative ureteral or bladder damage, the least possible rectal dissection will be employed and a stapled or hand-sutured end-to-side anastomosis on the anterior surface of the rectum will be performed [6, 11]. Difficulties will be much higher in the case of a very short rectal stump, in which situation a circular stapler must be available. Additionally, the initial positioning of the patient must permit access to the perineum (classic gynecologic position). In case of doubtful integrity of the created colorectal anastomosis, a covering ileostomy must be taken into consideration at the time of surgery.

Postoperative morbidity after open Hartmann's reversal is high, affecting over 40 % of the cases (48.5 % overall rate, with 43.8 % surgical complications in the study of Aydin et al.), with a mortality rate of 1.7 % in the same study [1].

References

1. Aydin N, Remzi F, Tekkis P, Fazio V. Hartmann's reversal is associated with high postoperative adverse events. Dis Colon Rectum. 2005;48(11):2117–26.
2. Biondo S, Parés D, Frago R, Marti-Ragué J, Kreisler E, De Oca J, Jaurrieta E. Large bowel obstruction: predictive factors for postoperative mortality. Dis Colon Rectum. 2004;47:1889–97.
3. Breitenstein S, Kraus A, Hahnloser D, Decurtins M, Clavien PA, Demartines N. Emergency left colon resection for acute perforation. Primary anastomosis or Hartmann's procedure? A case-matched control study. World J Surg. 2007;31:2117–24.
4. Dorudi S, Steele R, McArdle C. Surgery for colorectal cancer. Br Med Bull. 2002;64:101–18.
5. Eltinay O, Guraya S. Colorectal carcinoma: clinicopathological pattern and outcome of surgical management. Saudi J Gastroenterol. 2006;12(2):83–6.
6. Etala E. Atlas of gastrointestinal surgery. Baltimore: Lippincott Williams & Wilkins; 1997. p. 2186–93.
7. Fazio V. Indications and surgical alternatives for palliation of rectal cancer. J Gastrointest Surg. 2004;8(3): 262–5.
8. Gongaware R, Slanetz C. Hartmann procedure for carcinoma of the sigmoid and rectum. Ann Surg. 1973;178(1):28–30.
9. Hartmann H. Nouveau procédé d'ablation des cancers de la partie terminale du colon pelvien. Trentième Congrès de Chirurgie (procès-verbaux, mémoires et discussions), Strasbourg. 1921;30:411.
10. Heah S, Eu K, Ho Y, Leong A, Seow-Choen F. Hartmann's procedure vs abdominoperineal resection for palliation of advanced low rectal cancer. Dis Colon Rectum. 1997;40(11):1313–7.
11. Keighley M, Williams N. Surgery of the anus, rectum and colon. 3rd ed. Philadelphia: Saunders Elsevier; 2008.
12. Leong QM, Aung MO, Ho CK, Sim R. Emergency colorectal resections in Asian octogenarians: factors impacting surgical outcome. Surg Today. 2009;39: 575–9.

13. Liberman H, Adams D, Blatchford G, Ternent C, Christensen M, Thorson A. Clinical use of the self-expanding metallic stent in the management of colorectal cancer. Am J Surg. 2001;180:407–12.

14. Nash G, Saltz L, Kemeny N, Minsky B, Sharma S, Schwartz G, Ilson D, O'Reilly E, Kelsen D, Nathanson D, Weiser M, Guillem J, Wong D, Cohen A, Paty P. Radical resection of rectal cancer primary tumor provides effective local therapy in patients with stage IV disease. Ann Surg Oncol. 2002;9(10):954–60.

15. Ng KC, Law WL, Lee YM, Choi HK, Seto CL, Judy H. Self expanding metallic stent as a bridge to surgery emergency resection for obstructing left-sided colorectal cancer: a case matched study. J Gastrointest Surg. 2006;10(6):798–803.

16. Parc Y, Frileux P, Schmitt G, Dehni N, Olivier JM, Parc R. Management of postoperative peritonitis after anterior resection. Experience from a referral intensive care unit. Dis Colon Rectum. 2000;43(5):579–89.

17. Rohr S, Meyer C, Alvarez G, Abram F, Firtion O, de Manzini N. Résection-anastomose immédiate après lavage colique per-opératoire dans la cancer du côlon gauche en occlusion. J Chir (Paris). 1999;133(5): 195–200.

18. Schein M, Decker G. The Hartmann procedure. Extended indications in severe intra-abdominal infection. Dis Colon Rectum. 1988;31(2):126–9.

19. Tekkis P, Heriot A, Smith J, Thompson M, Finan P, Stamatakis J. Comparison of circumferential margin involvement between restorative and nonrestorative resections for rectal cancer. Colorectal Dis. 2005;7: 369–74.

20. Tøttrup A, Frost L. Pelvic sepsis after extended Hartmann's procedure. Dis Colon Rectum. 2005;48(2): 251–5.

21. Turan M, Ok E, Şen M, Koyuncu A, Aydin C, Erdem M, Güven Y. A simplified operative technique for single-staged resection of left sided colon obstructions: report of a 9-years experience. Surg Today. 2002;32:959–64.

22. Villar J, Martinez A, Villegas M, Muffak K, Mansilla A, Garrote D, Ferron H. Surgical options for malignant left-sided colonic obstruction. Surg Today. 2005;35:275–81.

Low Anterior Rectal Resection

8

Ionica Daniel Vilcea and Ion Vasile

Abstract

The surgical treatment remains the cornerstone in rectal cancer. Although many progresses have been made in the surgical treatment of rectal cancer in the recent years, starting with the developing of the total mesorectal excision by Heald, there are still some points of debate: how and when can we approximate the 2 cm limit from the lower border of the tumor: before or after the rectal mobilization? Is intraoperative rectoscopy mandatory? How laterally should the resection be extended? Is protective stoma necessary in all cases and if so, is ileostomy better than colostomy?

For upper rectal cancer, the anterior resection with partial mesorectal resection (at least 5 cm below the tumor), followed by a colorectal anastomosis, will be the preferred operation by most surgeons; still, there are opinions about total mesorectal excision, even for this high location of the rectal cancer. The most challenging decision will be in the middle rectal cancer: usually, a low or ultra-low anastomosis will be performed, but some points of debate persist especially related to the way in which the 2 cm limit between the tumor and the anal sphincter is determined.

Definition: Indication

A resection of the cancerous rectum followed by an anastomosis between the distal colon and rectum was originally performed by Cripps (1897) and Balfour (1910) [1], but the "father" of the end-to-end colorectal anastomosis following an anterior rectal resection for cancer is considered Claude Dixon (Dixon's procedure or Mayo clinic procedure, 1939) [2, 5, 18, 25].

The modern era of the anterior resection has been started by Bill Heald, who developed the technique of total mesorectal excision in rectal cancer [13, 14, 18]. This technique allows the removal of the entire fatty tissue surrounding the rectum along with perirectal lymph nodes and potentially tumoral deposits, ensuring a 4–8 % rate of local recurrence at 5 years [14, 35]. At the same time, performing a correct technique will allow to preserve the nervous plexus integrity, with a lower rate of functional (urinary or genital) disturbances [17, 24].

An anterior resection is considered low when colorectal anastomosis is performed and located below the peritoneal reflection of Douglas' pouch, involving opening the pelvic peritoneum, dividing the lateral ligaments, and freeing the rectum down to the anorectal junction; the

I.D. Vilcea, PhD (✉) • I. Vasile, PhD
The 7th Department (Surgical Specialities),
University of Medicine and Pharmacy of Craiova,
Craiova, Romania
e-mail: id.vilcea@yahoo.com;
vasileion52@yahoo.com

resection specimen will include the sigmoid with the inferior mesenteric pedicle and the rectum (at least 2 cm distal margin), with its attached mesorectum [14, 18, 35].

Low anterior rectal resection is performed for mid- and lower rectal cancers, leading to an increased number of sphincter-saving resection [6, 7, 18]. Of course, the lower the rectal cancer is, the higher difficulties will be encountered, both with the resection, but especially when fashioning the colorectal anastomosis.

Surgical Technique

In order to perform an anterior rectal resection for cancer, a good colorectal preoperative preparation, both mechanically and with antibiotics, is necessary to be made, at least for elective cases. The technique of mechanical preparation may differ among surgeons, but the option is relatively similar: a short period of solid food intake denial concomitant with an oral colonic lavage the day before surgery; the antibiotics used may also vary, but usually a combination of oral antibiotics (the day before surgery) and intravenous antibiotics (1 h before the operation commences) active against Gram-negative and anaerobe bacteria is used [7, 18, 21]. The prophylaxis of venous thrombosis must be taken into consideration (low-weight heparin just before surgery). The potentially stoma placement must be selected and the patient informed about the possibility of a temporary diverting stoma or a definitive one [18, 21].

The patient position on the operating table is usually in Trendelenburg position, but an easy access to the perineum must be granted, especially in low or very low anastomosis, or if an abdominoperineal resection is anticipated (Lloyd-Davies modified position) [7, 18, 21]. Just before the surgery, a urinary catheter must be inserted; although some surgeons use a suprapubic catheter during the intervention [21], the placement of a urethral Foley catheter has the advantage of making urethra easy to be identified if an abdominoperineal excision will be necessary to be performed.

The operation is made through a generous midline abdominal incision, having the advantage of simplicity, but more important, allowing a good access over the entire abdominal cavity and pelvis; the incision commences at the pubis and ends above the umbilicus (at least 5 cm above) [18, 21, 36]. In addition, the midline incision has the advantage of letting free the abdominal flanks, if stoma creation is necessary.

After the incision, the liver, peritoneum, and ovary must carefully be assessed, looking for metastasis (intraoperative ultrasound, biopsies from suspected lesion or enlarged lymph nodes with frozen-sections are very useful); also, the assessment of the large bowel frame is mandatory, especially when a preoperative pancolonoscopy is not available, looking for synchronous lesions, diverticular disease, and vascular distribution (continuity of the marginal arcade between proximal and distal colon). In pelvis, locoregional assessment (tumor extension, perirectal enlarged lymph nodes) will permit, along with a preoperative MRI, to anticipate the type of resection: R_0/R_1 or R_2; also, it is very important to establish that an anastomosis is possible to be made or, at the end, an abdominoperineal resection will be performed. A tumor located at or above the Douglas pouch is easy to be explored at this moment, but tumors located below the peritoneum are difficult to be assessed at this point, sometimes being inaccessible to palpation before the rectum is mobilized; hence, the final decision regarding the anastomosis will be made later, during the rectal mobilization [7, 36].

After careful intraoperative full exploration, the bowel loops will be removed from the abdominal cavity and packed in a moistened, worm drape; also, without a major inconvenient, the small bowel loops may be removed from the pelvis and kept in the upper abdomen by an assistant or, if available, by a third valve of the retractor [7, 18].

Starting from this point, the resection may evolve in two possible ways: from medial to lateral (initial discovery and ligation of the mesenteric pedicle, followed by colic mobilization – more specific to laparoscopic resection), or from lateral to medial approach (initial mobilization of the colon); there are not significant differences in terms of oncologic results between these two modalities, usually resection commencing with lateral mobilization of the sigmoid and descending colon, using the avascular plane of Toldt's fascia. The mobilization will be made medially till the aorta and aortic bifurcation, discovering the origin of the right common iliac artery, carefully not to injure the left ureter and genital vessels. Moreover, the extent of the mobilization will depend on the length of the sigmoid, the quality of the bowel wall, and, of course, the quality of the marginal arterial anastomosis between the superior and inferior mesenteric vessels. In the most favorable situation, the length will be enough to allow an anastomosis in pelvis, without a mobilization of the splenic flexure, but usually this is necessary in order to ensure a tension-free suture between the colon and rectal stump (especially in very low resections). Distal, the peritoneal sectioning continues on both sides of the rectum (a subperitoneal tumor may become palpable at this point); the incisions will meet on the anterior surface of the Douglas pouch, including 1–2 cm of the peritoneum from this level [13, 18, 21]. This is necessary for two reasons: to remove the possible malignant cells colonized peritoneum of Douglas pouch and also because the anterior plane of resection will include, for oncological reasons, the Denonvillier's fascia, to avoid entering into the very thin anterior mesorectum [14, 15, 21].

After careful colonic mobilization at the needed level, the vascular time will commence with the discovery of the inferior mesenteric artery on the aortic plane; (Fig. 8.1) the level of ligation will vary between the arterial origin and below the origin of the left colic artery [14] (the latter seems not to compromise the oncologic result, with the condition of no enlarged lymph node at this level; still, the high ligation of the inferior mesenteric artery will allow a better length of the colon, which will not be retracted above by the left colic artery string). After the ligation of the inferior mesenteric artery, the inferior mesenteric vein (Fig. 8.2) will be dissected and ligated below the pancreatic border, removing, at the same time, the lymph node from this level. Care must be taken at this point not

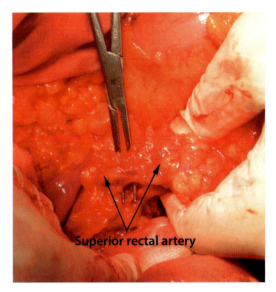

Fig. 8.1 Low tie of the inferior mesenteric artery (intraoperative aspect)

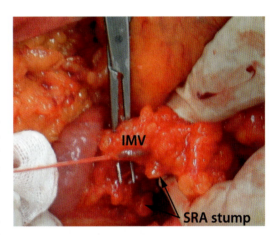

Fig. 8.2 Isolated and ligated inferior mesenteric vein (intraoperative aspect)

to damage the nervous fibers of the inferior mesenteric nervous plexus, one of the delicate points of nervous damage in anterior resection; still, in case of an enlarged lymph node at this level, in spite of an indicator of poor prognosis, the nerve will be sacrificed [18].

Regarding the vascular time of the anterior resection, there are surgeons who prefer the ligation of the inferior mesenteric vessels (vein and artery) before the mobilization of the left colon, in order to prevent mobilization of tumoral cells in portal

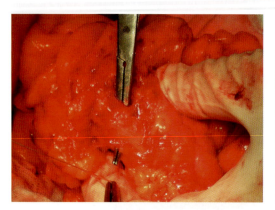

Fig. 8.3 Sigmoid mesentery sectioning (intraoperative aspect)

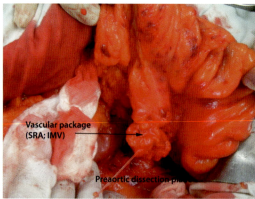

Fig. 8.4 Upper rectal vascular package prepared to enter the posterior mesorectum (intraoperative aspect)

venous system (no-touch isolation); even though after the surgery malignant cells were discovered in the portal vein blood stream, it was established that this approach (somehow more difficult and risky) does not influence the recurrence or the survival of the patients. The same conclusion is available for tumor's isolation between ties applied above and below the tumor, in order to prevent cancerous cells distal spillage and local anastomotic recurrences. For the latter reason, a good lavage with antiseptics (povidone-iodine) of pelvis and rectal stump will be more easy and efficient than a rectal untimely mobilization in order to isolate the tumor [7, 13, 14, 18].

After the main vascular trunks were divided, the left colonic mesentery will be carefully sectioned not to injure the left ureter and, also, not to interrupt the marginal vascular arcade up to the level chosen for sigmoid sectioning: at the descending-sigmoid junction or, if a long, healthy, sigmoid is available, a little more distal, preserving enough length for a low anastomosis (an approximation may be made at this point, descending the remaining colon until it reaches the pubis) (Fig. 8.3). At the chosen level, the vascular marginal arcade will be ligated and divided; also, the bowel wall will be sectioned at this point (in order to avoid a septic time of the surgery from this moment on, the colon may be sectioned after the rectal dissection, but with the sectioning, the next operative movements will be much more easier) [18]. If the colon is sectioned, the upper colon will be wrapped with povidone moistened swabs and put back in the peritoneal cavity, while

the resected sigmoid will be used for traction, in order to make mesorectal connections more evident with surrounding fascial and neurovascular structures.

Obviously, in case of cancer invasion in the anterior structures, an en bloc resection of the invaded portion must be taken into consideration, if a radical resection (R_0/R_1) seems probable (partial cystectomy, hysterectomy). Nowadays, such cases are usually diagnosed preoperatively, therefore these patient benefit from neoadjuvant chemoradiotherapy [10, 21, 30].

From this moment on, the most delicate part of the resection begins: discovering and maintaining a correct mesorectal plane and fashioning a delicate colorectal anastomosis deep in the pelvis. The pelvic dissection commences on the posterior aspect of the resection specimen: maintaining a moderate traction on the inferior mesenteric pedicle (already sectioned) (Fig. 8.4) and the sectioned sigmoid, the dissection will continue downward on the anterior surface of the aorta, looking for the "holly," avascular plane between the rectal fascia and presacral fascia [13, 14] (Fig. 8.5).

At this point, great care must be taken for two possible major risks: the risk of nervous damage (hypogastric nervous plexus, located just below the bifurcation of the aorta, and hypogastric nerve, which origins at this level and continues to both sides just under the presacral fascia); the other important risk is leaving the holly plane and

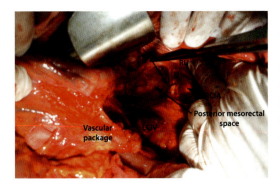

Fig. 8.5 Posterior mesorectal space dissected. The common risk on posterior dissection: *LU* left ureter, *RU* right ureter, *RCIA* right common iliac artery, *LCIV* left common iliac vein, *RHN* right hypogastric nerve (intraoperative aspect)

entering the rectal fascia (conning in) and leaving cancerous cell deposits or even lymph nodes in the pelvis, the source of local recurrence. Leaving the correct dissection plane and entering into the presacral fascia has another risk: lesions of the presacral veins, which tend to retract into the sacral foramen, hemostasis being very difficult to be achieved in such cases.

The posterior dissection is continued as deep as possible (until the tip of coccyx) with the rectum put on tension and careful sharp sectioning (diathermy or blunt scissors), keeping under direct vision the shinny mesorectal fascia and maintaining its integrity using only sharp dissections and avoiding blunt dissection which will tear the mesorectal fascia [13, 14].

When posterior dissection reached the desired level, low rectal resection will continue on the anterior plane, less risky in women, but with much more attention in men, in which leaving the correct plane may results in damage of the seminal vesicle, prostate, bladder, or genitourinary nerves, or penetrating in the rectum, increasing the risk of local recurrence. For these reasons, the anterior dissection will commence with peritoneal folds (already sectioned) put on tension and a good retraction of the bladder, using sharp scissors, until it reaches the seminal vesicle and the prostate; at this level, the Denonvillier's fascia will be sectioned, not too laterally to avoid damaging the nervi erigentes.

With posterior and anterior plane of dissections finished, the cylindrical mobilization of the rectum may be achieved now, by sectioning the lateral aspect of the mesorectum (lateral rectal ligaments). The lateral sectioning will be made maintaining contact with mesorectal fascia and a good tension on the rectosigmoid upward and to the opposite site of dissection, with care not to damage the ureters, or the pelvic plexus with its genitourinary nerves. On the lateral ligaments, in 15–20 % of cases, the middle rectal artery may be found, requiring careful diathermy or good isolation and ligation, in order to prevent bleeding (in case of bleeding the attempt to achieve the hemostasis increases the risk of autonomic pelvic plexus damage).

Obviously, a tumor extended beyond the mesorectal fascia will impose leaving this plane and removing all the surrounding tissue, regardless of the nerve damage, in order to ensure a good local clearance and prevent recurrence; still, in these advanced cases, a local recurrence is to be expected.

The level of rectal and surrounding mesorectum sectioning depends mainly on the level of the tumor; it is commonly agreed that mid-rectal and distal rectal cancer will impose total mesorectal excision, with sectioning of the rectal wall at least 2 cm below the macroscopic lower edge of the tumor (a much lower level of sectioning is recommended in case of an undifferentiated rectal cancer). For higher rectal cancers, it has been proved that total mesorectal excision is unnecessary, a level of the rectal and mesorectal sectioning located 5 cm below the tumor being sufficient (usually there are not cancerous mesorectal deposits beyond this limit) [15, 18, 21].

The distal limit of resection is, therefore, different, depending on the tumor topography: easier to be achieved in upper rectal cancer, but more difficult in case of a middle or lower rectal cancer. For the latter, there are two modalities of sectioning the mesorectum and rectal wall: in the Heald's vision, the posterior mesorectum will be removed from the pelvic wall until the anorectal angle, then it is removed back from the rectal muscle tube, leaving a 1–2 cm posterior rectal wall with a possible deficiency in the vascular

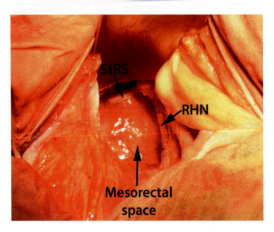

Fig. 8.6 Stapled rectal stump (StRS) and mesorectal postresectional space (*RHN* right hypogastric nerve) (intraoperative aspect)

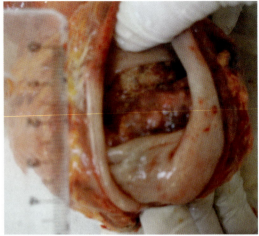

Fig. 8.8 Two centimeters safe distal margin in an anterior rectal resection specimen

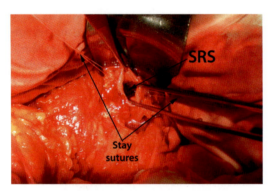

Fig. 8.7 Rectal stump sectioned (SRS) and prepared for hand-sutured anastomosis (intraoperative aspect)

supply, explaining the higher incidence of anastomotic dehiscence in this approach. The other possibility is to section the mesorectum and rectal wall at the lowest level of the mesorectum (2–3 cm above the dentate line) in all middle and lower rectal cancers [18, 21]. In case of a too lower tumor, the sectioning plane may be lowered to the intersphincteric plane (ultralow rectal resection).

After the distal desired limit of the dissection has been reached, the rectum will be transected (with scissors or transverse stapler) (Figs. 8.6 and 8.7). The resection specimen will be examined carefully to the distal resection limit (Fig. 8.8): a too close distal margin or even invaded distal margin will require a re-resection (usually it means transforming anterior resection

into an abdominoperineal resection), but the postoperative results may be compromised due to the risk of local recurrence (intraoperative contamination and inadequate circumferential margin).

Anastomosis

It is now the delicate moment of confectioning a colorectal anastomosis deep in the pelvis; the degree of difficulty is variable with respect to the local conformation: much easier in women (but not always), the difficulty increases in men with a deep and narrow pelvis. Before the anastomosis confectioning starts, a second control on mobilized colon length and, especially, on its quality of vascularization, is mandatory; if the length appears to be insufficient, a large mobilization may be performed, in order to avoid a tensioned anastomosis, by sectioning the gastrocolic ligament, but, in case of compromised vascularization, a re-resection (along with supplementary mobilization) is mandatory to be performed, in order to ensure a very good arterial blood supply and venous drainage of the anastomotic colon (arterial pulsation of the vasa recta in the vicinity of the section level, arterial bleeding from the sectioned colon, normal color of the bowel wall).

The anastomosis itself may be performed manually (hand-sutured anastomosis) or with a

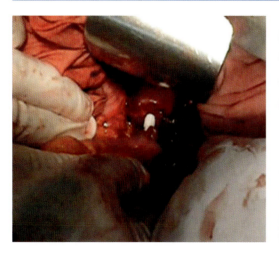

Fig. 8.9 The rectal and colonic stumps prepared for circular stapling (intraoperative aspect)

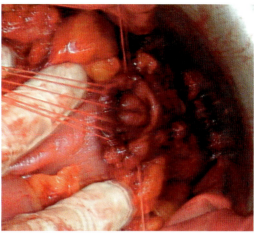

Fig. 8.11 Hand-sutured anastomosis (posterior aspect finalized)

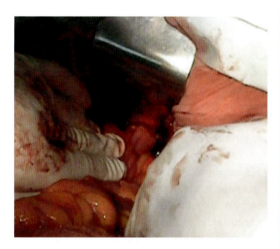

Fig. 8.10 Stapled anastomosis (final aspect)

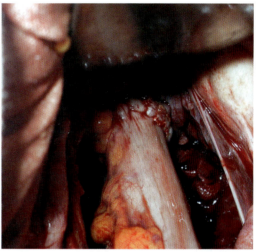

Fig. 8.12 Hand-sutured anastomosis (final aspect)

circular stapler; although there are several reports over an increase incidence in leakages and even local recurrence rate after stapled-anastomosis, no statistical significance has been reached, and, on the other hand, this conclusion may be affected by the conditions in which the anastomosis was performed: usually, a stapled anastomosis (Figs. 8.9 and 8.10) will be constructed in difficult conditions, hand-suture anastomosis being much more difficult in a narrow pelvis with a low rectal resection [4, 34].

Although considered possible, hand-sutured anastomosis (Figs. 8.11 and 8.12) will be much more difficult to be performed in low resections, especially in a narrow pelvis, therefore, in order to increase the number of sphincter-preserving resections, a stapler must be available when starting a presumed anterior resection; also, the initial positioning of the patient must allow a good access to the anal canal, regardless the type of anastomosis intended to be done. Of a greater importance is avoiding the rectal stump to retract after sectioning; for this reason, stay sutures or an L-shape clamp must be applied before rectal sectioning. The problem of the rectal stump remains even in case of an anticipated stapled anastomosis: in a narrow pelvis it will be difficult to insert a TA-stapler in order to transect the distal rectum, and also a purse-string suture may be very difficult to be performed. The modified double-stapling technique may be useful [27], but in a very low resection and great difficulty in performing the purse-string suture (even transanally in some cases!), a hand-sutured coloanal anastomosis may be preferable to a high risk colorectal anastomosis. Of course, in such difficult cases, a protective stoma is mandatory to be performed [21].

In order to ameliorate continence after a low anterior rectal resection, a series of modalities have been developed (side-to-end anastomosis, J-colonic pouches, coloplasty); still, in terms of long-distance dysfunctionalities, it is difficult to predict which one is the best fitted for every patient, and every one of them carry its morbidity. The most indicated situation which recommends the colonic J-pouch or at least a coloplasty, it seems to be after a very low resection, with less than 2 cm of the rectal stump for anastomosis, while in case of an anastomosis located above 8–9 cm from the anal verge, the postoperative results are similar between straight anastomosis and colonic J-pouches. In ultralow anastomosis (below 4 cm from the anal verge) and low anastomosis (5–8 cm from the anal verge), the colonic J-pouch has a better functional outcome than straight anastomosis and even coloplasty [8, 16].

The preoperative assessment of the anal sphincter quality is very important: a preoperative anal incontinence will be more severe postoperatively, regardless of the modality of colorectal or coloanal reconstruction; the same is available for intraoperative sphincteric trauma, in case of a difficult anastomosis, which may lead to a postoperative temporary (but sometimes permanent) incontinence [18]. Also, a preoperative or postoperative pelvic radiotherapy will lead to a number of cases with anal incontinence [3, 11, 12].

Anastomotic leakage represents the most fearful and unpredictable unfortunate postoperative event after a low anterior resection. The incidence of anastomotic leakage after low anterior resection with total mesorectal excision is high, between 5 and 15 % of the cases; although many of these leakages have little consequences, still a number of them will develop severe secondary morbidity, the most fearful being postoperative stercoral peritonitis, with a very high mortality. Therefore, in order to reduce the consequences of the anastomotic dehiscence, a diverting protecting stoma must be taken into consideration whenever the quality of the low colorectal anastomosis is doubtful, or if a preoperative chemoradiotherapy was employed [18, 22]; usually, an ileostomy [18, 21] (apparently easier to be performed and closed, with less postoperative complications), but also a transversostomy may be performed [7, 14, 15, 21]. In selected cases, even a virtual ileostomy may be performed [26]. Still, considering that the protecting stoma will need a new operation for closure, with its own morbidity and mortality, and especially considering that protecting stoma has no use in the majority of resected cases, there are authors who avoid this procedure or, at least, are trying to reduce its indications, with results similar to those who perform it [20, 26, 32, 34]. Still, in a recent meta-analysis, Tan et al. have found that defunctioning stomas decrease the clinical leakages and reoperation rate, hence recommended it in low rectal resections [31].

Also, in order to reduce the consequences of the anastomotic leakage and also to ensure the removal of the serosanguinolent collection around the anastomosis (source of pelvic infection and eventually anastomotic leakage), we drain the pelvic space after the low anterior resection [14, 15, 32].

Another postoperative specific problem of the low anterior rectal resection is represented by urinary and genital complication, favored by intraoperative lesions of the pelvic nervous plexuses, especially in anastomosis below 5–7 cm from the anal verge. Also, preoperative or postoperative radiotherapy may play a role, but with the use of the total mesorectal excision developed by Heald, the incidence of such complications decreased significantly [3, 14, 18]. Junginger et al. have found that previous pelvic surgery and intraoperative blood loss increase the risk of pelvic autonomic plexus lesions and subsequent postoperative urinary complications; also, urinary complications incidence was higher in men and locally advanced tumors [17]. Pocard et al. have found that a correct technique of total mesorectal excision with autonomic nerves identification and preservation has no effect on urinary and sexual functions [24].

Using the described surgical technique, the locoregional recurrence after low anterior resection with total mesorectal excision has significantly decreased to 8 % at 10 years, even when using only surgery [15]; thus, a good surgical technique is considered the most principal predictor for cure. The same lower local recurrence rate was also reproduced by other surgeons, using TME in combination with or without neoadjuvant therapies, even in nonspecialized centers [9, 21, 32].

Related to locoregional recurrence, another aspect must be mentioned: lateral lymph node involvement and, subsequently, the importance of extended lateral lymphadenectomy in rectal cancer. Considered very important in selected cases by the Eastern World (Japan, China, Korea) [19, 28, 29, 33], it is not considered necessary by the most developed Western countries (USA and Europe) [18, 23]. In addition, the lateral lymphadenectomy carries the risk of prolonging the operation, and increases the incidence of postoperative morbidity, especially lesions of the pelvic nervous plexus.

References

1. Balfour D. A method of anastomosis between sigmoid and rectum. Montreal Med J. 1910;51:239–41.
2. Breen R, Garnjobst W. Surgical procedures for carcinoma of the rectum. A historical review. Dis Colon Rectum. 1983;26(10):680–5.
3. Brennan T, Lipshutz G, Gibbs V, Norton J. Total mesenteric excision in the treatment of rectal carcinoma: methods and outcomes. Surg Oncol. 2002;10:171–6.
4. Chiappa A, Biffi R, Zbar A, Bertani E, Luca F, Pace U, Biela F, Grassi C, Zampino G, Fazio N, Pruneri G, Poldi D, Venturino M, Andreoni B. The influence of type of operation for distal rectal cancer: survival, outcomes, and recurrence. Hepatogastroenterology. 2007;54:400–6.
5. Corman M. Classic articles in colonic and rectal surgery. Claude F. Dixon 1893–1968. Dis Colon Rectum. 1984;27:419–29.
6. DiBetta E, D'Hoore A, Filez L, Penninckx F. Sphincter saving rectum resection is the standard procedure for low rectal cancer. Int J Colorectal Dis. 2003;18:463–9.
7. Etala E. Atlas of gastrointestinal surgery. Baltimore: Lippincott, Williams & Wilkins; 1997. p. 2049–211.
8. Fazio V, Zutshi M, Remzi F, Parc Y, Ruppert R, Fürst A, Celebrezze J, Galanduik S, Orangio G, Hyman N, Bokey L, Tiret E, Kirchdorfer B, Medich D, Tietze M, Hull T, Hammel J. A randomized multicenter trial to compare long-term functional outcome, quality of life, and complications of surgical procedures for low rectal cancers. Ann Surg. 2007;246(3):481–90.
9. Ferenschild F, Dawson I, de Wilt J, de Graaf E, Groenendijk R, Tetteroo G. Total mesorectal excision for rectal cancer in an unselected population: quality assessment in a low volume center. Int J Colorectal Dis. 2009;24:923–9.
10. Gambacorta MA, Valentini V, Coco C, Manno A, Doglietto G, Ratto C, Cosimelli M, Micciché F, Maurizi F, Tagliaferi L, Matini G, Balducci M, La Torre G, Barbaro B, Picciocchi A. Sphincter preserving in four consecutive PHASE II studies of preoperative chemoradiation: analysis of 247 T3 rectal cancer patients. Tumori. 2007;93:160–9.
11. Gervaz P, Coucke P, Gillet M. Irradiation du petit basin et function ano-rectale. Plaidoyer pour une radiothérapie d'épargne sphinctérienne. Gastroenterol Clin Biol. 2001;25:457–62.
12. Hassan I, Larson D, Wolff B, Cima R, Chua H, Hahnloser D, O'Byrne M, Larson D, Pemberton J. Impact of pelvic radiotherapy on morbidity and durability of sphincter preservation after coloanal anastomosis for rectal cancer. Dis Colon Rectum. 2008;51:32–7.
13. Heald R, Husband E, Ryall R. The mesorectum in rectal cancer surgery – the clue to pelvic recurrence? Br J Surg. 1982;69:613–6.
14. Heald R, Karanjia N. Results of radical surgery for rectal cancer. World J Surg. 1992;16:848–57.
15. Heald R, Moran B, Ryall R, Sexton R, MacFarlane J. Rectal cancer. The Basingstoke experience of total mesorectal excision, 1978–1997. Arch Surg. 1998;133:894–9.
16. Hida J, Yoshifuji T, Matsuzaki T, Hattori T, Ueda K, Ishimaru E, Tokoro T, Yasutom M, Shiozaki H, Okuno K. Long-term functional changes after low anterior resection for rectal cancer compared between a colonic J-pouch and a straight anastomosis. Hepatogastroenterology. 2007;54:407–13.
17. Junginger T, Kneist W, Heintz A. Influence of identification and preservation of pelvic autonomic nerves in rectal cancer surgery on bladder dysfunction after total mesorectal excision. Dis Colon Rectum. 2003;46:621–8.
18. Keighley M, Williams N. Surgery of the anus, rectum and colon. 3rd ed. Philadelphia: Saunders Elsevier; 2008.
19. Kim TH, Jeong SY, Choi DH, Kim DY, Jung KH, Moon SH, Chang HJ, Lim SB, Choi HS, Park JG. Lateral lymph node metastasis is a major cause of

locoregional recurrence in rectal cancer treated with preoperative chemoradiotherapy and curative resection. Ann Surg Oncol. 2007;15(3):729–37.

20. Koperna T. Cost-effectiveness of defunctioning stomas in low anterior resections for rectal cancer. A call for benchmarking. Arch Surg. 2003;138:1334–8.

21. Law WL, Chu KW. Anterior resection for rectal cancer with mesorectal excision. A prospective evaluation of 622 patients. Ann Surg. 2004;240:260–8.

22. Matthiessen P, Hallböök O, Rutegård J, Simert G, Sjödahl R. Defunctioning stoma reduces symptomatic anastomotic leakage after low anterior resection of the rectum for cancer – a randomized multicenter trial. Ann Surg. 2007;246:207–14.

23. Nelson H, Petrelli N, Carlin A, Couture J, Fleshman J, Guillem J, Miedema B, Ota D, Sargent D. Guidelines 2000 for colon and rectal surgery. J Natl Cancer Inst. 2001;93(8):583–94.

24. Pocard M, Zinzindohoue F, Haab F, Caplin S, Parc R, Tiret E. A prospective study of sexual and urinary function before and after total mesorectal excision with autonomic nerve preservation for rectal cancer. Surgery. 2002;131:368–72.

25. Ross H, Mahmoud N, Fry R. The current management of rectal cancer. Curr Probl Surg. 2005;42(2):78–127.

26. Sacchi M, Legge P, Picozzi P, Papa F, Giovani CL, Greco L. Virtual ileostomy following TME and primary sphincter-saving reconstruction for rectal cancer. Hepatogastroenterology. 2007;54:1676–8.

27. Sato H, Maeda K, Hanai T, Matsumoto M, Aoyama H, Matsuoka H. Modified double-stapling technique in low anterior resection for lower rectal carcinoma. Surg Today. 2006;36:30–6.

28. Shiozawa M, Akaike M, Yamada R, Godai T, Yamamoto N, Saito H, Sugimasa Y, Takemiya S, Rino Y, Imada T. Lateral lymph node dissection for

lower rectal cancer. Hepatogastroenterology. 2007; 54:1066–70.

29. Sugihara K, Kobayashi H, Kato T, Mori T, Mochizuki H, Kameoka S, Shirouzu K, Muto T. Indication and benefit of pelvic sidewall dissection for rectal cancer. Dis Colon Rectum. 2006;49:1663–72.

30. Synglarewicz B, Matkowski R, Kasprzak P, Sydor D, Forgacz J, Pudelko M, Kornafel J. Sphincter-preserving R0 total mesorectal excision with resection of internal genitalia combined with pre- or postoperative chemoradiation for T4 rectal cancer in females. World J Gastroenterol. 2007;13(16):2339–43.

31. Tan WS, Tang CL, Shi L, Eu KW. Meta-analysis of defunctioning stomas in low anterior resection for rectal cancer. Br J Surg. 2009;96:462–72.

32. Tocchi A, Mazzoni G, Lepre L, Liotta G, Costa G, Agostini N, Micini M, Scucchi L, Frati G, Tagliaccozo S. Total mesorectal excision and low rectal anastomosis for the treatment of rectal cancer and prevention of pelvic recurrences. Arch Surg. 2001;136:216–20.

33. Ueno H, Mochizuki H, Hashiguchi Y, Ishiguro M, Miyoshi M, Kajiwara Y, Sato T, Shimazak H, Hase K. Potential prognostic benefit of lateral pelvic node dissection for rectal cancer located below the peritoneal reflection. Ann Surg. 2007;245(1):80–7.

34. Vlot E, Zeebregts C, Gerritsen J, Mulder J, Mastboom W, Klaase J. Anterior resection of rectal cancer without bowel preparation and diverting stoma. Surg Today. 2005;35:629–33.

35. Zaheer S, Pemberton J, Farouk R, Dozois R, Wolff B, llstrup D. Surgical treatment of adenocarcinoma of the rectum. Ann Surg. 1998;227(6):800–11.

36. Zollinger Jr R, Zollinger Sr R. Zollinger's atlas of surgical operations. 8th ed. New York: The McGraw-Hill Co; 2006.

Abdominoperineal Resection of the Rectum (Miles Resection)

9

Ionica Daniel Vilcea and Ion Vasile

Abstract

Abdominoperineal resection has represented for almost one hundred years, the "gold standard" in the rectal cancer surgery. Nowadays, the indication for an abdominoperineal resection is limited to the distal rectal cancer, in case of anal sphincter involvement or invasion of the cancer in the levatorian plane, thus no sphincter-preserving surgery is possible anymore (no distal tumoral clearance is possible).

From the technical point of view, an abdominoperineal resection specimen will include the cancerous rectum, along with the distal part of the sigmoid, the anal canal, the mesorectum, the levators and the ischiorectal fat and perianal skin, followed by a definitive stoma formation. For this to be possible, two major ways of approach are necessary: a laparotomy and a perineal incision, which can be made by one or two surgical teams, simultaneously.

Multiple intraoperative or postoperative problems may be raised by this operation, from which the modality of solving the perineal wound and its complications continues to represent a difficult challenge.

I.D. Vilcea, PhD (✉) • I. Vasile, PhD
The 7th Department (Surgical Specialities),
University of Medicine and Pharmacy of Craiova,
Craiova, Romania
e-mail: id.vilcea@yahoo.com;
vasileion52@yahoo.com

Definition: Indications

Abdominoperineal resection (APR) of the rectum was the first truly oncological type of surgery in rectal cancer, dealing with the primary tumor-bearing organ and his lymphatic spread in every possible ways: upward (the most common spread), laterally, and downward (very rare). Although many attempts to remove the cancerous rectum had been already reported at that time, the abdominoperineal resection is attributed to Ernest Miles, who developed the technique, established its indications in rectal cancer, but, most important, had given a scientific basis for the procedure, in 1908. From that moment on, for almost 100 years, the abdominoperineal resection of the rectum was considered the "gold standard" in rectal cancer [10, 21, 27].

Abdominoperineal resection specimen includes the sigmoid (or the distal part of it), the entire rectum along with the anal canal, the mesorectum, the levators and the ischiorectal fat, and, in some authors' opinion, even the perianal skin [8, 19] (Fig. 9.1). The vascular ligation is recommended to be performed at the origin of the superior rectal artery, just below to the take-off of the left colic artery [17]. Due to its characteristics, the abdominoperineal resection will be finalized with a permanent left sigmoid colostomy, a difficult burden for the patient, determining a significant decrease in the quality of life [5, 7], hence being considered a "life-altering event" [21].

G. Baatrup (ed.), *Multidisciplinary Treatment of Colorectal Cancer*,
DOI 10.1007/978-3-319-06142-9_9, © Springer International Publishing Switzerland 2015

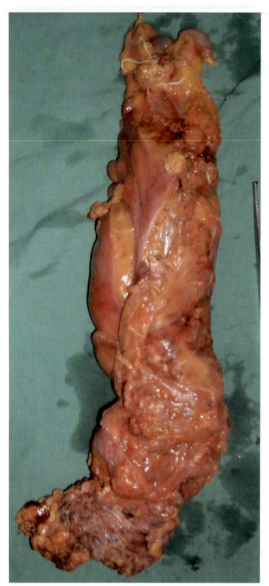

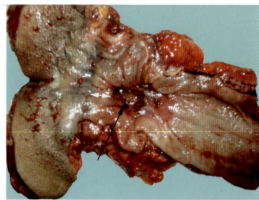

Fig. 9.2 Ulcerated cancer (*black arrow*) of the distal rectum located just above the dentate line (*white arrow*). No safe distal resection margin may be achieved – indication for abdominoperineal excision of the rectum (fresh resection specimen)

Fig. 9.1 Abdominoperineal fresh-resection specimen (sigmoid, rectum, and anal canal with mesorectal envelope and levator ani excised)

That is the reason why, over time, many surgeons tried to avoid this operation; in declining the number of the APR, there were several events: the paramount importance was the observation that rectal cancer rarely extended beyond 1–1.5 cm from the lower border of the tumor, thus a distal resection limit of 2 cm becoming sufficient oncologically [10, 17, 20]. Once with the development of the stapling devices and also of the neoadjuvant therapies, the feasibility of sphincter-saving procedure has been proved, even for low rectal cancers. Also nowadays, a percentage of the distal T_1 or even T_2 distal rectal cancer patients may be safely treated by a local excision. As a consequence, the incidence of abdominoperineal resection has started to decrease, limited most often to the distal rectal cancer, but now considered mandatory only in case of anal sphincter involvement by cancer or invasion of the cancer in the levatorian plane, thus no sphincter-preserving surgery is possible anymore (no distal tumoral clearance is possible) (Fig. 9.2).

Excepting for the local extension of the rectal cancer, there are several other factors influencing the decision of performing an APR; the preoperative anal sphincter dysfunction or intraoperative difficulties in performing a very low anastomosis with a high risk of leakage may lead to an APR. These factors have been already discussed by Rothenberger and Wong in their article and have been suffering very few modifications since then [22].

Another reason for that is represented by the postoperative results, with a significantly increased morbidity (55.4 % vs 34.2 %) [1] and a significantly higher length of the hospital stay after APR, when compared to low anterior resection. Also, a higher local recurrence rate and a worst long-distance survival have been reported after APR [8, 12, 14, 24] but these results have been contested by other studies [1, 16].

All of these considerations have made the APR to become an "endangered operation" [8]. This is due especially to Bill Heald and coll., who reported from 1997 only a 23 % of low rectal cancers (below 5 cm from the anal verge, or 1–1.5 cm from the dentate line) treated with APR [8]. The same decline in APR incidence was reported later, by Tilney and coll., who found in England that only 24.9 % of rectal cancers had been treated by APR from 1996 to 2004 [24].

In fact, sphincter-saving procedures became the standard procedure for low rectal cancer in many centers [5]; still, there are significant differences between different surgical centers, with a percentage of 24–38 % of rectal cancer cases requiring an APR [4, 8, 13, 14, 24, 26].

Surgical Technique

From the surgical technique point of view, by definition, the abdominoperineal resection requires an abdominal approach, for vascular ligation and removal of the most part of the sigmoid and rectum, and a perineal approach in order to remove the anal canal, the ischiorectal fat, and the lowest part of the rectum and mesorectum. The operation may be done in one team (as originally described by Miles) or in two synchronous teams (it has the advantage of shortening considerably the time of the operation – Lloyd-Davis) [10, 19].

The preoperative preparations are similar to those described in the anterior resection; maybe much consideration must be given to establish preoperatively the level of the tumor from the anal verge and the impossibility of a sphincter-saving procedure (fixed, bulky tumors, sphincteric or levator invasion on digital examination, rigid rectosigmoidoscopy, MRI, or endorectal ultrasound) and also an indication for neoadjuvant radio-chemotherapy; still, in some cases, the final intraoperative assessment will decide over the impossibility of preserving the anal sphincter. In any circumstances, the preoperative psychological implication of the stoma creation must be discussed with the patient, and the place where

stoma will be performed on the anterior abdominal wall must be noted, in order to ensure a good coverage by the colostomy device [19].

Abdominal Phase of the Operation

The abdominal phase of the operation is very similar to surgical elements presented at low anterior resection; therefore, in this chapter we will insist only on the particularities of the abdominal approach in APR.

The incision is a midline pubo-umbilical, extended above the umbilicus; some authors prefer a right transrectal or even a transverse infraumbilical incision [10, 22]. Exploration and mobilization of the colon is similar to low anterior resection, but the mobilization of the splenic flexure is not usually needed. The recommended level of vascular ligation is at the origin of the superior rectal artery, just below of the takeoff of the left colic artery [11, 17, 19, 22]; there is no strong evidence that high ligation has a benefit over the mentioned level [11]. Obviously, if enlarged lymph nodes are detected at the superior rectal artery origin, or along it, for oncological reasons are indicated to perform a high-tie, at the origin of the inferior mesenteric artery.

The pelvic dissection is somewhat different in APR: after the sigmoid was divided, the posterior dissection starts in a similar way, as it was described in low anterior resection (total mesorectal excision), using also the nerve-sparing technique. In the classic view, the pelvic dissection had to be as complete as possible, down to the pelvic floor, before the perineal sequence begins [19, 22]. In the modern APR it is better to avoid a very low dissection on the anterior and lateral mesorectum, the pelvic dissection being stopped once the level of the distal rectal tumor has been reached, in order to avoid tumoral cells spillage [4]. This is determined by the levatorian plane shape, which may lead to a conning-in the mesorectum if after the plane of the levator ani is reached, with an increased risk of local recurrent disease (Figs. 9.3 and 9.4). Therefore, after the levatorian plane is reached laterally and seminal vesicles or the prostate base [10] anterior, the dis-

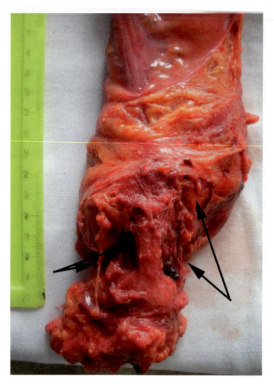

Fig. 9.3 Important coning-in the mesorectum (*black arrows*) due to the very low pelvic dissection in a distal rectal cancer (fresh resection specimen)

section must commence from the perineum, much more favorably to a correct dissection, favored by the shape of levator ani.

Perineal Phase of Surgery

The approach in the perineal sequence of the APR depends if the resection is performed by one team or synchronously, by two different surgical teams: in case of synchronous approach, the patient is positioned in modified Lloyd-Davis position (shorter operative time, no repositioning of the patient, and dissection from two planes in bulky tumors, but less visibility and difficult dissection in anterior plane from the abdomen). In case of one team APR, after the abdominal time is over (the colostomy is matured and the abdomen is closed), the patient is turned into the prone, jackknife position [10]. The rectum is irrigated with povidone-iodine solution, after which the anus is

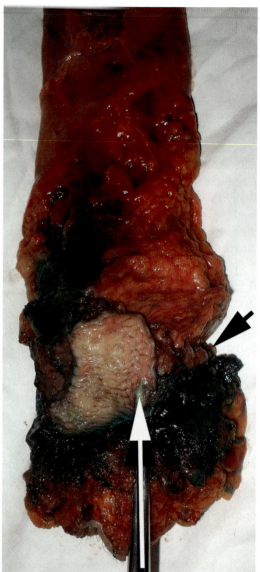

Fig. 9.4 APR with posterior partial colpectomy (*white arrow*). *Black arrow* indicates the presence of an area of coning-in the mesorectum due to distal pelvic resection in an inferior rectal cancer (fresh resection specimen)

closed in a purse-string suture (otherwise a source of perineal contamination with viable malignant cells and source of local recurrence) [8, 19, 22]. An ellipsoidal incision, 2–3 cm lateral the anal margin, is performed around the anal sphincter; the incision must encompass the entirely external anal sphincter [10, 19, 22]. The dissection starts posteriorly, with the sectioning of the ischiorectal fat, until the levatorian plane is reached; the inferior rectal vessels are ligated or electrocoagulated. Posterior dissection in ischiorectal fossae leads to the discovery of the ano-coccigian ligament, which will be sectioned sharply at the tip of the coccyx, thus entering into the retrorectal space. There is no consensus over the coccyx resection in order to enlarge the dissection space [12]. If the posterior mesorectal dissection was completed in pelvic phase, the two dissections plane will meet at this moment; in case of a bulky posterior tumor, if the posterior mesorectal excision was difficult through the abdomen, the dissection will progress from below, with care to avoid inadvertent perforation of the mesorectal fascia or the tumor. Along with the lateral resection of the levator ani, this is one of the delicate moments of perineal dissection, which could represent a source of local recurrence after APR; therefore, much consideration must be given at this point [2]. Also, care must be taken not to enter the presacral fascia and disrupt the presacral venous plexus.

The dissection continues with the lateral dissection which will permit to enlarge the latero-retrorectal space, by sectioning the levator ani as laterally as possible, close to their origin, and avoiding inadvertent perforation of the tumor, as recommended by Miles himself [4, 12, 14].

When posterior and lateral dissection is finished, the rectosigmoid is extracted through the perineal wound and the anterior dissection commences: less risky in women, in which the report between the anal sphincter and posterior vaginal wall will allow an easier dissection, and a lot riskier in men, due to the vicinity between anal sphincter and male urethra and bladder [19]. Maintaining a good plane is mandatory in order to avoid urinary lesions. After the ano-urethral plane is surpassed, the prostate must be dissected, and then, when the seminal vesicle is reached, the dissection is usually finished and the resection specimen is removed. If an anterior rectal cancer invades (or adheres) to the prostate or the vagina, an en bloc resection will be performed [4] (Figs. 9.4 and 9.5).

A good lavage and drainage of the presacral space is mandatory along with a good control of hemostasis [10, 19, 22]; if years ago the perineal wound was packed-up (for hemostasis) and left

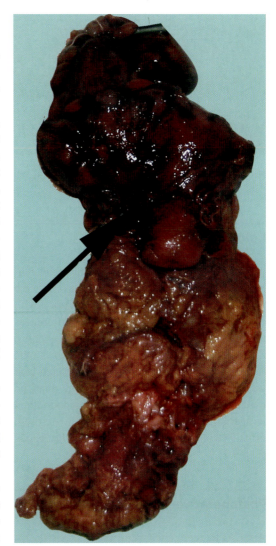

Fig. 9.5 APR specimen with total hysterectomy due to rectal cancer invasion in uterus (fresh resection specimen)

open to heal *per secundam intentionem* [18], nowadays this is an exceptional method, limited to very particular cases, in which hemostasis cannot be achieved otherwise. Hence, the perineal wound will be primarily closed in the majority of cases (over 90 % of cases) [4, 25] (Fig. 9.6). Still, due to the large muscular defect in the pelvic floor, an omentoplasty or sometimes a mesh may be used for "reconstruction"; also, using muscles flaps from the rectus abdominis or gracilis flaps may be used in order to prevent perineal herniation [6, 15, 18, 25].

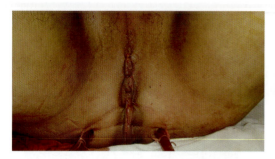

Fig. 9.6 Primary closure of the perineal wound after an APR

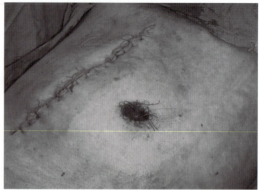

Fig. 9.7 Final abdominal aspect after APR: midline incision extended above the umbilicus and left colostomy

Colostomy Formation

After the resection is completed through combined abdominal and perineal approach, the abdominal surgeon will finish the operation with colostomy formation. There are no differences from the colostomy formation described at definitive Hartmann's resection chapter (Chap. 7); the same conditions are available: a well-vascularized with no tension exteriorized sigmoid must be used. After the colostomy is ended, an abdominal lavage is performed and the abdomen is closed, usually with a drain left deep in the pelvis (Fig. 9.7).

Postoperative-Specific Morbidity

After APR, there are several specific postoperative complications: urinary complications (chronic bladder retention, urinary tract infections, urethral, bladder or ureteral lesions, urinary fistula formation), genital disturbances (impotence, retrograde ejaculation), stoma complications (necrosis, stenosis or prolapse), and perineal wound complications (hemorrhage, abscess, local recurrence) [6, 10, 22].

Many of these complications are also encountered after an anterior rectal resection, therefore they did not weight against one or another procedure; besides these, there are a few who need a further discussion, being more specifically to APR, therefore contributing to the declining of this procedure. Genitourinary complications are relatively similar between these two types of resection; also stoma-related complications may

weight against APR; still they are somehow counterbalanced by anastomotic leakages following an anterior resection.

More specifically, it seems to be perineal wound-related complications, which are absent in case of an anterior resection; also, urethral lesions are specific to APR [19], while the ureters may be injured in both operations. Intraoperative bleeding also seem to be more important and frequent after APR, requiring, in some cases, even a temporary packing of the perineal wound and pelvis; of course, this will increase the risk of further infectious complications [18, 22].

Management of the perineal wound represents a great challenge [6]. Infectious complications and delayed healing of the perineal wound with the persistence of a perineal sinus may represent a troublesome problem, which may also delay the adjuvant therapies in case they are needed, and also in other cases require surgical reinterventions, not always easy to be performed or even successful [15, 22] (Fig. 9.8). Perineal wound complications increase the patient's sufferance, prolong hospital stay and need for home care, and also may contribute to the increase of local recurrence incidence [25]. The incidence of the perineal wound dehiscence after APR was 24.3 %, with a 14.4 % of cases with a persistent perineal fistula, in the study of Ishikawa and col., in which the high-dose preoperative radiotherapy may have also played a role [9, 18, 25]. In one study the incidence of infection of the perineal wound has significantly decreased and primary closure of the wound was significantly more

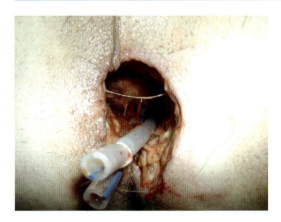

Fig. 9.8 Dehiscent, infected perineal wound after a complicated postoperative evolution of the perineal wound (perineal abscess drained) after APR

often obtained using collagen resorbable sponge impregnated with gentamicin, applied into the sacral cavity after APR [3]. Other perineal wound complications, also difficult to treat, and creating a great discomfort for the patient are represented by perineal pain and perineal hernia [18].

Local recurrence rate is maybe the most important "enemy" of the nowadays APR, a higher rate of local recurrence (both pelvic and perineal) being reported after the APR vs low or very low anterior resections. The local recurrence rate varies from 22.3 to 33 % after APR (vs 1–13.5 % local recurrence rate for anterior resection) [8, 12]. This is due especially to the effect of coning-in when dissecting the mesorectum, with an increased rate of circumferential margin involvement (16.7–41 %) [12, 14, 23, 26], and even intraoperative perforation (13.7–16 %) [14, 16] after APR due to inadequate dissection. Using a correct surgical but also a multimodal therapeutic approach, a local recurrence rate below 10 % could be obtained after APR with mesorectal excision [4].

References

1. Chiappa A, Biffi R, Zbar A, Bertani E, Luca F, Pace U, Biela F, Grassi C, Zampino G, Fazio N, Pruneri G, Poldi D, Venturino M, Andreoni B. The influence of type of operation for distal rectal cancer: survival, outcomes, and recurrence. Hepatogastroenterology. 2007;54:400–6.

2. Chuwa E, Seow-Choen F. Outcomes for abdominoperineal resections are not worse than those of anterior resections. Dis Colon Rectum. 2005;49(1):41–9.

3. De Bruin AF, Gosselink M, Wijffels NA, Coene PP, van der Harst E. Local gentamicin reduces perineal wound infection after radiotherapy and abdominoperineal resection. Tech Coloproctol. 2008;12:303–7.

4. Dehni N, McFadden N, McNamara DA, Guiguet M, Tiret E, Parc R. Oncologic results following abdominoperineal resection for adenocarcinoma of the low rectum. Dis Colon Rectum. 2003;46:867–74.

5. DiBetta E, D'Hoore A, Filez L, Penninckx F. Sphincter saving rectum resection is the standard procedure for low rectal cancer. Int J Colorectal Dis. 2003;18:463–9.

6. Efron J. Surgical outcomes of abdominoperineal resection for low rectal cancer in a Nigerian tertiary institution. Invited commentary. World J Surg. 2009; 33:240–1.

7. Engel J, Kerr J, Schlesinger-Raab A, Eckel R, Sauer H, Hölzel D. Quality of life in rectal cancer patients. A four-year prospective study. Ann Surg. 2003;238: 203–13.

8. Heald R, Smedh R, Kald A, Sexton R, Moran B. Abdominoperineal excision of the rectum – an endangered operation. Dis Colon Rectum. 1997;40(7): 747–51.

9. Ishikawa H, Fujii H, Koyama F, Mukogawa T, Matsumoto H, Morita T, Hata M, Terauchi S, Kobayashi T, Nakao T, Nishikawa T, Yoshimura H, Ohishi H, Nakajima Y. Long-term results after high-dose extracorporeal and endocavitary radiation therapy followed by abdominoperineal resection for distal rectal cancer. Surg Today. 2004;34:510–7.

10. Keighley M, Williams N. Surgery of the anus, rectum and colon. 3rd ed. Philadelphia: Saunders Elsevier; 2008.

11. Lange M, Buunen M, van de Velde C, Lange J. Level of arterial ligation in rectal cancer surgery: low tie preferred over high tie. A review. Dis Colon Rectum. 2008;51:1139–45.

12. Marr R, Birbeck K, Garvican J, Macklin C, Tiffin N, Parsons W, Dixon M, Mapstone N, Sebag-Montefiore D, Scott N, Johnsto D, Sagar P, Finan P, Quirck P. The modern abdominoperineal excision: the next challenge after total mesorectal excision. Ann Surg. 2005;242(1):74–82.

13. Marusch F, Koch A, Schmidt U, Wenisch H, Ernst M, Manger T, Wolff S, Pross M, Tautenhahn J, Gastinger I, Lippert H. Early postoperative results of surgery for rectal carcinoma as a function of the distance of the tumor from the anal verge: results of a multicenter prospective evaluation. Langenbecks Arch Surg. 2002;387:94–100.

14. Nagtegaal I, van de Velde C, Marijnen C, van Krieken J, Quirke P. Low rectal cancer: a call for a change of approach in abdominoperineal resection. J Clin Oncol. 2005;23(36):9257–64.

15. Nakafusa Y, Matsuhita S, Shimonishi T, Uemura T, Tomiyama Y, Miyazaki K. Successful wound management of infected perineum in recurrent rectal cancer

by a two-step operation using muscle flaps: a case report. Hepatogastroenterology. 2007;54:1679–81.

16. Nakagoe T, Ishikawa H, Sawai T, Tsuji T, Tanaka K, Hidaka S, Nanashima A, Yamaguchi H, Yasutake T. Survival and recurrence after a sphincter-saving resection and abdominoperineal resection for adenocarcinoma of the rectum at or below the peritoneal reflection: a multivariate analysis. Surg Today. 2004;34:32–9.

17. Nelson H, Petrelli N, Carli A, Couture J, Fleshman J, Guillem J, Miedema B, Ota D, Sargent D. Guidelines 2000 for colon and rectal surgery. J Natl Cancer Inst. 2001;93(8):583–94.

18. Ogilvie J, Ricciardi R. Complications of perineal surgery. Clin Colon Rectal Surg. 2009;22:51–9.

19. Perry WB, Connaughton JC. Abdominoperineal resection: how is it done and what are the results? Clin Colon Rectal Surg. 2007;20(3):213–20.

20. Philips R. Adequate distal margin of resection for adenocarcinoma of the rectum. World J Surg. 1992; 16:463–6.

21. Ross H, Mahmoud N, Fry R. The current management of rectal cancer. Curr Probl Surg. 2005;42(2):78–127.

22. Rothenberger D, Wong D. Abdominoperineal excision for adenocarcinoma of the low rectum. World J Surg. 1992;16(3):478–85.

23. Tekkis P, Heriot A, Smith J, Thompson M, Finan P, Stamatakis J. Comparison of circumferential margin involvement between restorative and nonrestorative resections for rectal cancer. Colorectal Dis. 2005;7: 369–74.

24. Tilney H, Heriot A, Purkayastha S, Antoniou A, Aylin P, Darzi A, Tekkis P. A national perspective on the decline of abdominoperineal resection for rectal cancer. Ann Surg. 2008;247(1):77–84.

25. Wiatrek R, Thomas S, Papaconstantinou H. Perineal wound complications after abdominoperineal resection. Clin Colon Rectal Surg. 2008;21:76–86.

26. Wibe A, Syse A, Andersen E, Tretli S, Myrvold H, Søreide O, Norwegian Rectal Cancer Group. Oncological outcomes after total mesorectal excision for cure for cancer of the lower rectum: anterior vs. abdominoperineal resection. Dis Colon Rectum. 2004;47(1):48–58.

27. Zbar A. Pioneers in colorectal surgery: Sir W. Ernest Miles. Tech Coloproctol. 2007;11:71–4.

T. Wiggers and K. Havenga

Abstract

A successful treatment of locally advanced and recurrent rectal cancer is based on the responsibility of the surgeon to perform a radical of the resection. Planning of treatment starts with imaging with an MRI of the pelvis and a CT scan of the abdomen. Neoadjuvant chemoradiation is given to achieve downstaging and downsizing. After a waiting period of at least 6 weeks, a total mesorectal excision is performed with often an extra-anatomical extension based on the initial imaging. Reconstruction using several types of pedicled flaps is often necessary to close the defect of the pelvis floor.

Primary Advanced Rectal Cancer

Introduction

A local recurrence is one of the worst outcomes of the treatment of rectal cancer. After the introduction of the total mesorectal excision (TME) technique with or without a short course of preoperative radiotherapy, the local recurrence rate may not exceed 5 % [1, 2]. The surgeon has become the most important prognostic factor in the successful treatment of rectal cancer [3]. This makes him responsible for the result. Every attempt should be made to achieve an R0 resection (complete macroscopic and microscopic removal of the tumor including its lateral and caudal lymphatic spread in the mesorectum). There is no role for debulking surgery.

In case of a threatened circumferential margin, primary resection of the tumor will result in a high percentage of an involved margin with a subsequent high local recurrence rate [4]. The TNM classification is not sufficient to make the distinction between primary resectable cases and patients needing neoadjuvant treatment [5]. The following definition will be used for locally advanced rectal cancers: any T4, any T3 with a predicted margin of less than 1 mm to the endopelvic fascia, and any lymph node outside the TME field. A special challenge is the management of the tumors with

T. Wiggers (✉) • K. Havenga
Department of Surgery, University Medical Center
Groningen, P.O. Box 30 001, Groningen 9700 RB,
The Netherlands
e-mail: t.wiggers@umcg.nl; k.havenga@umcg.nl

G. Baatrup (ed.), *Multidisciplinary Treatment of Colorectal Cancer*,
DOI 10.1007/978-3-319-06142-9_10, © Springer International Publishing Switzerland 2015

the synchronous presence of distant metastases since most of these tumors are locally advanced as well.

Modern imaging techniques are necessary for accurate assessment of the extent of the tumor. Digital examination only is inferior [6]. This staging should include an abdominal CT scan (see Chap. 14) and an MRI of the pelvis.

After staging, three groups of tumors can be distinguished: tumors with extensive tumor growth toward the endopelvic fascia but within the mesorectal envelope (including pathological lymph nodes), tumors invading adjacent structures but with growth limited to the pelvis, and tumors with metastatic extra-pelvic disease (liver, lung, para-aortic, and/or inguinal). In the first two situations, neoadjuvant radiotherapy (dose between 45 and 50 Gray) combined with chemotherapy as a radiosensitizer should be considered as standard therapy (Chap. 14). Neoadjuvant therapy with the goal of increasing the rate of sphincter-saving procedures has not been successful [7].

Evaluation of the effect of the neoadjuvant treatment is difficult. Reporting the rate of R0 resections gives a better insight in the aimed effect of the treatment and should be considered as a substitute of the complete response rate. Imaging with MRI after the induction treatment is difficult since it may be impossible to distinguish between scar and remaining tumor. However, a visible endopelvic fascia of the post-treatment MRI has a high predictive value for the radicality of the resection [8].

It is the best option to start with induction chemotherapy if a patient presents himself with synchronous metastases. A short course (5×5 Gy) of radiotherapy preceding the chemotherapy is necessary to achieve similar results for local control as in patients without distant metastases [9]. The technical details for the rectal resection are the same as in cases without metastases. If technically feasible, a combined resection of the primary tumor and the rectum is advocated. An extensive liver should be performed first followed by the rectal resection after 1–2 months.

Any T3 with a Predicted Margin of Less Than 1 mm to the Endopelvic Fascia

After a waiting period of at least 6 weeks to allow for downsizing and downstaging, a TME resection may be performed in case of tumor confined to the pelvic envelope (even with sparing of the autonomic plexus and saving of the sphincter) (see Chap. 5).

T4

In case of T4 tumors, the operative procedure should exist in more extensive "en bloc" resections. The extent of the resection is mainly based on the primary imaging. This may include removal of the lateral side wall, pelvic floor, and involved organs.

Lateral Side Wall

The pelvis consists of two compartments: a parietal outer compartment and a visceral inner compartment. The parietal compartment is built around the skeletal part of the pelvis (sacrum, pubic, iliac, and ischial bone). Muscles on the inside of the pelvis are the piriformis muscle, coccygeal muscle, levator ani muscle, and obturator muscle. The common internal and external iliac artery and vein belong to the parietal compartment as well as the lumbosacral nerve plexus.

If the tumor is close to the inferior hypogastric plexus (by means of palpation or MRI scan), or if a total pelvic exenteration is performed, a plane lateral to the inferior hypogastric plexus can be chosen. Resection of the internal iliac artery and vein creates laterally another few millimeters of extra margin. Resection of muscles is demanding and technical difficult. Some surgeons even advocate resection of bony structures and sacrificing the lumbosacral plexus (partially) [10].

Sometimes enlarged obturator lymph nodes are seen on the pretreatment MRI. The obturator space is cleared if the nodes are still visible on the MRI after the chemoradiation. This resection is not en bloc with the primary tumor and usually vessels do not have to be sacrificed. The obturator nerve is spared during this dissection.

Pelvic Floor

A complete removal of the levator muscle has become standard (extralevator resection) if an abdominoperineal resection with a wide local resection is necessary [11]. The prone position may facilitate this procedure especially if the os coccyx or even a part of the sacrum has to be removed. The patient is turned in the jackknife or knee-chest position. Special care has to be given to this positioning. A detailed description of the knee-chest position is as follows. Gravity will cause flexion of hip and the knees. To prevent sliding away, a roll is put under the upper legs. The operation table is tilted some degrees of anti-Trendelenburg to balance the patient in a way that most of the weight is transferred to the upper legs. The chest is supported with a large, firm but soft roll. In this way the abdomen is hanging freely, facilitating ventilation. Performing the perineal phase in the knee-chest position instead of the standard position in stirrups has several advantages: (a) exposure to the operative field is better; (b) hydrostatic venous pressure is lower, reducing bleeding; (c) assistance and tutoring is feasible; and (d) gravity will pull the perineum downward, flattening the pelvic floor. Contraindications for this position are instability of circulation, stiff hip joints, above-knee amputation, and severe overweight (>100 kg).

The perineal phase is started with closure of the anus with a purse string stitch. The perineal skin is incised in an ellipse extending to the perineum ventrally and extending some centimeters lateral to the anus. Dorsally the incision extends below the coccyx. In selected cases this incision is extended to include the coccyx or distal sacrum. Ventrally, the posterior vaginal wall in female patients may be included in the resection. The ischiorectal fat is then divided using diathermia. Some branches of the inferior rectal artery and vein are encountered. During the continuation of this dissection, the inferior outer surface of the levator ani muscle and its insertion to the obturator muscle will be exposed. Ventrally the perineal muscle will be divided. This will expose the bulbus of the penis in male patients or the posterior vaginal wall in female patients. In male patients the ventral plane leads from the

bulbus to the urethra. A transurethral catheter is helpful to identify the urethra by palpation. After identifying the urethra, it may be difficult to continue in the correct plane on the prostate because of a sharp dorsal angle in the dissection plane. During dissection on the bulbus, urethra, and prostate, the left and right levator muscles stand out as vertical columns which can be divided. Step by step the prostate is dissected and the levator is divided on its origin. The levator should be cut above the horizontal plan of the dorsal site of the prostate in order to prevent damage of the autonomic nerves entering the prostate laterodorsally. On the posterior side the dissection plane created during the laparotomy will be met. In some cases some upward dissection has to be made to reach this plane. Some authors advocate entering the retro rectal plane below the tip of the coccyx. This technique of the perineal phase ensures that the levator ani muscle is resected en bloc with the specimen, avoiding a positive margin in distal T3/T4 tumors because of a thin distal mesorectal layer. It is called the extralevator resection. The removed specimen has less perforations and a wider margin in comparison with the conventional technique [12]. As the levator is completely resected, the perineal wound presents as a large defect in the pelvic floor. An omentoplasty is used to close this perineal defect. If it is not possible to make an omentoplasty, a rectus abdominis flap and in rare cases the gluteus flap will be used. After fixating the omentoplasty or rectus flap in the perineal defect, the subcutaneous fascia is approximated. In cases with preoperative fistula to the pelvic floor, a large skin defect has to be created. Under these circumstances a rectus abdominis flap with skin island is used [13]. Finally, the skin is closed with interrupted sutures.

Involved Organs

The rectal cancer extends sometimes to the anterior compartment of the pelvis. Organs within this internal compartment are the rectum and bladder and the genitourinary organs: in females the uterus; the round ligament of the uterus, tube, and ovaries; and the vagina and in males the seminal vesicles, the ductus deferens, and the prostate.

Radical resection of the tumors invading one of these structures requires resection of the affected organs. This may result in partial bladder resection, selective resection of the seminal vesicles, and resection of the uterus or posterior vaginal wall en bloc with the total mesorectal excision. After resection of the vagina, a reconstruction should be offered to a patient whom is sexually active. Several techniques are available such as the rectus abdominis flap, split skin on a mold [14].

Resection of both the prostate and bladder is called a total pelvic exenteration. Pelvic exenteration is in the initial phase similar to a standard low anterior resection or abdominoperineal resection. The patient's position in stirrups, the midline incision from the pubic bone to just above the umbilicus, the careful inspection of the abdomen and liver for metastatic disease, and the exposition of the pelvis by installing a self-retaining retractor keeping the small bowel and omentum away are all the same. After mobilizing and dividing the sigmoid, the superior rectal artery is divided close to the inferior mesenteric artery. The presacral plane is developed. It is helpful to identify the hypogastric nerves at this stage and find the plane posterior to these nerves, contrary to the regular rectal resection. This outward plane follows the outer layer of the visceral pelvic compartment. It is filled with loose areolar tissue; some small vessels cross the layer. Often, this plane is edematous by the neoadjuvant radiation therapy. The ureter is encountered at its crossing of the iliac artery. The ureter is divided at this point, putting a temporarily small (Chap. 8) silicone catheter in the ureter to allow observation of diuresis. Dividing the ureter at this point allows for an anastomosis to the Bricker loop at the promontory. A longer ureter could allow a Bricker anastomosis deeper in the pelvis, at risk for leakage in the pelvis as it is not covered with tissue and for obstruction in the case of recurrent disease. On the ventral side, the loose areolar tissue of Retzius' space is divided. The remaining bridge to the pelvic sidewall is now divided. This dissection is carried out close to the internal iliac artery and vein and its subsequent branches and just outside the pelvic autonomic nerve plexus. A bipolar vessel sealing device may facilitate dis-

section in the narrow working space in this part of the operation. At the caudal edge of the pubic bone, firm attachments of the prostate to the bone are found: the puboprostatic ligament. Under and lateral to this ligament is an extensive venous plexus. It can be the cause extensive bleeding if the dissection is carried forward into this plexus. After bilateral incision of the endopelvic fascia, the branches of the vesicoprostatic plexus are ligated and the dissection is continued within the prostatic capsule toward the pelvic floor. The urethra is then encountered and divided. The final part of the resection has two options. In case of a distal tumor, a perineal resection is mandatory (see perineal resection). In case of a more proximal tumor, future herniation is prevented by leaving the pelvic floor intact.

Locally Recurrent Cancer

Introduction

The treatment strategy for locally recurrent cancer is based on staging and a discussion in a multidisciplinary team to define the maximal multimodality treatment.

Imaging focuses on establishing the local extent of the tumor and on detecting distant metastases. At least 50 % of the patients with a recurrence have detectable distant metastases at the time of diagnosis making them nearly always unsuitable for curative treatment [15]. A helical CT or a high-resolution MRI with a phase array coil can assess local tumor extension. Due to its various pulse sequence techniques, MRI has better soft tissue resolution than CT. This is useful in assessing the extent of local recurrent disease, as it can better distinguish tumor from scar tissue due to a higher signal on the T2-weighted images. Tumor extent must be measured in ventral, dorsal, lateral, caudal, and cranial directions. Reconstruction of the images in several planes is helpful in determining resection margins and the level of sacral transection. Introduction of the PET scan has been useful in distinguishing scar tissue from recurrence and in finding unsuspected metastatic disease especially in retroperitoneal lymph nodes and liver [16]. Patients with a previous anterior or Hartmann resection should undergo a pelvic examination. In female patients this has to be extended with a gynecological examination and in some cases with a cystoscopy. A laparotomy can be part of the staging procedure. It may exclude extra pelvic disease, divert the bowel in case of a preceding low anterior resection, and fill the superior part of the pelvis with a (biological) spacer, such as omentum, to prevent irradiation of the small bowel. Diverting the colon in the presence of a low anterior reconstruction can be difficult with regard to both mobilization and vascularization of the afferent loop of the bowel. In these circumstances, it may be wise to divert via a loop ileostomy or a transversostomy. A practical algorithm for the initial approach has been published recently [17].

Most surgeons consider the following features as (relative) contraindications for local resection: extensive pelvic sidewall involvement, sacral invasion above S2–S3 junction, encasement of external iliac vessels, extension of tumor through the sciatic notch, and presence of gross lower limb edema from lymphatic or venous obstruction. Deep infiltration into the lumbosacral plexus or sacrum can never result in an R0 or R1 resection without severe mutilation. A predicted R2 resection, distant metastases (which cannot be resected radically), and a poor performance status are absolute contraindications.

A practical system is the classification from the Leeds group [18] since it can be used in planning the operative treatment strategy: central (tumor confined to the pelvic organs or connective tissue without contact onto or invasion into bone), sacral (tumor present in the presacral space and abuts onto or invades into the sacrum), sidewall or lateral (tumor involving the structures on the pelvic sidewall, including the greater sciatic foramen and sciatic nerve through to piriformis and the gluteal region), and composite (sacral and sidewall recurrence combined).

Multimodality Approach

As with primary rectal cancer, the aim of the treatment is an R0 resection. Debulking has no place in the surgical strategy for these cases since postoperative radiotherapy cannot compensate for macroscopic residual disease. Inadequate surgery has the disadvantages of an extensive operative procedure without any beneficial palliative effect since the tumor causing the symptoms is not removed. Radiotherapy only has an effect on symptom control and is, depending if previous radiation was delivered, more effective with increasing dose. The duration of this symptom relief is usually between 6 and 9 months [19]. Surgery is beneficial especially for, so-called, central recurrences with limited or no pelvic sidewall involvement. The introduction of standard high-dose preoperative radiotherapy (usually 50.4 Gy in 28 1.8 Gy fractions) in combination with extensive surgery has resulted in long-term survivors with an acceptable re-recurrence rate [20]. Additional intraoperative radiotherapy, by either an electron beam irradiation (IOERT) at a dose of 10–17.5 Gy or a high-dose-rate brachytherapy (HDR-IORT) of 10 Gy, has resulted in a cure rate not far below that achieved in locally advanced primary rectal cancer [21]. The combination of chemotherapy with a long course of radiotherapy is promising, as it may increase the R0 resection rate.

Treatment has now become more difficult after the introduction of TME surgery and preoperative radiotherapy since the anatomy is obliterated and the toxicity of more radiotherapy is cumulative. Increasing experience has been gained using preoperative re-irradiation of 30 Gy followed directly by resection and intraoperative radiotherapy of another 10 Gy [22]. Toxicity is considerable including radio necrosis and neuropathy by either the resection or the radiotherapy, but oncological outcome is comparable with primarily nonirradiated patients [23]. After TME the recurrence may be located low in the pelvis with infiltration of the pelvic floor relatively far from the nervous pelvic plexus making this location suitable for an abdominoperineal (sacral) approach.

Treatment of recurrent disease after transanal endoscopic microsurgery (TEM) is in the absence of metastatic disease feasible. Salvage surgery after chemoradiation follows the planes of the TME resection as in primary cases. In nearly all cases, an R0 resection can be achieved. The main problem is the high percentage of metastatic disease during follow-up [24].

Surgical Treatment

General

A multidisciplinary team depending on the individual experience of the members is needed and may include colorectal, urological, gynecological, plastic surgery, and in rare cases neurosurgery and/or orthopedic surgery. The procedure begins with an exploratory laparotomy. Peritoneal seedings and unexpected not locally treatable liver metastases are in general a contraindication for continuing with the procedure. The aim of the technical approach is the development of a free circumferential margin.

Central

A centrally located recurrence is treated with an abdominoperineal resection or low anterior resection. The central dissection is comparable with the resection in primary cases. Most cases are after a low anterior resection, and there is always an adhesion at the dorsal site at the spot of the transection of the mesorectum. If in doubt about the nature of this adhesion, a sacral resection has to be included in the procedure. A new anastomosis can be made if a safe distal margin can be obtained. Since the percentage of re-recurrence is considerable and there is a lot of fibrosis due to the radiotherapy and repeated surgery, it may be wise to end up with a permanent fecal diversion by means of a permanent colostomy.

Sacral

Extensive dorsal and dorsolateral invasion requires an abdominosacral approach with transaction of the sacrum. This part of the operation is done in the prone position (knee-chest or jackknife). A long dorsal midline sacral incision is used including the anus or anal scar. The gluteal muscles are mobilized laterally. The sacrotuberous and sacrospinous ligaments have to be sacrificed. The level of transection of the sacrum is assessed after palpation of the cut of the chisel which was performed in the abdominal phase [25]. The highest level is mid S3. Resections above this level require additional measures to stabilize the pelvis and closure of the dural sac. Under these circumstances there is usually an extensive lateral spread with infiltration of the lumbosacral plexus.

Lateral

If during the first operation the endopelvic fascia was the anatomical limit of the dissection, a plane outside including resection of the vessels is still possible [26]. In general it follows the same principle as an advanced primary tumor. Due to retraction of the vessels medially after the irradiation, dissection can be cumbersome and sometimes leading to substantial blood loss. Before intraoperative irradiation of the lateral pelvic wall, the internal iliac vessels are ligated with nonabsorbable sutures to prevent later blowout in case of an infection with radio necrosis. Ventrally, dissection beyond the bladder or the internal genital organs is sometimes necessary for creation of a free resection margin. This will result in a pelvic exenteration.

After the resection the area at risk for possible tumor residue is determined and preferably quantified by frozen sections to define the spots with minimal residual disease.

Either by electron beam irradiation or by high-dose-rate brachytherapy, a boost of irradiation is given in a shielded operating room.

After this extensive surgery filling the dead space left by the resection is essential. It serves several purposes. There is often diffuse venous bleeding and although it may be necessary to pack the pelvic cavity, a tissue flap can help to achieve hemostasis. The second reason for putting vital tissue in the pelvis is the prevention of radio necrosis. Omitting this part of the operation may result in a blowout of the vessels in the postoperative phase. Finally reconstruction of the pelvic floor prevents the development of a perineal hernia. An omentoplasty, due to the pliability and the strong hemostatic capacity, is the best option for filling the pelvic cavity [27]. A pedicled rectus abdominis flap is a good solution in case with extensive resection of the pelvic floor. It can even be used when two stomas are constructed at the site of the urinary stoma. An alternative in this situation is a mesh graft covered on the abdominal side by the omentum or the cecum and from the perineal side by a (double) graciloplasty [28].

The treatment of a local recurrence has certain disadvantages. The perioperative mortality is low (around 3 %) in experienced hands, but the short-term morbidity, although similar whether or not IORT is applied, is high. It includes wound infection (perineal), sacral plexus neuropathy, voiding problems, and fistula formation [29]. The long-term morbidity is considerable but should be put in the perspective of uncontrolled tumor growth in the pelvis with severe pain, infection, and fistula often experienced for a long period in the absence of disseminated disease [30].

Summarizing it has become clear that identification of locally advanced rectal tumors is based on imaging guided staging. Presently effective neoadjuvant treatment is available after which in most cases radical surgery aiming on an R0 resection is still possible. In recurrent cancers the strategy is useful with the drawback that in most cases full preoperative treatment is no longer possible and that anatomical plane are distorted making standard resection impossible.

References

1. Peeters KC, Marijnen CA, Nagtegaal ID, et al. Dutch Colorectal Cancer Group. The TME trial after a median follow-up of 6 years: increased local control but no survival benefit in irradiated patients with resectable rectal carcinoma. Ann Surg. 2007;246: 693–701.
2. Sebag-Montefiore D, Stephens RJ, Steele R, et al. Preoperative radiotherapy versus selective postoperative chemoradiotherapy in patients with rectal cancer (MRC CR07 and NCIC-CTG C016): a multicentre, randomised trial. Lancet. 2009;373:811–20.
3. Wiggers T, van de Velde CJ. Reduction 'by half'. The need for standardised surgical technique in radiotherapy studies for rectal cancer. Eur J Surg. 1999;165: 407–9.
4. den Dulk M, Marijnen CAM, Putter H, et al. Risk factors for adverse outcome in patients with rectal cancer treated with an abdominoperineal resection in the TME trial. Ann Surg. 2007;246:83–90.
5. Nagtegaal ID, Gosens MJ, Marijnen CA, et al. Combinations of tumor and treatment parameters are more discriminative for prognosis than the present TNM system in rectal cancer. J Clin Oncol. 2007; 25:1647–50.
6. Brown G, Davies S, Williams GT, et al. Effectiveness of preoperative staging in rectal cancer: digital rectal examination, endoluminal ultrasound or magnetic resonance imaging? Br J Cancer. 2004;91:23–9.
7. Bujko K, Kepka L, Michalski W, et al. Does rectal cancer shrinkage induced by preoperative radio(chemo)therapy increase the likelihood of anterior resection? A systematic review of randomised trials. Radiother Oncol. 2006;80:4–12.
8. Engelen SM, Beets-Tan RG, Lahaye MJ, et al. MRI after chemoradiotherapy of rectal cancer: a useful tool to select patients for local excision. Dis Colon Rectum. 2010;53:979–86.
9. van Gijn W, Marijnen CA, Nagtegaal ID, et al. Dutch Colorectal Cancer Group. Preoperative radiotherapy combined with total mesorectal excision for resectable rectal cancer: 12-year follow-up of the multicentre, randomised controlled TME trial. Lancet Oncol. 2011;12:575–82.
10. Austin KK, Solomon MJ. Pelvic exenteration with en bloc iliac vessel resection for lateral pelvic wall involvement. Dis Colon Rectum. 2009;52: 1223–33.
11. Holm T, Ljung A, Haggmark T, et al. Extended abdominoperineal resection with gluteus maximus flap reconstruction of the pelvic floor for rectal cancer. Br J Surg. 2007;94:232–8.
12. West NP, Anderin C, Smith KJ, et al. European Extralevator Abdominoperineal Excision Study Group. Multicentre experience with extralevator abdominoperineal excision for low rectal cancer. Br J Surg. 2010;97:588–99.
13. Kroll SS, Pollock R, Jessup JM, et al. Transpelvic rectus abdominis flap reconstruction of defects following abdominal-perineal resection. Am Surg. 1989;55: 632–7.
14. Pusic AL, Mehrara BJ. Vaginal reconstruction: an algorithm approach to defect classification and flap reconstruction. J Surg Oncol. 2006;94:515–21. Review.
15. van den Brink M, Stiggelbout AM, van den Hout WB, et al. Clinical nature and prognosis of locally recurrent rectal cancer after total mesorectal excision with or without preoperative radiotherapy. J Clin Oncol. 2004;22:3958–64.
16. Franke J, Rosenzweig S, Reinartz P, et al. Value of positron emission tomography (18F-FDG-PET) in the diagnosis of recurrent rectal cancer. Chirurg. 2000;71: 80–5.
17. Mirnezami AH, Sagar PM, Kavanagh D, et al. Clinical algorithms for the surgical management of locally recurrent rectal cancer. Dis Colon Rectum. 2010;53:1248–57.
18. Boyle KM, Sagar PM, Chalmers AG, et al. Surgery for locally recurrent rectal cancer. Dis Colon Rectum. 2005;48:929–37.
19. Knol HP, Hanssens PE, Rutten HJ, et al. Effect of radiation therapy alone or in combination with surgery and / or chemotherapy on tumor and symptom control of recurrent rectal cancer. Strahlenther Onkol. 1997;173:43–9.

20. Wiggers T, de Vries MR, Veeze-Kuypers B. Surgery for local recurrence of rectal carcinoma. Dis Colon Rectum. 1996;39:323–8.

21. Kusters M, Valentini V, Calvo FA, et al. Results of European pooled analysis of IORT-containing multi-modality treatment for locally advanced rectal cancer: adjuvant chemotherapy prevents local recurrence rather than distant metastases. Ann Oncol. 2010;21: 1279–84.

22. Valentini V, Morganti AG, Gambacorta MA, et al. Study Group for Therapies of Rectal Malignancies (STORM). Preoperative hyperfractionated chemora-diation for locally recurrent rectal cancer in patients previously irradiated to the pelvis: a multicentric phase II study. Int J Radiat Oncol Biol Phys. 2006;64:1129–39.

23. Rutten HJ, Mannaerts GH, Martijn H, et al. Intraoperative radiotherapy for locally recurrent rectal cancer in The Netherlands. Eur J Surg Oncol. 2000;26(Suppl A):S16–20.

24. Doornebosch PG, Ferenschild FT, de Wilt JH, et al. Treatment of recurrence after transanal endoscopic microsurgery (TEM) for T1 rectal cancer. Dis Colon Rectum. 2010;53:1234–9.

25. Mannaerts GH, Rutten HJ, Martijn H, et al. Abdominosacral resection for primary irresectable and locally recurrent rectal cancer. Dis Colon Rectum. 2001;44:806–14.

26. Enker WE, Kafka NJ, Martz J. Planes of sharp pelvic dissection for primary, locally advanced, or recurrent rectal cancer. Semin Surg Oncol. 2000;18:199–206.

27. Logmans A, van Lent M, van Geel AN, et al. The pedi-cled omentoplasty, a simple and effective surgical tech-nique to acquire a safe pelvic radiation field; theoretical and practical aspects. Radiother Oncol. 1994;33:269–71.

28. Borel Rinkes IH, Wiggers T. Gracilis muscle flap in the treatment of persistent, infected pelvic necrosis. Eur J Surg. 1999;165:390–1.

29. Mannaerts GH, Rutten HJ, Martijn H, et al. Effects on functional outcome following IORT-containing multi-modality treatment for locally advanced primary and locally recurrent rectal cancer. Int J Radiat Oncol Biol Phys. 2002;54:1082–8.

30. Mannaerts GH, Schijven MP, Hendrikx A, Martijn H, et al. Urologic and sexual morbidity following multi-modality treatment for locally advanced primary and locally recurrent rectal cancer. Eur J Surg Oncol. 2001;27:265–72.

Reconstructions After Neoadjuvant and Abdominoperineal Resection

11

Søren Laurberg and Marie-Louise Feddern

Abstract

Reconstruction after abdominoperineal resection for low rectal cancer is an ongoing challenge. Perineal wound complications have a significant impact on postoperative morbidity. The use of neoadjuvant therapy may increase the risk of wound complications. Intraoperative perineal wound management has evolved from open wound packing to primary closure. Tissue transfer techniques are used as filling of the dead space and reconstruction of large perineal defects. This chapter describes the management strategy of perineal reconstruction at our clinic.

Introduction

Abdominoperineal resection (APR) is still the most common resectional procedure in patients with very low rectal cancer.

Perineal wound complications are common and include wound infections, abscess formations, delayed healing, and a persistent perineal sinus [1].

The lack of primary perineal healing is associated with a significant morbidity and prolonged hospital stay.

The high rate of infections is due to a large dead space in an irradiated field.

The reported incidence of infectious complications varies substantially 0–44 % [2–7] – most likely due to different definitions of infection, variation in patient population and surgical technique.

In the long term APR may be associated with development of a perineal hernia in 1.4–6 % [2, 4, 7]. APR has not been standardised, and part of the reported variation in infection and perineal hernia might be due to differences in the extent of surgery. Variation in use of neoadjuvant irradiation/chemo irradiation might also contribute to the variation in complication rates [8, 9].

Recently more standardised APR techniques have been promoted, subdividing APRs into intersphincteric, extralevatory and ischioanal APR. At our clinic we use these three well-defined types of APRs depending upon the tumour location and extent.

Several techniques including omentoplasty [10], gracilis transposition [11, 12], mesh repair [13–16], rectus abdominis flap [2, 17, 18] and

S. Laurberg (✉) • M.-L. Feddern, MD
Department of Surgery P, Aarhus University Hospital,
Tage-Hansens Gade 2, Aarhus 8000, Denmark
e-mail: soerlaur@rm.dk; ml_feddern@hotmail.com

G. Baatrup (ed.), *Multidisciplinary Treatment of Colorectal Cancer*,
DOI 10.1007/978-3-319-06142-9_11, © Springer International Publishing Switzerland 2015

gluteal flaps [5, 19, 20] have been used to improve the perineal healing and reduce the risk of a perineal hernia.

At our clinic we have never used omentoplasty and only very selectively gracilis flap, since the muscle is small and the blood supply to its skin unreliable.

Below I will describe our strategy for reconstruction of the perineum following standardised APR surgery.

Perineal Reconstruction Following Intersphincteric APR (In-APR)

At our clinic we use an In-APR after TME surgery when we abstain from performing a colo-anal anastomosis in patients with poor sphincter function, severe co-morbidity or disseminated disease.

In In-APR the pelvic floor is intact, the tissue loss in perineum is minimal and the irradiation field will not include the external sphincter.

In these cases we perform a layered approximation of the puborectal muscle, the external anal sphincter and the perianal skin.

Perineal Reconstruction Following Extralevatory APR (E-APR)

In the E-APR the perineal dissection follows the peripheral/lower border of the external sphincter and pelvic floor, and a major portion of the levator plate is removed en bloc with the specimen. Compared to the conventional nonstandardised APR, there will be a larger defect in the pelvic floor, while the loss of tissue in the perineum is less extensive.

The defect in the pelvic floor cannot be adapted.

Results from our clinic indicate that the defect must be repaired since 21 % (7 out of 33 patients) will develop a clinical perineal hernia within 1 year, if the perineal dead space is filled with a fasciocutaneous gluteal flap without reconstruction

of the pelvic floor. Our infection rate with this flap was only 6 % and all except one perineum were healed within 3 months [14]. Recognising this unacceptable high rate of perineal hernia, we changed strategy and reconstructed the pelvic floor defect with a biological mesh. A 10×10 cm porcine dermal collagen mesh was sutured to the cut edges of levator ani muscle and the paracoccyx ligaments with interrupted monofilament absorbable sutures. A suction drain was placed superficial to the mesh and a layered approximation of the subcutaneous tissue was performed.

In our first consecutive 24 cases, we have observed no perineal hernia, the infection rate was 17 % and all except 1 perineum were healed within 3 months. No mesh was removed [14].

The main advantages of the mesh technique are that it is technical simple and can easily be performed by a colorectal surgeon. Furthermore, the theatre time is shorter, there is no restriction in patient mobilisation and there is no donor site morbidity.

The main disadvantage is the cost of the mesh. We and others have used the costly biological mesh. A randomised trial is needed to show its advantage.

Torbjörn Holm has promoted the use of a musculocutaneous gluteal flap to cover the defect of the pelvic floor and the dead space in the perineum. For larger defects he has used bilateral flaps and he has also used the flap for vaginal reconstruction. In 28 cases the perineal infection rate was 11 % (3/28) [5]. The surgical procedure takes longer time, it is more complicated and there are restrictions in the early perioperative period. The long-term donor site morbidity is unknown. Only a randomised trial will be able to decide whether a mesh or the musculocutaneous gluteal flap is the most optimal procedure after an E-APR.

Selectively we have used the VRAM flap (see below) following E-APR for the reconstruction of the vagina and to cover the pelvic catheters when we have treated patients with advanced or recurrent rectal cancer with postoperative brachytherapy.

Perineal Reconstruction Following Ischioanal Abdominoperineal Resection (Ia-APR)

We perform the Ia-APR procedure for anal cancer salvage surgery and when a rectal cancer has penetrated or perforated into the ischioanal fossa (Figs. 11.1 and 11.2).

With this procedure, there is an extensive tissue loss of the levator plate and the perineum within an irradiated field.

In these cases we always reconstruct the perineum with a vertical rectus abdominis myocutaneous flap (VRAM), to cover the defect in the pelvic floor and perineum. This flap is large and bulky and has a safe blood supply to the skin and subcutaneous tissue.

Generally the VRAM flap has been harvested from the right site of the abdominal wall. If there is a transverse incision on the right site of the abdominal wall, we perform Doppler ultrasonography to document that the inferior epigastric arteries are patent, since the flap is depending on its blood supply (Figs. 11.3 and 11.4).

The harvest of flap and the perineal reconstruction have always been performed by a dedicated plastic surgeon. The VRAM flap has several advantages:

1. The muscular part can cover catheters in the pelvic cavity and thereby protect the small bowel against irradiation damage if postoperative brachytherapy is used.
2. It can be used for reconstruction of the vagina.
3. It can cover a large defect in the perineum. In cases where there is very extensive loss of skin, the peripheral part can be left open and secondarily repaired by a split skin transplant.
4. The reported primary healing rate of the perineum is very high, and in a consecutive series of Ia-APR for anal cancer salvage surgery, no perineal surgical intervention was needed in 49 cases [21].

The main drawback of this flap is that it prolongs the operation time and that a plastic surgeon has to be involved.

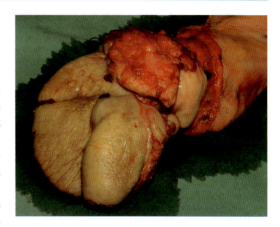

Fig. 11.1 Ia-APR specimen

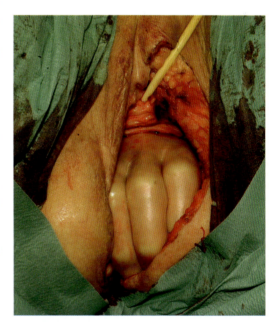

Fig. 11.2 Defect following Ia-APR. Notice that the entire posterior wall of the vagina has been removed

Furthermore, there are some donor site morbidities with herniation.

The flap is denervated and this might lead to atrophy of the muscle and sensory disturbances of the skin.

An alternative would be the use of one or two myocutaneous gluteal flaps, but we have never used it in these cases due to our good results with the VRAM flap (Fig. 11.5).

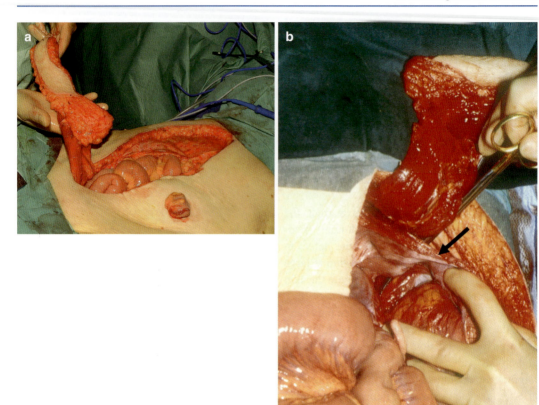

Fig. 11.3 (**a**) VRAM flap harvest. The flap includes skin paddle, subcutaneous fat, a cuff of anterior rectus sheath fascia and one rectus abdominis muscle. (**b**) The rectus sheath is divided caudally to the pubic bone raised on inferior epigastric artery (*arrow*) serving as the vascular pedicle for the VRAM flap

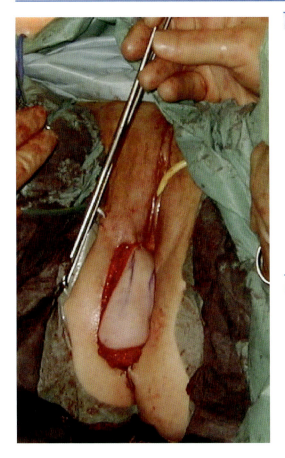

Fig. 11.4 The large VRAM flap inserted for reconstruction of the posterior vaginal wall and perineum

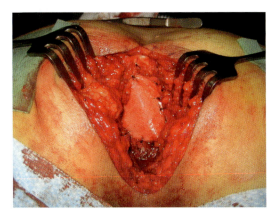

Fig. 11.5 Use of a Permacol mesh for reconstruction of the pelvic floor following E-APR

Conclusion

I would recommend standardised APR procedures.

For In-APR no pelvic floor reconstruction is needed.

Following E-APR we prefer a mesh reconstruction, but an alternative might be a myocutaneous gluteal flap. Randomised studies are needed to document which procedure is best and whether a biological mesh has an advantage.

In the author's experience, the VRAM flap is the method of choice when extensive defects of the perineum have to be repaired.

References

1. El-Gazzaz G, Kiran RP, Lavery I. Wound complications in rectal cancer patients undergoing primary closure of the perineal wound after abdominoperineal resection. Dis Colon Rectum. 2009;52(12):1962–6.
2. Buchel EW, Finical S, Johnson C. Pelvic reconstruction using vertical rectus abdominis musculocutaneous flaps. Ann Plast Surg. 2004;52(1):22–6.
3. Burke TW, Morris M, Roh MS, Levenback C, Gershenson DM. Perineal reconstruction using single gracilis myocutaneous flaps. Gynecol Oncol. 1995; 57(2):221–5.
4. Butler CE, Gundeslioglu AO, Rodriguez-Bigas MA. Outcomes of immediate vertical rectus abdominis myocutaneous flap reconstruction for irradiated abdominoperineal resection defects. J Am Coll Surg. 2008;206(4):694–703.
5. Holm T, Ljung A, Haggmark T, Jurell G, Lagergren J. Extended abdominoperineal resection with gluteus maximus flap reconstruction of the pelvic floor for rectal cancer. Br J Surg. 2007;94(2):232–8.
6. Houvenaeghel G, Ghouti L, Moutardier V, et al. Rectus abdominis myocutaneous flap in radical oncopelvic surgery: a safe and useful procedure. Eur J Surg Oncol. 2005;31(10):1185–90.
7. Vermaas M, Ferenschild FT, Hofer SO, et al. Primary and secondary reconstruction after surgery of the irradiated pelvis using a gracilis muscle flap transposition. Eur J Surg Oncol. 2005;31(9):1000–5.
8. Bullard KM, Trudel JL, Baxter NN, Rothenberger DA. Primary perineal wound closure after preoperative radiotherapy and abdominoperineal resection has a high incidence of wound failure. Dis Colon Rectum. 2005;48(3):438–43.

9. Chadwick MA, Vieten D, Pettitt E, Dixon AR, Roe AM. Short course preoperative radiotherapy is the single most important risk factor for perineal wound complications after abdominoperineal excision of the rectum. Colorectal Dis. 2006;8(9):756–61.

10. Hultman CS, Sherrill MA, Halvorson EG, et al. Utility of the omentum in pelvic floor reconstruction following resection of anorectal malignancy: patient selection, technical caveats, and clinical outcomes. Ann Plast Surg. 2010;64(5):559–62.

11. Persichetti P, Cogliandro A, Marangi GF, et al. Pelvic and perineal reconstruction following abdominoperineal resection: the role of gracilis flap. Ann Plast Surg. 2007;59(2):168–72.

12. Shibata D, Hyland W, Busse P, et al. Immediate reconstruction of the perineal wound with gracilis muscle flaps following abdominoperineal resection and intraoperative radiation therapy for recurrent carcinoma of the rectum. Ann Surg Oncol. 1999;6(1):33–7.

13. Cui J, Ma JP, Xiang J, et al. Prospective study of reconstructing pelvic floor with GORE-TEX Dual Mesh in abdominoperineal resection. Chin Med J (Engl). 2009;122(18):2138–41.

14. Christensen HK, Nerstrøm P, Tei T, Laurberg S. Perineal repair after extralevatory abdominoperineal excision for low rectal cancer. Dis Colon Rectum. 2011;54(6):711–7.

15. Han JG, Wang ZJ, Gao ZG, et al. Pelvic floor reconstruction using human acellular dermal matrix after cylindrical abdominoperineal resection. Dis Colon Rectum. 2010;53(2):219–23.

16. Wille-Jorgensen P, Pilsgaard B, Moller P. Reconstruction of the pelvic floor with a biological mesh after abdominoperineal excision for rectal cancer. Int J Colorectal Dis. 2009;24(3):323–5.

17. Bell SW, Dehni N, Chaouat M, et al. Primary rectus abdominis myocutaneous flap for repair of perineal and vaginal defects after extended abdominoperineal resection. Br J Surg. 2005;92(4):482–6.

18. Lefevre JH, Parc Y, Kerneis S, et al. Abdominoperineal resection for anal cancer: impact of a vertical rectus abdominis myocutaneous flap on survival, recurrence, morbidity, and wound healing. Ann Surg. 2009;250(5):707–11.

19. Boccola MA, Rozen WM, Ek EW, et al. Inferior gluteal artery myocutaneous island transposition flap reconstruction of irradiated perineal defects. J Plast Reconstr Aesthet Surg. 2010;63(7):1169–75.

20. Wagstaff MJ, Rozen WM, Whitaker IS, et al. Perineal and posterior vaginal wall reconstruction with superior and inferior gluteal artery perforator flaps. Microsurgery. 2009;29(8):626–9.

21. Sunesen KG, Buntzen S, Tei T, et al. Perineal healing and survival after anal cancer salvage surgery: 10-year experience with primary perineal reconstruction using the vertical rectus abdominis myocutaneous (VRAM) flap. Ann Surg Oncol. 2009;16(1): 68–77.

Part III

Oncology

Introduction to Oncology

12

Per Pfeiffer

Abstract

Over the past decade, the efficacy of modern chemotherapy, with or without targeted therapy, has been markedly improved. Systemic therapy generates substantial tumour regression in around 50 % of patients with metastatic colorectal cancer, median progression-free survival is prolonged to around 9 months, median overall survival approaches 2 years and the chance for resection is increased. The optimal strategy must be decided on by a multidisciplinary team.

Over the past two decades, the survival of patients with colorectal cancer (CRC) has increased constantly, not only due to better selection of patients and better surgical techniques but also due to an increased use of effective chemotherapy in the adjuvant and the metastatic situation.

Establishment of multidisciplinary teams with participation of colorectal surgeons, medical and radiation oncologist, radiologists and pathologist as a minimum has probably been the most important concept on its own perhaps in sharp competition with introduction of TME and resection of solitary metastasis.

Since the introduction of 5-fluorouracil (FU) in 1957, numerous well-conducted phase III studies have proven efficacy, although modest, of FU. For almost 40 years, FU, often biomodulated with folinic acid (FA), was the only available drug for patients with CRC, and therefore, numerous different treatment schedules were developed and compared. It was soon established that FA increased the efficacy of FU, but the optimal combination of FU and FA was still a matter of great debate – the dose of 5-FU and FA, bolus or infusion, one or several days of therapy and FA or FU first were some of the many questions that were asked and discussed. A combination of FU and FA is even nowadays the backbone of systemic therapy in patients with CRC. Presently, the most widely FU/FA schedule is a combination of FU bolus and infusion with high-dose FA (often called the "de Gramont" regimen).

The era of modern combination therapy started when it was shown that irinotecan prolonged median survival in patients with 5-FU-resistant disease. Since then, several new drugs have been approved for therapy in patients with CRC:

P. Pfeiffer, MD, PhD
Department of Oncology, Odense University Hospital, Sdr Boulevard 29, Odense DK – 5000, Denmark
e-mail: per.pfeiffer@ouh.regionsyddanmark.dk

G. Baatrup (ed.), *Multidisciplinary Treatment of Colorectal Cancer*,
DOI 10.1007/978-3-319-06142-9_12, © Springer International Publishing Switzerland 2015

irinotecan and oxaliplatin, three oral formulations of FU (capecitabine, uftoral and S-1) and three targeted drugs – bevacizumab (targeting vasculature), cetuximab and panitumumab (both targeting EGF receptor). However, since 2005, no new drugs have been approved for patients with CRC.

Modern combination chemotherapy with irinotecan or oxaliplatin generates tumour regression in 50 % of patients with metastatic CRC. Progression-free survival is prolonged to 9 months, and median overall survival (OS) is approaching 24 months but only in fit selected patients who are potential candidates for inclusion in clinical trials. The addition of novel biologic agents (e.g. cetuximab or bevacizumab), especially in patients with liver-only disease, further increases response rates to almost 70 % and subsequently, the proportion of patients who are candidates for supplementary local therapy with curative intent. It is very important that the oncologist regularly considers the possibility for resection because even with response rates around 70 %, the number of complete pathological response is still less than 10 %.

Approximately 30 % of patients with colorectal cancer (CRC) will develop hepatic metastases at some point during the course of the disease. Surgical resection is the golden standard for patients with resectable CRLM. After microscopic radical resection (R0), the expected 5-year survival is around 35 % and even higher in recent selected series. Peri-operative systemic therapy is used to reduce the risk of recurrence in patients with resectable CRLM, but major tumour regression has also permitted salvage surgery in 10–30 % of patients with initially un-resectable CRLM. It is again important to notice that chemotherapy alone is not administered with curative intent but as downsizing therapy or neo-adjuvant therapy in patients with liver-only CRC.

Presently, around 10 % of patients with CRLM are candidates for local treatment. This number will definitely grow up due to introduction of newer surgical and ablative techniques and markedly enhanced efficacy of systemic chemotherapy. The optimal combination of these different modalities must be decided on by a multidisciplinary team (MDT), as a minimum including liver surgeons, oncologists and interventional radiologists.

Disclosure Part of the information in this introduction has been previously published in *Acta Radiol.*, Sept 2009;50(7):707–708. doi:10.1080/028418509031722515.

Systemic Therapy for Patients with Colorectal Cancer: State of the Art

13

Per Pfeiffer, Camilla Qvortrup, and Josep Tabernero

Abstract

Recent modalities and strategies have increased the complexity of treatment choice in patients with colorectal cancer (CRC), and therefore all cases should be assessed at a multidisciplinary conference.

Adjuvant chemotherapy for 6 months increases the chance of cure by absolutely 5 % in stage II and 10–15 % in stage III. Targeted therapy is not recommended in the adjuvant setting.

Treatment options in patients with non-resectable CRC are based on the extent of disease (resectable/potential resectable/non-resectable) and symptoms. Surgery first or chemotherapy first in patients with synchronous metastasis is one of several yet unsolved questions which should be discussed at a MDT in each case taking into account patients symptoms and performance.

Introduction

Worldwide, it is estimated that more than 1 million patients are diagnosed with colorectal cancer (CRC) each year and that more than half a million will die due to the disease [1]. At the time of diagnosis, approximately 20 % of the patients have synchronous metastases, but totally nearly 50 % of patients will at some point develop metastatic disease (mCRC).

P. Pfeiffer, MD, PhD (✉) • C. Qvortrup
Department of Oncology,
Odense University Hospital,
Sdr. Boulevard 29, DK – 5000, Odense, Denmark
e-mail: per.pfeiffer@ouh.regionsyddanmark.dk;
camilla.qvortrup@ouh.regionsyddanmark.dk

J. Tabernero
Department of Medical Oncology,
Vall d'Hebron University Hospital,
Vall d'Hebron Institute of Oncology,
Barcelona, Spain
e-mail: jtabenero@vhio.net

Chemotherapeutics and Regimens Used in the Treatment of Colorectal Cancer

Fluoropyrimidines

For more than 50 years, 5-fluorouracil (FU) has been the cornerstone in the treatment of patients with CRC [2]. The antitumour activity arises from several mechanisms (Fig. 13.1) including

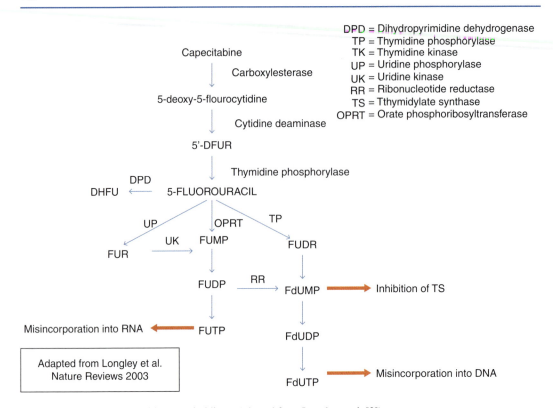

Fig. 13.1 The metabolism of fluoropyrimidines (Adapted from Longley et al. [3])

Table 13.1 Most important FU/FA regimens used in patients with colorectal cancer

Regimen	Doses of 5-flourouracil	Doses of folinic acid	Cycles
De Gramont	400 mg/m² bolus (2 h) followed by 600 mg/m² infusion days 1–2	200 mg/m² days 1–2 (2 h inf.)	2 weeks
Mayo	425 mg/m² bolus days 1–5	20 mg/m² bolus days 1–5	4 weeks
AIO	2,600 mg/m² (24 h inf.)	500 mg/m² (24 h inf.)	Weekly
Roswell Park	600 mg/m² bolus	500 mg/m² bolus	Weekly
Nordic	500 mg/m² bolus (3 min) days 1–2	60 mg/m² days 1–2	2 weeks

FU/FA 5-fluorouracil and folinic acid

inhibition of the thymidylate synthase (TS) and incorporation of FU metabolites into RNA and DNA [3]. It has been proposed that the mechanisms of action are dependent on the treatment schedule: bolus administration primarily results in inhibition of RNA synthesis, whereas prolonged venous infusion (PVI) inhibits TS and thereby DNA synthesis [4].

For many years, the best administration schedule for FU has been debated, and many efforts have been made in order to improve the efficacy

of FU. These include different ways of administration (e.g. bolus injection, PVI and a combination of bolus injection and PVI (Table 13.1)) as well as biochemical modulation of FU [5]. Traditionally FU was administered as a bolus injection; when using bolus regimens, a rapid intravenous injection produced higher response rates than short-time infusion of 15–30 min [6]. However, experimental data indicated that prolonged infusion time resulted in a longer exposure to FU, thereby increasing the cytotoxic effects [7, 8]. PVI has been tested in mCRC without any final conclusion; however, a meta-analysis demonstrated that PVI increased response rates (22 % vs. 14 %) and prolonged median overall survival (OS) marginally [9]. Preclinical studies showed that folinic acid (FA or leucovorin) added to FU resulted in a more stable binding to TS and improved growth inhibition in cell lines [10], which in the clinical setting was translated into a significantly improved efficacy in terms of increased response rate (from 11 to 23 %) and OS (from 10.5 to 11.7 months) [11, 12]. Therefore, FU, when given as intravenous infusion, should always be administered in combination with Lv.

FU is catabolised primarily in the liver by dihydropyrimidine dehydrogenase (DPD) (Fig. 13.1), which is the rate-limiting enzyme in the catabolism [6]. However, DPD is also found in high concentrations in the gastrointestinal (GI) tract making oral administration of FU impossible.

Capecitabine is an oral prodrug of FU, which is absorbed directly from the GI tract. After absorption, capecitabine is activated to FU by three enzymatic steps (Fig. 13.1). The last step is catalysed by thymidine phosphorylase (TP), which has been shown to have a higher activity in GI cancer tissue compared to the surrounding normal tissue [13, 14] indicating a preferential activation of capecitabine in tumour tissue. This has been confirmed by the finding of higher concentration of FU in tumour compared to normal tissue after administration of capecitabine [15].

As described, the efficacy of FU is improved by modulation with FA, so naturally it has also been tested whether FA modulation of capecitabine would also improve efficacy. This was investigated in a small randomised phase II study [16], where three different regimens were tested – a continuous regimen (capecitabine 1,331 mg/m^2 days 1–21), an intermittent regimen (capecitabine 2,510 mg/m^2 days 1–14 every 3 weeks) and an intermittent regimen in combination with FA (capecitabine 1,657 mg/m^2 and oral FA 60 mg, days 1–14 every 3 weeks). The addition of FA did not improve efficacy but increased toxicity. This resulted in the establishment of a regimen with capecitabine as single agent

2,500 mg/m^2/day in 14 days followed by 1 week rest.

Capecitabine as single agent has been compared to bolus FU/FA in two randomised phase III trials. Both studies demonstrated that capecitabine was as efficient as bolus FU/FA [17, 18].

A second available oral fluoropyrimidine is UFT, which is a combination of uracil and Ftorafur, a prodrug of FU. Uracil reversibly inhibits DPD, thereby increasing the bioavailability of FU [3]. In contrast to capecitabine, UFT is most often combined with FA. UFT/FA had equivalent efficacy and was safer than bolus administration of FU/FA [19, 20]. In recent years, UFT/FA is seldom used in Europe and the USA, but UFT with or without FA or the related drug S1 is predominantly used and investigated in Japan.

Patient Preference

An obvious question is if the patients prefer oral or intravenous therapy. When chemo-naive patients were asked before they have received any treatment, the majority of patients would prefer oral therapy [21], and these results were confirmed in a randomised crossover trial [22]. However, the Mayo regimen is probably the most toxic FU regimen, and consequently side effects are not comparable to side effects of the low-toxic UFT.

A Danish randomised study demonstrated that the administration route was of only minor importance compared to the toxicity of the treatment [23], and these data were confirmed in an English crossover study [24].

Oxaliplatin

Oxaliplatin is a third-generation platinum compound, which is rapidly activated by nonenzymatic hydrolysis to form platinum derivates and oxalate. Newer studies suggest that not only the platinum derivates but also the intact oxaliplatin may exert cytotoxic effects [25]. The cytotoxicity of oxaliplatin arises from DNA damage by several mechanisms as DNA adducts formation, inter- and intra-strand DNA cross-link and DNA protein cross-links [26]. In preclinical studies oxaliplatin as single agent has been shown to have antitumour activity against colon cancer cell lines [27], and adding FU/FA to oxaliplatin has been shown to result in a synergistic cytotoxicity. A clinical study confirmed this, showing that oxaliplatin as single agent only had modest activity compared to the combination of oxaliplatin and FU/FA [28], and therefore oxaliplatin should preferably be delivered in combination with a fluoropyrimidine.

The dose-limiting toxicity of oxaliplatin is neuropathy and is seen in two forms – an acute and a chronic form.

The acute form is usually transient and resolves within days and is seen in most patients treated with oxaliplatin and is characterised by cold-induced paraesthesias and dysaesthesias during or shortly after the infusion [29]. The probability and severity of acute neuropathy are claimed to be dependent on the infusion rate so that prolongation of infusion with lower peak plasma concentrations of oxaliplatin will reduce acute neuropathy.

The chronic form of oxaliplatin-induced neuropathy is characterised by sensory paraesthesias and dysaesthesias primarily in the extremities. The most important factor for chronic persistent neuropathy is still the total cumulative dose of oxaliplatin [30].

In order to reduce neuropathy, a delivery time of 2 h of oxaliplatin is recommended; however, in the daily clinical practice with limited existing resources, a lower overall treatment time may be of importance. Therefore and inspired by a small study in patients with ovarian cancer [31], delivery of oxaliplatin as a 30 min infusion has been tested in several prospective trials in order to reduce overall treatment time. A 30-min infusion of oxaliplatin is feasible and apparently does not increase the severity of sensory neuropathy [32–37]. However, an infusion time of 30 min has never been directly compared to the standard 120 min infusion in a randomised study.

Irinotecan

Irinotecan is a derivate of camptothecin and an inactive prodrug, which is converted to the active metabolite SN-38 by carboxylesterases [38, 39]. The cytotoxicity results from inhibition of the topoisomerase [40]. The active metabolite SN-38 is primarily inactivated in the liver by the UDP-glucuronosyltransferase (UGT) – primarily by the isoenzyme 1A1 [41], which also glucuronidates bilirubin. The inactivated SN-38 is mainly excreted in the bile.

The main severe adverse events of irinotecan are diarrhoea and neutropenia. The irinotecan-induced diarrhoea is seen in two forms – an early-onset and a late-onset form – and is caused by different mechanisms. The acute form is cholinergic and occurs during or shortly after administration of irinotecan and can be prevented by administration of atropine prior to treatment.

In recent years, genetic polymorphisms in UGT1A1 have been linked to the severity of adverse events of irinotecan. Patients with reduced UGT1A1 activity – primarily caused by the UGT1A1*28 polymorphism – have more severe reactions to irinotecan, and therefore in patients who are known homozygotes for the UGT1A1*28 genotype, a reduced starting dose of irinotecan is recommended [42].

Targeted Therapy

In recent years a number of biologically active substances attacking specific signalling pathways in cancer cells (targeted therapy) have been developed and included in the treatment of patients with CRC. Three monoclonal antibodies have by now been approved for therapy in mCRC.

Angiogenesis is essential in tumour development and controlled in part by the vascular endothelial growth factor (VEGF) system. VEGF-A has the greatest impact on angiogenesis, and specifically VEGF-A is inhibited by bevacizumab (Avastin®).

Cetuximab (Erbitux®) and panitumumab (Vectibix®) block the extracellular portion of the epidermal growth factor receptor (EGFR).

Adjuvant Therapy After Radical Resection for Colon Cancer

In the adjuvant situation, patients with colon and rectal cancer are treated differently. Pre- and postoperative radiotherapy and chemoradiation for rectal cancer will be discussed in Chap. 12. The scientific support for adjuvant chemotherapy in patients with rectal cancer is much less than in colon cancer, but – similar to the situation in colon cancer – adjuvant chemotherapy may be provided. However, in the metastatic situation, patients with colon and rectal cancer are treated as one group.

Summary

- Adjuvant single-agent chemotherapy increases the chance of cure by absolutely 5 % in stage II and 10 % in stage III.
- Stage II patients can be divided into high and low risk of recurrence, according to the presence of at least one of the following factors: lymph nodes sampling <12, poorly differentiated tumour, vascular or lymphatic or perineural invasion, obstruction or perforation or pT4 stage.
- Adjuvant chemotherapy should be offered to all medically fit patients with high-risk stage II and stage III disease, should be started as early as possible (3–8 weeks after surgery) and should be given for 6 months.
- Fluoropyrimidine and oxaliplatin combinations are superior compared to single-agent 5-FU in terms of DFS and OS in stage III patients.
- Fluoropyrimidine and oxaliplatin combinations might be considered in high-risk stage with multiple risk factors.
- The use of targeted therapy should be avoided outside clinical trials.

Since the publication of Moertel's study in 1990 [43] demonstrating superiority in terms of disease-free survival (DFS) and OS of FU compared to surgery alone in patients with stage III colon cancer, FU has been the cornerstone in the adjuvant treatment. The efficacy of biochemically FA-modulated FU as adjuvant therapy has subsequently been confirmed in several studies [44]. Originally, adjuvant therapy was administered for 12 months, but the duration of treatment can safely be reduced to 6 months without compromising efficacy.

Oral prodrugs of FU (capecitabine and tegafur/FA) are alternatives to intravenous treatment with FU/FA as it has been demonstrated that these oral agents have at least similar efficacy compared to intravenous FU-based regimens [45, 46].

Adjuvant FU/FA for 6 months increases the chance of cure by absolutely 5 % in stage II and 10 % in stage III [44] and was therefore the golden standard until the MOSAIC study was published in 2004 [47].

The MOSAIC trial was the first study to show that addition of oxaliplatin further improved efficacy beyond FU/FA (Table 13.2). In a recent update of MOSAIC data, it was found that in patients with stage III disease, 6-year OS was increased from 68.7 to 72.9 % [48].

The efficacy and tolerability of oxaliplatin (Table 13.2) have since been confirmed in NSABP C-07 [49], and recently it was demonstrated that capecitabine in combination with oxaliplatin (CapOx) increased 3-year DFS [50].

As described above, adjuvant fluoropyrimidine-based chemotherapy is the standard of care in patients with radical resected stage III colon cancer, whereas it is more controversial in patients with stage II colon cancer. Only modest but definite benefits of 4–5 % benefit in 5-year OS have been demonstrated in pooled analyses and in the Quasar study [44, 51–53] in patients treated with FU-based therapy. There is no significant benefit of adding oxaliplatin in an unselected group of patients with stage II disease. However, in the MOSAIC trial, patients with high-risk stage II had a nonsignificant reduction in the risk of relapse of 26 %, but no tendency for improvement in survival.

There is a great variability in survival within patients with stage II disease [54], and probably the choice of adjuvant therapy should be individualised and based on the risk of recurrence and the expected relative reduction in recurrence (Table 13.3).

Table 13.2 Single-agent fluoropyrimidines versus oxaliplatin-based adjuvant chemotherapy in patients with colon cancer stage 3

	Stage	3 year DFS (%)			5 year OS (%)		
		Fp	+oxaliplatin	Δ	Fp	+oxaliplatin	Δ
MOSAIC	3	65.3	72.2	6.9*	68.7	72.9	4.2*
C-07	3	71.5	76.1	4.6*	78.3	80.3	2.0
XELOXA	3	66.5	70.9	4.5*	74.2	77.6	3.4

MOSAIC: Andre et al. [48]; C-07: Kuebler et al. [49]; XELOXA: Haller et al. [50]. Δ = difference
Fp fluoropyrimidine, i.e. *FU/FA* 5-fluorouracil and folinic acid or *Cap* capecitabine * = significant difference

Table 13.3 TNM 7th edition – correlation with Dukes classification and 5-year survival for patients with colon cancer based on SEER data [54]

Stage	T	N	Dukes	% of TxNxM0	5-year survival (%)	
					Relative	Absolute
I	T1–T2	N0	A	21.4	**97.1**	**76.3**
II	T3–T4	N0	B	43.9	**84.8**	**64.7**
IIA	T3	N0		36.6	87.5	66.7
IIB	T4a	N0		4.5	79.6	60.6
IIC	T4b	N0		2.8	58.4	45.7
III	Any T	N1–2	C	34.7	**60.3**	**47.8**
IIIA				3.1	86.8	70.5
	T1–T2	N1a		1.7	90.7	73.7
	T1–T2	N1b		1.1	83.0	67.2
	T1	N2a		0.3	79.0	64.7
IIIB				24.1	65.4	51.6
	T3	N1a		8.0	74.2	58.2
	T4a	N1a		1.5	67.6	52.2
	T3	N1b		8.3	65.3	51.7
	T1–T2	N2b		0.1	62.4	51.8
	T4a	N1b		1.3	54.0	42.1
	T3	N2a		4.9	53.4	42.8
IIIC				7.5	32.9	26.5
	T4a	N2a		0.9	40.9	32.5
	T3	N2b		3.0	37.3	30.4
	T4b	N1a		0.8	38.5	30.6
	T4b	N1b		0.9	31.2	25.4
	T4b	N2a		0.7	23.3	18.3
	T4a	N2b		0.6	21.8	17.5
	T4b	N2b		0.6	15.7	12.9

Most clinical guidelines [55, 56] recommend adjuvant chemotherapy to patients with high risk of recurrence (poorly differentiated adenocarcinoma, T4 tumour, perineural/perivenous tumour growth, perforation, acute resection due to ileus or a yield of less than 12 lymph nodes). However, still additional markers to selected patients for adjuvant therapy are warranted.

The status of the DNA mismatch repair system (MMR) is suggested to be a predictor of benefit of adjuvant therapy. Approximately 15 % of sporadic colorectal cancers have defective MMR (dMMR), and these patients have a lower risk of recurrence. Several studies have reported that FU therapy alone is of no value in dMMR patients [57]. It should be considered to assess MMR status in patients considered for FU as single-agent therapy in the adjuvant setting.

So far only few data on the effect of the MMR status in patients treated with combination chemotherapy are available [58].

The recommended treatment duration of oxaliplatin based is currently 6 months, but several ongoing international phase III studies are investigating whether treatment time can be reduced to 3 months. The purpose of IDEA (International Duration Evaluation of Adjuvant Chemotherapy) is to conduct a single, pooled analysis of all studies to test whether 3 months of oxaliplatin-based adjuvant therapy is non-inferior for disease-free survival (DFS) to 6 months of the identical therapy. The IDEA pooled analysis will consist only of stage III colon patients randomised to 3 or 6 months of a FOLFOX regimen (FOLFOX4 or mFOLFOX6) or CapOx.

In contrast to the improvement in efficacy by oxaliplatin-containing combination chemotherapy regimens, it has not been possible to demonstrate that irinotecan enhances the effect of FU/FA as adjuvant therapy [59–61].

The new targeted drugs (bevacizumab and cetuximab) have also been tested in the adjuvant setting. The first study of several studies was presented in 2009. In NSABP C-08 study, patients were randomised to adjuvant FOLFOX for 6 months with or without bevacizumab and then bevacizumab as maintenance therapy for additional 6 months. Unfortunately, preliminary data could not demonstrate an improvement in DFS by addition of bevacizumab [62].

A similar phase III study (AVANT) is also evaluating the use of adjuvant bevacizumab. A press release September 2010 stated that 'unlike the C-08 results, preliminary efficacy data from AVANT numerically favour chemotherapy alone (the control arm)'.

N0147 assessed the potential benefit of cetuximab added to FOLFOX in patients with colon cancer stage III. The primary end point was 3-year DFS. Initially patients were enrolled regardless of KRAS status, but when the impact of KRAS status on the effect of anti-EGFR antibodies in the metastatic setting was established, the study was amended to include only patients with KRAS wild-type tumours. In patients with KRAS mutations, both 3-year DFS and OS favoured FOLFOX alone [63]. It was planned to include 2.070 patients with KRAS wild type, but NO147 closed after accrual of 1.760 patients when a pre-planned interim analysis demonstrated no benefit of addition of cetuximab – in any subgroup. Cetuximab only added to toxicity [64].

Data from ongoing or completed adjuvant trials are awaited, but currently targeted therapy should be avoided outside trials.

Systemic Treatment of Metastatic Colorectal Cancer

Summary

Systemic Therapy

- The optimal strategy for every patient should be discussed in a multidisciplinary team.
- FU/FA single-agent treatment prolongs median OS from 6 to 12 months.
- Combination chemotherapy prolongs median OS further to around 20 months for medically fit patients.
- It is important that fit patients are exposed to all active drugs.
- A sequential strategy (single agent immediately followed by combination upon progression) in patients with unresectable disease and no tumour-related symptoms initially seems to be a safe strategy.
- Fit elderly patients tolerate combination chemotherapy and have the same benefit as younger patients.
- Targeted therapy enhances efficacy of chemotherapy, but in the general population, the benefit is not as high as anticipated from the original trials.

Surgery

- The optimal strategy for every patient should be discussed in a multidisciplinary team.
- Surgery first or chemotherapy first in patients with synchronous metastasis should be

discussed at an MDT in each case and taking into account symptoms (primary, metastasis) and performance.

- Patients with resectable metastases should receive perioperative treatment for 3 months preoperatively followed by resection followed by 3 months postoperatively.
- Good prognosis patients with a single small (<2 cm) metachronous liver metastasis should be considered for upfront surgery.
- If preoperative chemotherapy was not administered, adjuvant chemotherapy with fluoropyrimidines with or without oxaliplatin for 6 months should be the standard of care.

Patients with mCRC may be grouped according to the resectability of their metastases: resectable at diagnosis and initially unresectable. Patients with initially unresectable mCRC can be further subdivided into two groups: potential resectable mCRC which is defined as disease that may become resectable after tumour shrinkage and non-resectable which is defined as disease remaining unresectable despite major tumour regression [65]. Treatment strategies depend on the resectability of the disease. For patients with non-resectable mCRC, therapy is primarily of palliative character.

Monotherapy with FU/FA

Palliative chemotherapy improves quality of life [66] and prolongs OS [67] in patients with mCRC.

For several years, FU/FA was the only available therapy in patients with mCRC producing response rates of 20 % and prolonging median OS from 6 to 12 months compared to best supportive care (BSC) [2].

Second-Line Therapy After FU/FA

Irinotecan and oxaliplatin were implemented in the treatment of CRC in the late 1990s. Irinotecan was introduced in the second-line setting in patients with mCRC resistant to FU/FA. In this setting, it was demonstrated that irinotecan significantly prolonged median OS from 6.5 to 9.2 months compared to BSC [68] and from 8.5 to 10.8 months compared to FU/FA alone [69].

A recently published study comparing oxaliplatin and FU/FA (FOLFOX) and irinotecan as single agent in patients with mCRC resistant to FU/FA demonstrated similar survival in the two treatment groups; however, the oxaliplatin-containing regimen produced significant higher response rate and longer PFS than irinotecan as single agent [70].

When oxaliplatin is given in combination with the 'de Gramont schedule' of FU/FA, the combination is generally is termed FOLFOX. This regimen has been modified several times, but in this review we will not distinguish between the different FOLFOX variations.

Rothenberg and colleagues performed a large study in patients resistant to irinotecan-based treatment, in which it was demonstrated that FOLFOX was superior to both oxaliplatin single agent and FU/FA in terms of response (9.9 % vs. 1.3 % vs. 0 %) and PFS (4.6 months vs. 1.6 months vs. 2.7 months); however, this benefit was not translated into a significant OS benefit (9.8 months vs. 8.7 months vs. 8.1 months) [28].

Combination Regimens as First-Line Therapy

First-line therapies with fluoropyrimidines combined with either oxaliplatin [71, 72] or irinotecan [73–75] are effective regimens (Table 13.4) producing response rates of up to 50 %, a PFS of 6–8 months and an OS of 14–16 months. Some of the studies performed failed to demonstrate a significant improvement in OS, which may be explained by crossover to the combination regimen after progressive disease to single-agent therapy.

Many patients maintain an excellent performance status despite progressive disease on second-line therapy. However, no chemotherapeutic has proven efficacy in the third-line settings after progression to irinotecan and oxaliplatin and FU/FA [76, 77].

Several studies have compared the different combinations head to head (summarised in Table 13.4). Efficacy of the different regimens is similar – only the US IFL regimen is definite inferior and should not be used [78–80]. It is of minor

Table 13.4 Selected phase III studies evaluating efficacy of first-line combination chemotherapy in patients with mCRC

Author, year	Regimen	No. of patients	RR (%)	Median PFS (months)	Median OS (months)
5FU/FA versus combination therapy with irinotecan					
Saltz et al. *NEJM* 2000 [75]	FU/FA	226	21	4.3	12.6
	IFL	231	39*	7.0*	14.8*
Douillard et al. *Lancet* 2000 [73]	FU/FA	187	22	4.4	14.1
	FOLFIRI	198	35*	6.7*	17.4*
Köhne et al. *JCO* 2005 [74]	FU/FA	216	32	6.4	16.9
	'FOLFIRI'	214	54*	8.5*	20.1
5FU/FA versus combination therapy with oxaliplatin					
de Gramont et al. *JCO* 2000 [71]	FU/FA	210	22	6.2	14.7
	FOLFOX	210	51*	9.0*	16.2
Giacchetti et al. *JCO* 2000 [72]	FU/FA	100	12	6.1	19.9
	FOLFOX	100	34*	8.7*	19.4
Combination versus combination					
Tournigand et al. *JCO* 2004 [80]	FOLFOX	111	54	10.9	20.6
	FOLFIRI	111	56	14.2	21.5
Goldberg et al. *JCO* 2004 [79]	IFL	264	31	6.9	15.0
	FOLFOX	267	45*	8.7*	19.5*
Glimelius et al. *Ann Oncol* 2008 [78]	FLIRI	281	35	9.4	19.4
	FOLFIRI	286	49*	9.0	19.0
Cassidy et al. *JCO* 2008 [85]	CapOx	1,017	47	8.0	19.8
	FOLFOX	1,017	48	8.5	19.6

Abbreviations: *Bev* bevacizumab, *BSC* best supportive care, *Cet* cetuximab, *FLIRI* FU/FA with folinic acid + irinotecan (Nordic bolus regimen), *Fp* fluoropyrimidine, *FU/FA* 5-fluorouracil/folinic acid, FOLFOX = oxaliplatin + FU/FA (combined bolus and infusion), *FOLFIRI* irinotecan + FU/FA (combined bolus and infusion) *IFL* Irinotecan + FU/FA (US bolus regimen), *Iri* irinotecan, *'Iri'* irinotecan regime, *MUT* mutated KRAS, *OS* overall survival, *'Ox'* oxaliplatin regimen, *Pan* panitumumab, *PFS* progression-free survival, *RR* response rate, *WT* wild-type KRAS, *CapOx* capecitabine + oxaliplatin, *** = significant difference

importance in which sequence the different regimens are used; however, it is important that patients are exposed to all three active drugs [81].

Different treatment strategies have been tested in two large randomised trials, either starting with single-agent capecitabine or FU/FA (sequential therapy) or initiating therapy with combination chemotherapy. It was demonstrated that there were no differences in OS between the different strategies [82, 83]; however, higher response rates were obtained with initial use of combination chemotherapy. This has led to a conclusion that in patients where response is of importance – e.g. in patients with a potentially curative resection of tumour after shrinkage or in patients with tumour-related symptoms – treatment with combination chemotherapy should be used initially. However, in patients with unresectable disease and no tumour-related symptoms, initially treatment with

single-agent fluoropyrimidine (either oral or intravenous) seems to be a safe strategy.

Capecitabine in Combination with Oxaliplatin

Different schedules of CapOx have been developed, but the most widely used regimen of CapOx is the 3-week schedule with oxaliplatin 130 mg/m^2 day 1 and capecitabine 2,000 mg/m^2 days 1–14 every 3 weeks, even though a randomised phase II study showed that oxaliplatin in combination with dose-intensified capecitabine may be beneficial in terms of improved response rate (54.4 % vs. 42.2 %) and longer PFS (10.5 months vs. 6.0 months) compared to the 'standard' CapOx regimen [84]. The dose-intensified regimen did not increase the risk of toxicity.

The CapOx regimen has been compared to combination treatment with infusional FU/FA

Table 13.5 Phase III trials comparing CapOx to infusional FU/FA + oxaliplatin

Author	No	Regimen	mPFS (months)	mOS (months)	RR (%)
First-line therapy					
Porschen et al. *JCO* 2007 [88]	474	CapOx	7.1	16.8	48
		FUFOX	8.0	18.8	54
Diaz-Rubio et al. *JCO* 2007 [86]	348	CapOx	8.9	18.1	37
		FUOX	9.5	20.8	46
Cassidy et al. *JCO* 2008 [85]	2,034	CapOx	8.0	19.8	47
		FOLFOX	8.5	19.6	48
Ducreux et al. *IJC* 2011 [87]	306	CapOx	8.8	19.9	42
		FOLFOX6	9.3	20.5	46
Second-line therapy					
Rothenberg et al. *Ann Oncol* 2008 [90]	627	CapOx	4.7	11.9	20
		FOLFOX	4.8	12.5	18

Abbreviations: *Bev* bevacizumab, *BSC* best supportive care, *Cet* cetuximab, *FLIRI* FU/FA with folinic acid + irinotecan (Nordic bolus regimen), *Fp* fluoropyrimidine, *FU/FA* 5-fluorouracil/folinic acid, FOLFOX = oxaliplatin + FU/FA (combined bolus and infusion), *FOLFIRI* irinotecan + FU/FA (combined bolus and infusion), *IFL* Irinotecan + FU/FA (US bolus regimen), *Iri* irinotecan, *'Iri'* irinotecan regime, *MUT* mutated KRAS, *OS* overall survival, *'Ox'* oxaliplatin regimen, *Pan* panitumumab, *PFS* progression-free survival, *RR* response rate, *WT* wild-type KRAS, *CapOx* capecitabine + oxaliplatin, * = significant difference

and oxaliplatin in several randomised non-inferiority phase III trials (Table 13.5). The majority of the studies conducted in the first-line setting [85–87] have demonstrated non-inferiority of CapOx compared to infusional-based regimens. However, in a study conducted by the German AIO group [88], in which an alternative CapOx regimen was used (spilt course of oxaliplatin), a slightly inferior efficacy of CapOx was found. A pooled analysis of data from studies comparing CapOx to infusional FU/FA and oxaliplatin regimens concluded that CapOx had similar PFS and OS compared to infusional regimens; however, CapOx resulted in significant lower response rates with an absolute difference of 6.6 % [89]. In second-line efficacy, CapOx is comparable to FOLFOX [90].

Duration of Combination Chemotherapy and Complete Chemotherapy-Free Intervals

When FU/FA was the only available drug, median PFS – and thus median duration of treatment – was around 4–5 months. Chemotherapy was regularly maintained until progression of disease, because there is no cumulative dose-limiting

toxicity. This approach was frequently carried on with the introduction of modern combination chemotherapy. However, this policy must be revised as recent studies have shown that different stop-and-go strategies compared with continuous use of chemotherapy until progression do not necessarily reduce efficacy [91].

In a Medical Research Council trial, patients with mCRC started monotherapy (de Gramont, continuous infusional 5-FU or raltitrexed), and patients without progression at 12 weeks were randomised to continue therapy or to stop. There was no evidence of a difference in OS between the intermittent or the continuous group, and furthermore patients on intermittent chemotherapy had significantly less toxicity [92].

The major issue with continuous oxaliplatin regimens is the risk of chronic neuropathy, and as a consequence the majority of patients will discontinue therapy before progression. The French GERCOR group has evaluated different stop-and-go strategies to optimise the use of oxaliplatin. First a 'stop-and-go strategy with dose-intensive FOLFOX for 6 cycles followed by maintenance therapy with FU/FA alone until progression and reintroduction of oxaliplatin at progression' (OPTIMOX approach) was compared with 'standard FOLFOX until

Table 13.6 Selected randomised studies evaluating a stop-and-go strategy in patients with mCRC

Author, year	Regimen	No. of patients	RR (%)	Median PFS (months)	Median OS (months)
Continuous FOLFOX versus stop-and-go strategy					
Tournigand et al. JCO 2006 [93]	FOLFOX	311	58.5	9.0	19.3
	Stop-and-go[a]	309	59.2	8.7	21.2
Chibaudel et al. *JCO* 2009 [94]	FOLFOX	98	59.2	8.6	23.8
	CFI[b]	104	59.6	6.6*	19.5
Adams et al. *ECCO* 2009, *ASCO* 2010 [97]	Continuous Ox-Fp	815	–	–	15.6
	Intermittent Ox-Fp CFI[b]	815	–	–	14.3
Labianca et al. *ASCO* 2006 [91]	Continuous FOLFIRI	168	36.5	6.5	17.6
	Intermittent FOLFIRI [b]	163	33.6.5	6.2	16.9

Abbreviations: *Bev* bevacizumab, *BSC* best supportive care, *Cet* cetuximab, *FLIRI* FU/FA with folinic acid+irinotecan (Nordic bolus regimen), *Fp* fluoropyrimidine, *FU/FA* 5-fluorouracil/folinic acid, FOLFOX=oxaliplatin+FU/FA (combined bolus and infusion), *FOLFIRI* irinotecan+FU/FA (combined bolus and infusion), *IFL* Irinotecan+FU/FA (US bolus regimen), *Iri* irinotecan, 'Iri' irinotecan regime, *MUT* mutated KRAS, *OS* overall survival, 'Ox' oxaliplatin regimen, *Pan* panitumumab, *PFS* progression-free survival, *RR* response rate, *WT* wild-type KRAS, *CapOx* capecitabine+oxaliplatin, *=significant difference
[a]Stop and go: FOLFOX 3 months → FU/FA 3 months → FOLFOX 3 months
[b]CFI: complete chemo-free interval: FOLFOX 3 months → pause → FOLFOX reintroduction after progression

progression' strategy. Patients receiving the OPTIMOX approach experienced less neurotoxicity and without any loss of efficacy (Table 13.6) [93].

Subsequently it was therefore natural to investigate whether patients could stay away from maintenance therapy with FU/FA, but a chemotherapy-free interval (CFI) after just 3 months of FOLFOX and reintroduction after progression resulted in loss of efficacy [94, 95].

A follow-up of the two OPTIMOX studies concluded that if patients received chemotherapy for at least 6 months, a treatment pause is fully acceptable [96].

In the Medical Research Council COIN trial, 2,415 patients with mCRC received oxaliplatin-fluoropyrimidine-based (Ox-Fp) first-line chemotherapy according to three different strategies. In arms A and C, patients were randomised to continuous versus intermittent therapy (3 months of therapy, break and 3 months of therapy upon progression) [97].

Patients receiving intermittent Ox-Fp (iOx-Fp) had significantly less toxicity (fatigue, anorexia and diarrhoea) and spent a median of 15 weeks on treatment compared to 25 weeks on continuous Ox-Fp (cOx-Fp). Median OS was

only 15.6 months on cOx-Fp and 14.3 months on iOx-Fp. In a recent correspondence, the authors declared that they could exclude a survival difference of more than 10 weeks with continuous chemotherapy, and they concluded – as the GERCOR group – that discontinuation of chemotherapy can be safely considered in selected patients [98].

The Spanish MACRO study evaluated bevacizumab as maintenance therapy in 480 previously untreated patients with mCRC [99]. After 6 courses of CapOx+bevacizumab, patients were randomised to maintenance therapy with bevacizumab or CapOx+bevacizumab until PD. The primary end point was PFS. There were no statistically significant differences in PFS, RR or OS, and as expected bevacizumab was better tolerated, especially relating to reduced neuropathy. The authors concluded that bevacizumab as a maintenance therapy following induction CapOx-bevacizumab was not inferior to continuation CapOx-bevacizumab. However, lack of a control arm makes a final conclusion difficult, but hopefully the questions of 'bevacizumab after discontinuation of chemotherapy' and 'bevacizumab after progression' will be answered by ongoing phase III studies.

How Can We Best Integrate These Results into Daily Practice?

Whether an intermittent approach will prove best remains unanswered; however, clearly no patient should receive continuously first-line therapy for more than 4–6 months without a definite objective. Most often intermittent treatment breaks are necessary, but this determination will require clinical assessment and individualisation. Some patients will benefit from less toxic or biologic maintenance. In the future, we will identify, clinically or by biomarker parameters, meaningful ways to tailor the optimal strategy.

Elderly Patients Tolerate and Benefit from Combination Chemotherapy

Fit elderly patients (70+ years) enrolled in trials have benefits and toxicities of single-agent fluoropyrimidines and FOLFOX comparable to younger patients [100]. The only exception is thrombocytopenia and especially neutropenia, which is significantly worse in older patients [101, 102].

In a recent combined analysis of more than 2,500 patients treated with different irinotecan/FU schedules in four first-line phase III trials, the authors concluded that elderly patients (70+ years) who fulfilled the inclusion criteria of these trials had similar benefits and similar risk of toxicity as younger patients, and these results have been confirmed in systematic reviews [103, 104].

Nevertheless, a large community-based study demonstrated that elderly patients (age 65+ years) were less likely to receive first-line doublet chemotherapy and also less likely to receive irinotecan, oxaliplatin and bevacizumab during the entire course of the disease. In this unselected group of patients, the elderly had a shorter median survival (19.1 months vs. 24.5 months) and more toxicity-related hospitalisations (21 % vs. 11 %) than the younger patients. This discrepancy between the results from subgroup analyses in randomised clinical trials and this community-based study is probably due to a higher proportion of patients with co-morbidities and poorer performance status in the unselected

community-based study than reported in randomised clinical trials [105].

The MOSAIC study showed that adjuvant FOLFOX significantly improved 5-year DFS and 6-year OS in patients with stage II colon cancer [48]. However, subgroup analysis indicated that patients above 65 years did not benefit from FOLFOX. This tendency was confirmed in a recent update of the MOSAIC study [106]. These data are in contrast to the XELOXA study where benefit of CapOx (compared to FU) was maintained in elderly patients [107].

It is very important to distinguish between the frail elderly patients with co-morbidity and poor performance status and the fit elderly patient – as fit elderly tolerate combination chemotherapy and have the same benefit as younger patients.

Targeted Therapy

Inhibition of VEGF

Bevacizumab should be considered in patients with mCRC, as it increases the activity of many active cytotoxic regimens. It increases OS, PFS and RR in first-line treatment in combination with IFL and in combination with FU/FA or capecitabine alone. In addition, bevacizumab improves also OS and PFS in combination with FOLFOX in second-line treatment (Table 13.7).

Bevacizumab (Table 13.7) was approved (presently approved in combination with FU-containing chemotherapy) in Europe and America after the first phase III study showed that bevacizumab increased the efficacy of IFL [108]. In the fundamental Hurwitz study, improvement was seen in every efficacy parameters, and the prolongation of OS was one of the largest ever seen in mCRC. Unfortunately, IFL has significantly lower efficacy and higher toxicity than other combination regimens [79], and therefore IFL is not recommended any longer. However, this principal first-line study in mCRC created huge expectations for the future, and it was immediately anticipated that median OS easily would surpass 24 months if patients received optimal chemotherapy in combination with

Table 13.7 Selected phase III studies evaluating efficacy of bevacizumab and chemotherapy in patients with mCRC

Author, year	Regimen	No. of patients	RR (%)	Median PFS (months)	Median OS (months)
Combination ± bevacizumab, first-line treatment					
Hurwitz et al. *NEJM* 2004 [108]	IFL	411	35	6.2	15.6
	IFL+Bev	402	45*	10.6*	20.3*
Tebbutt et al. *JCO* 2010 [111]	Cap	156	30	5.7	18.9
	Cap+Bev	157	38	8.5*	18.9
	Cap+MMC+Bev	158	46*	8.4*	16.4
Saltz et al. *JCO* 2008 [112]	IFL+Bev	701	38	8.0	19.9
	'Ox'+Bev	699	38	9.2*	21.3
Combination ± bevacizumab, second-line treatment					
Giantonio et al. *JCO* 2007 [113]	FOLFOX	286	9	4.7	10.8
	FOLFOX+Bev	291	23*	7.3*	12.9*

Abbreviations: *Bev* bevacizumab, *BSC* best supportive care, *Cet* cetuximab, *FLIRI* FU/FA with folinic acid+irinotecan (Nordic bolus regimen), *Fp* fluoropyrimidine, *FU/FA* 5-fluorouracil/folinic acid, FOLFOX=oxaliplatin+FU/FA (combined bolus and infusion), *FOLFIRI* irinotecan+FU/FA (combined bolus and infusion), *IFL* Irinotecan+FU/FA (US bolus regimen), *Iri* irinotecan, *'Iri'* irinotecan regime, *MUT* mutated KRAS, *OS* overall survival, *'Ox'* oxaliplatin regimen, *Pan* panitumumab, *PFS* progression-free survival, *RR* response rate, *WT* wild-type KRAS, *CapOx* capecitabine+oxaliplatin, *=significant difference

targeted therapy. This view was supported by two randomised phase II studies evaluating addition of bevacizumab to FU/FA as first-line therapy in mCRC [109, 110]. In a recent Australasian study (MAX), adding bevacizumab to capecitabine significantly improved PFS but did not prolong OS [111].

However, in combination with CapOx or FOLFOX, the expectations were not met. Bevacizumab significantly prolonged PFS [112], but surprisingly there was no significant improvement in confirmed response rate (38 % vs. 38 %) or OS (19.9 vs. 21.3 months). One and all had imagined a much larger benefit in combination with oxaliplatin-based therapy. However, there is no doubt that bevacizumab has a clinically significant activity, but oncologists must learn to select the right treatment to the right patients. Unfortunately, until now there is no valid predictive marker for efficacy of bevacizumab.

Bevacizumab improves also the survival and progression-free survival in combination with FOLFOX as second-line treatment [113].

Bevacizumab has a number of specific but rare side effects (hypertension, proteinuria, arterial thrombosis, bleeding) with gastrointestinal perforation (1–2 % patients) as the most serious.

Inhibition of EGFR

EGFR Inhibition in Patients with Chemoresistant mCRC

There are no established cytotoxic drugs or combination in the third-line settings after progression to irinotecan and oxaliplatin and FU/FA, but this has changed when efficacy of EGFRi was proven in patients with chemoresistant mCRC [100, 114].

The promising activity observed in phase I and II studies was first confirmed in the pivotal BOND study [115] where 329 patients with irinotecan-resistant mCRC were randomised to receive either weekly single-agent cetuximab alone or cetuximab in combination with irinotecan. The combination (CetIri) significantly increased response rate from 11 to 23 % and prolonged PFS from 1.5 to 4.1 months. OS was not significantly prolonged, perhaps due to crossover and use of CetIri as salvage therapy. As a result of the BOND study, CetIri was approved for patients with irinotecan-resistant disease in the USA and Europe in 2004.

One of the criticisms of the BOND study was the lack of a control group, and therefore NCIC-CO.17 was planned and completed [116], in which patients pretreated with irinotecan and

Table 13.8 Selected randomised studies evaluating efficacy of EGFR inhibition (cetuximab or panitumumab) in patients with mCRC

Author, year	Regimen	KRAS	No. of patients	RR (%)	Median PFS (months)	Median OS (months)
Third-line therapy						
Jonker et al. *NEJM* 2007 [116]	BSC	?	285	0	1.8	4.6
	Cet	?	287	7*	1.9*	6.1*
Karapetis et al. *NEJM* 2008 [132]	BSC	WT	113	0	1.9	4.8
	Cet	WT	117	13*	3.8*	9.5*
Van Cutsem et al. *JCO* 2007 [117]	BSC	?	232	0	1.7	6.5
	Pan+BSC	?	231	10*	1.8*	6.5
Amado et al. *JCO* 2008 [131]	BSC	WT	119	0	1.7	7.6
	Pan+BSC	WT	124	17*	2.8*	8.1
Cunningham et al. *NEJM* 2004 [115]	Cet	?	111	11	1.5	6.9
	Cet+Iri	?	218	23*	4.1*	8.5
Di Fiore et al. *ASCO* 2008 [133]	Weekly Cet+Iri	MUT	281	0	2.7	8.0
	Weekly Cet+Iri	WT		43*	5.5*	13.2*
Jensen et al. *ASCO* 2010 [124]	Biweekly Cet+Iri	MUT	165	3	3.9	7.9
	Biweekly Cet+Iri	WT		23*	5.5*	12.1*
Second-line therapy						
Sobrero et al. *JCO* 2008 [120]	Iri	?	650	4	2.6	10.0
	Cet+Iri	?	648	16*	4.0*	10.7

Abbreviations: *Bev* bevacizumab, *BSC* best supportive care, *Cet* cetuximab, *FLIRI* FU/FA with folinic acid+irinotecan (Nordic bolus regimen), *Fp* fluoropyrimidine, *FU/FA* 5-fluorouracil/folinic acid, FOLFOX=oxaliplatin+FU/FA (combined bolus and infusion), *FOLFIRI* irinotecan+FU/FA (combined bolus and infusion), *IFL* Irinotecan+FU/FA (US bolus regimen), *Iri* irinotecan, 'Iri' irinotecan regime, *MUT* mutated KRAS, *OS* overall survival, 'Ox' oxaliplatin regimen, *Pan* panitumumab, *PFS* progression-free survival, *RR* response rate, *WT* wild-type KRAS, *CapOx* capecitabine+oxaliplatin, *=significant difference

oxaliplatin were randomised to receive best supportive care (BSC – no crossover upon progression) or cetuximab monotherapy (Table 13.8). Compared to BSC, cetuximab prolonged OS from 4.6 to 6.1 months (Table 13.8).

In a similar study using the fully human anti-EGFR monoclonal antibody panitumumab, the value of EGFRi was confirmed [117]. Panitumumab was approved for monotherapy of refractory mCRC by the US Food and Drug Administration in September 2006 and conditionally approved in patients with tumours harbouring wild-type KRAS by the European Medicines Agency (EMEA) in December 2007. Presently there is insufficient data on the combination of panitumumab and chemotherapy as salvage therapy. In patients with allergic reactions to cetuximab, retreatment with cetuximab is possible if patients receive premedication, but panitumumab is a good alternative in these patients [118, 119]. Indirectly these data suggest that CetIri increases response rate to more than 20 % and prolongs PFS from less than 2 months to more than 4 months and that OS is prolonged from around 5 to 9 months.

The EPIC and '181' studies (Tables 13.8 and 13.10) showed that second-line CetIri or FOLFIRI+panitumumab, respectively, significantly increased response rate and prolonged PFS [120, 121].

Originally cetuximab was administered as a weekly infusion; however, cetuximab may also be administered as double dose every second week without compromising the efficacy [122, 123]. For the convenience of the patient, CetIri may be infused as cetuximab 500 mg/m^2 in only 60 min, immediately followed by

Table 13.9 Recent studies evaluating EGFR inhibition as first-line therapy according to KRAS status

Author, year	Regimen	KRAS	No. of patients	RR (%)	Median PFS (months)	Median OS (months)
First-line therapy						
Crystal	FOLFIRI	WT	350	40	8.4	20.0
van Cutsem et al.	FOLFIRI+Cet	WT	316	57*	9.9*	23.5*
NEJM 2009 &	FOLFIRI	MUT	183	40	7.7	16.7
ECCO 2009 [126]	FOLFIRI+Cet	MUT	214	36	7.4	16.2
Prime	FOLFOX	WT	331	48	8.0	19.7
Siena et al.	FOLFOX+Pan	WT	325	55	9.6*	23.9
ASCO GI 2010	FOLFOX	MUT	219	40	8.8*	18.7*
	FOLFOX+Pan	MUT	221	40	7.3	15.1
Coin	'Ox'	WT	367	50	8.6	17.9
Maughan et al.	'Ox'+Cet	WT	362	59*	8.6	17.0
ECCO 2009 [129]	'Ox'	MUT	268	41	6.9	14.8
	'Ox'+Cet	MUT	297	40	6.5	13.6
Second-line therapy						
181	FOLFIRI	WT	294	10	3.9	12.5
Peeters et al.	FOLFIRI+Pan	WT	303	35*	5.9*	14.5
ECCO 2009	FOLFIRI	MUT	248	14	4.9	11.1
	FOLFIRI+Pan	MUT	238	13	5.9	11.8

Abbreviations: *Bev* bevacizumab, *BSC* best supportive care, *Cet* cetuximab, *FLIRI* FU/FA with folinic acid+irinotecan (Nordic bolus regimen), *Fp* fluoropyrimidine, *FU/FA* 5-fluorouracil/folinic acid, FOLFOX=oxaliplatin+FU/FA (combined bolus and infusion), *FOLFIRI* irinotecan+FU/FA (combined bolus and infusion), *IFL* Irinotecan+FU/FA (US bolus regimen), *Iri* irinotecan, *'Iri'* irinotecan regime, *MUT* mutated KRAS, *OS* overall survival, *'Ox'* oxaliplatin regimen, *Pan* panitumumab, *PFS* progression-free survival, *RR* response rate, *WT* wild-type KRAS, *CapOx* capecitabine+oxaliplatin. *=significant difference

irinotecan 180 mg/m^2 in 30 min resulting in a total treatment time of only 90 min. In a large phase II study, it was concluded that activity, feasibility and safety of biweekly CetIri are comparable to results of weekly CetIri [124]. Panitumumab may be given every second or third week.

EGFR Inhibition as First-Line Therapy

Several phase II studies have shown promising activity for chemotherapy-cetuximab or panitumumab combinations as first-line therapy with response rates as high as 80 %, high liver resection rates and long OS [125]. Recently the first phase III data (Table 13.9) confirmed efficacy of EGFRi in combination with irinotecan or oxaliplatin regimens.

In the CRYSTAL study, more than 1,200 patients with EGFR-expressing mCRC were randomised to FOLFIRI or FOLFIRI+cetuximab [126]. Response rate and resection rate

were higher, and PFS was longer. Higher response rate and longer PFS were also observed in the OPUS and PRIME studies [127, 128], but in the COIN study only response rate was increased [129].

Predicting Efficacy of EGFRi

High costs of targeted therapies warrant the selection of patients that actually benefit from the therapy. Until recently, the development of skin rash during cetuximab therapy was the most promising predictive factor, but focus has changed towards assessment of tumour tissue [114, 130].

EGFR expression cannot be used to predict efficacy because there is no difference in activity in patients with EGFR-positive and EGFR-negative tumours.

The extracellular epidermal growth factor receptor has an impact in stimulating growth in cancer. A number of intracellular downstream

Table 13.10 Recent studies evaluating double targeted therapy (inhibition of VEGF and EGFR) according to KRAS status

Author, year	Regimen	KRAS	No. of patients	RR (%)	Median PFS (months)	Median OS (months)
CAIRO2	CapOx + Bev	WT	156	50	10.6	22.4
Tol et al. NEJM	CapOx + Bev + Cet	WT	158	61	10.5	21.8
2009 [137]	CapOx + Bev	MUT	108	59*	12.5*	24.9*
	CapOx + Bev + Cet	MUT	98	46	8.3	17.2
PACCE	'Ox' + Bev	WT	203	56	11.5*	24.5*
Hecht et al. JCO	'Ox' + Bev + Pan	WT	201	50	9.8	20.7
2009 [136]	'Ox' + Bev	MUT	125	44	11.0	19.3
	'Ox' + Bev + Pan	MUT	135	47	10.5	19.3
	'Ir' + Bev	WT	58	48	12.5	19.8
	'Ir' + Bev + Pan	WT	57	54	10.0	NR
	'Ir' + Bev	MUT	39	38	11.9	20.5
	'Ir' + Bev + Pan	MUT	47	30	8.3	17.8

Abbreviations: *Bev* bevacizumab, *BSC* best supportive care, *Cet* cetuximab, *FLIRI* FU/FA with folinic acid + irinotecan (Nordic bolus regimen), *Fp* fluoropyrimidine, *FU/FA* 5-fluorouracil/folinic acid, FOLFOX = oxaliplatin + FU/FA (combined bolus and infusion), *FOLFIRI* irinotecan + FU/FA (combined bolus and infusion), *IFL* Irinotecan + FU/FA (US bolus regimen), *Iri* irinotecan, 'Iri' irinotecan regime, *MUT* mutated KRAS, *OS* overall survival, 'Ox' oxaliplatin regimen, *Pan* panitumumab, *PFS* progression-free survival, *RR* response rate, *WT* wild-type KRAS, *CapOx* capecitabine + oxaliplatin, * = significant difference

regulating molecules including KRAS reinforce this signal. Mutation in KRAS results in persisting growth signal even though the extracellular receptor is inhibited. Consequently, KRAS mutant status, which is the case with approximately 40 % of mCRC patients, is a predictive marker for lack of efficacy of EGFRi, but KRAS mutation in itself is not a prognostic factor [131, 132].

In patients with normal KRAS (KRAS wild type), CetIri has extraordinary efficacy in patients with chemoresistant tumours [124, 133], PFS is almost 6 months, and OS is prolonged from around 4–5 months to around 12 months.

In the CRYSTAL study, 1,200 patients were randomised, and the authors succeeded to collect and evaluate KRAS status in tumour tissue from 1,063 patients (Table 13.9). In patients with KRAS wild type, response rate (40 % vs. 57 %), PFS (8.4 months vs. 9.9 months) and OS (20.0 months vs. 23.5 months) were significantly improved in patients receiving FOLFIRI and cetuximab [134]. Based on data from the CRYSTAL trial [134] and the OPUS trial [127], the European Commission has extended its cetuximab licence to first-line treatment of mCRC patients with KRAS wild-type tumours, in combination with chemotherapy.

Comparable efficacy for panitumumab (Table 13.9) has been observed in the PRIME study (first line) and '181' study (second line) even though the difference in OS was not significant [121, 128].

The efficacy of cetuximab and panitumumab therapy is confined to patients with KRAS wild type, and data suggest that KRAS status should be analysed in all patients with mCRC before therapy with EGFRi is commenced. However, it must also be stressed that presently, there are no available phase III results of studies comparing efficacy of bevacizumab and cetuximab or panitumumab in patients with KRAS wild-type tumours.

Combinations of Targeted Therapies

In vitro studies have shown that simultaneous inhibition of VEGF and EGFR systems has additive and perhaps even synergistic effect, but surprisingly this advantage could not be confirmed in first-line randomised studies (Table 13.10).

In a small randomised phase II study (BOND2), a triple combination of CetIri and bevacizumab (CIB) was more effective than cetuximab + bevacizumab alone [135]. Even more interesting, PFS and OS for the CIB combination were considerably longer than the historical control of CetIri in BOND1 trial. It was therefore expected that a similar combination would increase efficacy also as first-line therapy.

In the PACCE study, more than 1,000 patients were randomised to a combination of chemotherapy with bevacizumab (optional oxaliplatin-based regimen ($n = 823$) or irinotecan-based regimen ($n = 230$)) with or without panitumumab [136]. The four-drug combination of oxaliplatin-based therapy with bevacizumab and panitumumab resulted in several serious adverse events and also a shorter PFS and OS, while there was no significant difference in efficacy data in the smaller group where therapy was based on irinotecan. Even in patients with KRAS wild type, there was evidence of a harmful effect of double targeted therapy (Table 13.10).

In the CAIRO-2 study, 734 patients were randomised to CapOx + bevacizumab with or without cetuximab. Similar to PACCE study, PFS was significantly shorter in patients receiving double targeted therapy, and subgroup analysis of patients with KRAS mutations showed that efficacy (RR, PFS and OS) was significant worse [137].

Double targeted therapy against VEGF and EGFR should not be used as first-line treatment outside of controlled studies.

Conclusion

It was hoped that the new targeted drugs would add considerably to efficacy of chemotherapy and perhaps even replace standard chemotherapy. There is no doubt that the new drugs add to efficacy, but the overall benefit must be described as modest and in the near future combination chemotherapy will continue to be the backbone of systemic therapy. The search for predictive markers, such as KRAS status, will continue to protect patients – with little or no likelihood of success – from toxicity.

Treatment Algorithm in Metastatic CRC

In daily practice, it is very important to realize the goal of therapy for each individual patient when the treatment strategy is planned. The objective of therapy depends on the classification of the disease – are metastases regarded as initial resectable, potentially resectable or never resectable? This classification has to be done in a close collaboration between surgeons, oncologists, radiologist and pathologist – in a multidisciplinary team (MDT).

Of course the treatment decision is also dependent on local conditions – which treatment is available and convenient – and on the expected individual patient tolerance.

Initially Resectable Metastases

Around 30 % of patients with colorectal cancer (CRC) will develop hepatic metastases (CRLM) at some point during the course of the disease. Despite lack of randomised, controlled trials (RCT), resection is the golden standard for patients with resectable CRLM. After microscopic radical resection (R0), the expected 5-year survival is around 35 % and even higher in recent selected series [138, 139].

Presently, around 10 % of patients with CRLM are candidates for local treatment. This number will definitely grow up due to introduction of newer surgical (e.g. preoperative portal vein embolisation and 2-stage resection) and ablative techniques, markedly enhanced efficacy of systemic and regional chemotherapy. The optimal combination of these different modalities must be decided on by a multidisciplinary team (MDT), as a minimum including liver surgeons, oncologists and interventional radiologists. In the same way, the possibility of resection of metastases limited to lungs should be continually assessed.

Peri-operative oxaliplatin-based therapy increases 3-year PFS with 7–8 % in patients with resectable CRLM [140]. A recent subgroup analysis showed that only patients with elevated CEA and excellent performance status may benefit from perioperative chemotherapy [141].

If not given, preoperative chemotherapy patients should be considered for adjuvant chemotherapy [142]. It has been not demonstrated that combination therapy is more effective than FU/FA alone, but many oncologists will nevertheless choose an oxaliplatin regimen based on experience from stage III colon cancer.

Potentially Resectable

In patients with potential resectable metastases (10–30 % of patients with initially unresectable CRLM), major tumour regression will permit salvage surgery, and the likelihood of resection increases when the response rate is increased [143]. Therefore, patients with potential resectable metastases must always be offered combination chemotherapy often with targeted therapy. Modern combination chemotherapy generates tumour regression in at least 50 % of patients with CRLM. The addition of novel targeted agents (e.g. cetuximab, panitumumab or bevacizumab) further increase response rates – perhaps to 70 % – and subsequently the proportion of patients who are candidates for cure, but new effective systemic therapies have also increased the complexity. It is very important that the oncologist regularly considers the possibility for local therapy because even with response rates around 70 %, the number of complete pathological response is still less than 10 %. Furthermore, metastases should be resected before they may become radiological invisible.

In 2001, radio frequency ablation (RFA) was approved by the FDA in patients with unresectable CRLM, and since then, an increasing number of patients have received RFA as an adjunct to resection and as an alternative to resection in unfit non-operable patients but unfortunately an increasing number of operable patients with resectable CRLM have been treated with local ablative techniques (LAT) even in the absence of phase III data and absence of a proper evaluation by a MDT [138].

Based on an excellent review, Mulier et al. proposed a phase 3 study comparing RFA (or microwave ablation) to surgical resection in patients with resectable CRLM less than 3 cm [144]. However, others argue that it is not yet time for randomised studies in patients with resectable CRLM [145].

Several chemotherapy regimens are known to induce hepatic injury such as hepatic steatosis and sinusoidal obstruction syndrome [146].

In such cases, surgical morbidity is increased, but mortality is not higher if duration of preoperative chemotherapy is limited to 3 months.

A major dilemma is how to treat patients with synchronous CRLM – resection of primary first or metastases first. For decades, the traditional approach to the management of the asymptomatic primary in patients with synchronous CRLM was to resect the primary to prevent obstruction, perforation or bleeding. However, the primary is as responsive as metastases, and consequently these complications are very seldom, and recent data supports the use of chemotherapy as initial therapy [147].

Never Resectable

In this group of patients, it is important to realise whether the patient have symptoms relating from tumour and therefore is in need of obtaining a high/rapid response in order to achieve the best palliation – and therefore a treatment strategy as described in section above (potentially resectable) must be chosen. However, if no tumour-related symptoms exit, then a less aggressive strategy – FU/FA or capecitabine followed by combination therapy upon progression – may be chosen in order to achieve the best palliation with a lesser amount of side effects.

Conclusion

Every patient with CRLM or lung-limited metastases must be carefully evaluated by MDT and the optimal treatment chosen in respect to type, extent and location of tumour and co-morbidity.

RFA is not an alternative to surgery [138], but RFA can be combined with surgery if resection alone is not technically feasible and RFA may be the only local treatment in patients who are not candidates for resection.

During recent years, antibodies directed against the vascular endothelial growth factor (VEGF), bevacizumab, and against the epidermal growth factor receptor (EGFR), panitumumab and cetuximab, have been implemented in the treatment of patients with mCRC and have added further to the benefit of treatment [114].

However, the largest benefits have been achieved with modern chemotherapy, which remains the backbone of treatment of patients with mCRC. Modern systemic therapy has resulted in a marked improvement in OS [148] as well as in the rate of long-term survivors (defined as patients alive after 5 years from initiating of systemic treatment for mCRC). In a study, including patients enrolled into clinical trials investigating the efficacy of FU (in the period 1972–1995), the rate of long-term survivors was 1.3 % [149]. In another recent publication – which was an update of a randomised trial investigating combination chemotherapy as first-line treatment in patients with mCRC – a 5-year survival rate of 9.8 % was seen in patients treated with FOLFOX [150]. Of the patients (from all treatment arms) surviving 5 years, only 7 % underwent resection, thereby indicating that most patients survived due to drug therapy alone.

However, these survival data are from patients included in clinical trials. In a recent population-based study including more than 700 unselected patients with mCRC, there was a clear difference in characteristics as well as OS between patients enrolled into clinical trials and patients receiving chemotherapy outside protocol [151].

Concluding Remarks

Optimal therapy of patients with CRC has increased in complexity, and unfortunately our expectations for new targeted drugs have not quite been settled. Targeted therapy has clinically significant effect, but we must learn to identify the correct regimes for the right patients. KRAS status is currently the most important predictive marker for efficacy of anti-EGFR therapy. To ensure the optimal treatment strategy, every patient with mCRC must be assessed by a MTD.

References

1. Parkin DM, Bray F, Ferlay J, et al. Global cancer statistics, 2002. CA Cancer J Clin. 2005;55:74–108.
2. Meyerhardt JA, Mayer RJ. Systemic therapy for colorectal cancer. N Engl J Med. 2005;352:476–87.
3. Longley DB, Harkin DP, Johnston PG. 5-Fluorouracil: mechanisms of action and clinical strategies. Nat Rev Cancer. 2003;3:330.
4. Sobrero AF, Aschele C, Bertino JR. Fluorouracil in colorectal cancer–a tale of two drugs: implications for biochemical modulation. J Clin Oncol. 1997;15: 368–81.
5. Ragnhammar P, Hafstrom L, Nygren P, et al. A systematic overview of chemotherapy effects in colorectal cancer. Acta Oncol. 2001;40:282–308.
6. Glimelius B, Jakobsen A, Graf W, et al. Bolus injection (2–4 min) versus short-term (10–20 min) infusion of 5-fluorouracil in patients with advanced colorectal cancer: a prospective randomised trial. Nordic Gastrointestinal Tumour Adjuvant Therapy Group. Eur J Cancer. 1998;34:674–8.
7. Fischel JL, Etienne MC, Formento P, et al. Search for the optimal schedule for the oxaliplatin/5-fluorouracil association modulated or not by folinic acid: preclinical data. Clin Cancer Res. 1998;4:2529–35.
8. Lokich J, Anderson N. Dose intensity for bolus versus infusion chemotherapy administration: review of the literature for 27 anti-neoplastic agents. Ann Oncol. 1997;8:15–25.
9. Meta-analysis Group in Cancer. Efficacy of intravenous continuous infusion of fluorouracil compared with bolus administration in advanced colorectal cancer. J Clin Oncol. 1998;16:301–8.
10. Rustum YM, Trave F, Zakrzewski SF, et al. Biochemical and pharmacologic basis for potentiation of 5-fluorouracil action by leucovorin. NCI Monogr 1987;5:165–70.
11. Advanced Colorectal Cancer Meta-Analysis Project. Modulation of fluorouracil by leucovorin in patients with advanced colorectal cancer: evidence in terms of response rate. J Clin Oncol. 1992;10:896–903.
12. The Meta-Analysis Group. Modulation of fluorouracil by leucovorin in patients with advanced colorectal cancer: an updated meta-analysis. J Clin Oncol. 2004; 22:3766–75.
13. Choong YS, Lee SP, Alley PA. Comparison of the pyrimidine nucleoside phosphorylase activity in human tumours and normal tissues. Exp Pathol. 1988; 33:23–5.
14. Miwa M, Ura M, Nishida M, et al. Design of a novel oral fluoropyrimidine carbamate, capecitabine, which generates 5-fluorouracil selectively in tumours by enzymes concentrated in human liver and cancer tissue. Eur J Cancer. 1998;34:1274–81.
15. Schüller J, Cassidy J, Dumont E, et al. Preferential activation of capecitabine in tumour following oral administration to colorectal cancer patients. Cancer Chemother Pharmacol. 2000;45:291–7.
16. Van Cutsem E, Findlay M, Osterwalder B, et al. Capecitabine, an oral fluoropyrimidine carbamate with substantial activity in advanced colorectal cancer: results of a randomized phase II study. J Clin Oncol. 2000;18:1337–45.
17. Hoff PM, Ansari R, Batist G, et al. Comparison of oral capecitabine versus intravenous fluorouracil plus

leucovorin as first-line treatment in 605 patients with metastatic colorectal cancer: results of a randomized phase III study. J Clin Oncol. 2001;19:2282–92.

18. Van Cutsem E, Twelves C, Cassidy J, et al. Oral capecitabine compared with intravenous fluorouracil plus leucovorin in patients with metastatic colorectal cancer: results of a large phase III study. J Clin Oncol. 2001;19:4097–106.

19. Carmichael J, Popiela T, Radstone D, et al. Randomized comparative study of tegafur/uracil and oral leucovorin versus parenteral fluorouracil and leucovorin in patients with previously untreated metastatic colorectal cancer. J Clin Oncol. 2002;20:3617–27.

20. Douillard JY, Hoff PM, Skillings JR, et al. Multicenter phase III study of uracil/tegafur and oral leucovorin versus fluorouracil and leucovorin in patients with previously untreated metastatic colorectal cancer. J Clin Oncol. 2002;20:3605–16.

21. Liu G, Franssen E, Fitch MI, et al. Patient preference for oral versus intravenous palliative chemotherapy. J Clin Oncol. 1997;15:110–5.

22. Borner M, Schöffski P, de Wit R, et al. Patient preferences and pharmacokinetics of oral modulated UFT versus intravenous fluorouracil and leucovorin: a randomised crossover trial in advanced colorectal cancer. Eur J Cancer. 2002;38:349–58.

23. Pfeiffer P, Mortensen JP, Bjerregaard B, et al. Patient preference for oral or intravenous chemotherapy: a randomised cross-over trial comparing capecitabine and Nordic fluorouracil/leucovorin in patients with colorectal cancer. Eur J Cancer. 2006;42:2738–43.

24. Twelves C, Gollins S, Grieve R, Samuel L. A randomised cross-over trial comparing patient preference for oral capecitabine and 5-fluorouracil/leucovorin regimens in patients with advanced colorectal cancer. Ann Oncol. 2006;17:239–45.

25. Jerremalm E, Wallin I, Ehrsson H. New insights into the biotransformation and pharmacokinetics of oxaliplatin. J Pharm Sci. 2009;98:3879–85.

26. Woynarowski JM, Faivre S, Herzig MCS, et al. Oxaliplatin-induced damage of cellular DNA. Mol Pharmacol. 2000;58:920–7.

27. Raymond E, Lawrence R, Izbicka E, et al. Activity of oxaliplatin against human tumour colony-forming units. Clin Cancer Res. 1998;4:1021–9.

28. Rothenberg ML, Oza AM, Bigelow RH, et al. Superiority of oxaliplatin and fluorouracil-leucovorin compared with either therapy alone in patients with progressive colorectal cancer after irinotecan and fluorouracil-leucovorin: interim results of a phase III trial. J Clin Oncol. 2003;21:2059–69.

29. Gamelin E, Gamelin L, Bossi L, et al. Clinical aspects and molecular basis of oxaliplatin neurotoxicity: current management and development of preventive measures. Semin Oncol. 2002;29:21–33.

30. Grothey A. Clinical management of oxaliplatin-associated neurotoxicity. Clin Colorectal Cancer. 2005; 5 Suppl 1:S38–46.

31. Chollet P, Bensmaine MA, Brienza S, et al. Single agent activity of oxaliplatin in heavily pretreated advanced epithelial ovarian cancer. Ann Oncol. 1996;7:1065–70.

32. Pfeiffer P, Hahn P, Jensen HA. Short time infusion of oxaliplatin (Eloxatin®) in combination with capecitabine (Xeloda®) in patients with advanced colorectal cancer. Acta Oncol. 2003;42:832–6.

33. Pfeiffer P, Sørbye H, Ehrsson H, et al. Short-time infusion of oxaliplatin in combination with capecitabine (XELOX$_{30}$) as second line therapy in patients with advanced colorectal cancer after failure to irinotecan and 5-fluorouracil. Ann Oncol. 2006;17:252–8.

34. Dupont J, Jensen HA, Jensen BV, et al. Phase I study of short-time oxaliplatin, capecitabine and epirubicin (EXE) as first line therapy in patients with non-resectable gastric cancer. Acta Oncol. 2007;46:330–5.

35. Schonnemann KR, Jensen HA, Yilmaz M, et al. Phase II study of short-time oxaliplatin, capecitabine and epirubicin (EXE) as first-line therapy in patients with non-resectable gastric cancer. Br J Cancer. 2008;99:858–61.

36. Qvortrup C, Yilmaz M, Ogreid D, Berglund A, Balteskard L, Ploen J, Fokstuen T, Starkhammar H, Sørbye H, Tveit K, Pfeiffer P. Chronomodulated capecitabine in combination with short-time oxaliplatin: A Nordic phase II study of second-line therapy in patients with metastatic colorectal cancer after failure to irinotecan and 5-flourouracil. Ann Oncol. 2008;19:1154–9.

37. Qvortrup C, Jensen BV, Fokstuen T, Nielsen SE, Keldsen N, Glimelius B, Bjerregaard B, Mejer J, Larsen FO, Pfeiffer P. A randomized study comparing short-time infusion of oxaliplatin in combination with capecitabine XELOX30 and chronomodulated XELOX30 as first-line therapy in patients with advanced colorectal cancer. Ann Oncol. 2010;21:87–91.

38. Kaneda N, Nagata H, Furuta T, et al. Metabolism and pharmacokinetics of the camptothecin analogue CPT-11 in the mouse. Cancer Res. 1990;50:1715–20.

39. Kawato Y, Furuta T, Aonuma M, et al. Antitumour activity of a camptothecin derivative, CPT-11, against human tumour xenografts in nude mice. Cancer Chemother Pharmacol. 1991;28:192–8.

40. Hsiang YH, Hertzberg R, Hecht S, et al. Camptothecin induces protein-linked DNA breaks via mammalian DNA topoisomerase I. J Biol Chem. 1985;260:14873–8.

41. Iyer L, Hall D, Das S, et al. Phenotype-genotype correlation of in vitro SN-38 (active metabolite of irinotecan) and bilirubin glucuronidation in human liver tissue with UGT1A1 promoter polymorphism. Clin Pharmacol Ther. 1999;65:576–82.

42. Kweekel D, Guchelaar HJ, Gelderblom H. Clinical and pharmacogenetic factors associated with irinotecan toxicity. Cancer Treat Rev. 2008;34:656–69.

43. Moertel CG, Fleming TR, Macdonald JS, et al. Levamisole and fluorouracil as adjuvant therapy of resected colon carcinoma. N Engl J Med. 1990;322:352–8.

44. Sargent D, Sobrero A, Grothey A, et al. Evidence for cure by adjuvant therapy in colon cancer: observations based on individual patient data from 20,898 patients on 18 randomized trials. J Clin Oncol. 2009;27:872–7.

45. Twelves C, Wong A, Nowacki MP, et al. Capecitabine as adjuvant treatment for stage III colon cancer. N Engl J Med. 2005;352:2696–704.

46. Lembersky BC, Wieand HS, Petrelli NJ, et al. Oral uracil and tegafur plus leucovorin compared with intravenous fluorouracil and leucovorin in stage II and III carcinoma of the colon: results from National Surgical Adjuvant Breast and Bowel Project Protocol C-06. J Clin Oncol. 2006;24:2059–64.

47. Andre T, Boni C, Mounedji-Boudiaf L, et al. Oxaliplatin, fluorouracil, and leucovorin as adjuvant treatment for colon cancer. N Engl J Med. 2004;350: 2343–51.

48. Andre T, Boni C, Navarro M, et al. Improved overall survival with oxaliplatin, fluorouracil, and leucovorin as adjuvant treatment in stage II or III colon cancer in the MOSAIC trial. J Clin Oncol. 2009;27:3109–16.

49. Kuebler JP, Wieand HS, O'Connell MJ, et al. Oxaliplatin combined with weekly bolus fluorouracil and leucovorin as surgical adjuvant chemotherapy for stage II and III colon cancer: results from NSABP C-07. J Clin Oncol. 2007;25:2198–204.

50. Haller D, Tabernero J, Maroun J et al. First efficacy findings from a randomized phase III trial of capecitabine + oxaliplatin vs bolus 5-FU/LV for stage III colon cancer (NO16968/XELOXA study). ECCO 2009. Abstr 5LBA.

51. Gill S, Loprinzi CL, Sargent DJ, et al. Pooled analysis of fluorouracil-based adjuvant therapy for stage II and III colon cancer: Who benefits and by how much? J Clin Oncol. 2004;22:1797–806.

52. Gray R, Barnwell J, McConkey C, Hills RK, Williams NS, Kerr DJ. QUASAR Collaborative Group: Adjuvant chemotherapy versus observation in patients with colorectal cancer: a randomised study. Lancet 2007; 370: 2020–9.

53. QUASAR Collaborative Group. Adjuvant chemotherapy versus observation in patients with colorectal cancer: a randomised study. Lancet. 2007;370: 2020–9.

54. Gunderson LL, Jessup JM, Sargent DJ, et al. Revised TN categorization for colon cancer based on national survival outcomes data. J Clin Oncol. 2010;28:264–71.

55. Labianca R, Nordlinger B, Beretta GD. Primary colon cancer: ESMO Clinical Practice Guidelines for diagnosis, adjuvant treatment and follow-up. Ann Oncol. 2010;21 Suppl 5:v70–7.

56. NCCN Clinical Practice Guidelines in Oncology (NCCN Guidelines™). Colon cancer, version 1.2011, NCCN.org.

57. Sargent DJ, Marsoni S, Monges G, et al. J Clin Oncol. 2010;28:3219–26.

58. Zaanan A, Cuilliere-Dartigues P, Guilloux A, et al. Impact of p53 expression and microsatellite instability on stage III colon cancer disease-free survival in patients treated by 5-fluorouracil and leucovorin with or without oxaliplatin. Ann Oncol. 2010;21:772–80.

59. Van Cutsem E, Labianca R, Bodoky G, et al. Randomized phase III trial comparing biweekly infusional fluorouracil/leucovorin alone or with irinotecan in the adjuvant treatment of stage III colon cancer: PETACC-3. J Clin Oncol. 2009;27:3117–25.

60. Ychou M, Raoul JL, Douillard JY, et al. A phase III randomised trial of LV5FU2 + irinotecan versus LV5FU2 alone in adjuvant high-risk colon cancer (FNCLCC Accord02/FFCD9802). Ann Oncol. 2009;20:674–80.

61. Saltz LB, Niedzwiecki D, Hollis D, et al. Irinotecan fluorouracil plus leucovorin is Not superior to fluorouracil plus leucovorin alone as adjuvant treatment for stage III colon cancer: results of CALGB 89803. J Clin Oncol. 2007;25:3456–61.

62. Wolmark N, Yothers G, O'Connell MJ, et al. A phase III trial comparing mFOLFOX6 to mFOLFOX6 plus bevacizumab in stage II or III carcinoma of the colon: results of NSABP protocol C-08. ASCO 2009; LBA4.

63. Goldberg RM, Sargent DJ, Thibodeau SN, et al. Adjuvant mFOLFOX6 plus or minus cetuximab (Cmab) in patients (pts) with KRAS mutant (m) resected stage III colon cancer (CC): NCCTG Intergroup Phase III Trial N0147. ASCO 2010; abstract 3508.

64. Alberts SR, Sargent DJ, Smyrk TC, et al. Adjuvant mFOLFOX6 with or without cetuxiumab (Cmab) in KRAS wild-type (WT) patients (pts) with resected stage III colon cancer (CC): results from NCCTG Intergroup Phase III Trial N0147. ASCO 2010; abstract CRA 3507.

65. Poston GJ, Figueras J, Giuliante F, et al. Urgent need for a New staging system in advanced colorectal cancer. J Clin Oncol. 2008;26:4828–33.

66. Glimelius B, Hoffman K, Graf W, et al. Quality of life during chemotherapy in patients with symptomatic advanced colorectal cancer. The Nordic Gastrointestinal Tumour Adjuvant Therapy Group. Cancer. 1994;73: 556–62.

67. Scheithauer W, Rosen H, Kornek GV, et al. Randomised comparison of combination chemotherapy plus supportive care with supportive care alone in patients with metastatic colorectal cancer. BMJ. 1993;306:752–5.

68. Cunningham D, Pyrhonen S, James RD, et al. Randomised trial of irinotecan plus supportive care versus supportive care alone after fluorouracil failure for patients with metastatic colorectal cancer. Lancet. 1998;352:1413–8.

69. Rougier P, Van Cutsem E, Bajetta E, et al. Randomised trial of irinotecan versus fluorouracil by continuous infusion after fluorouracil failure in patients with metastatic colorectal cancer. Lancet. 1998;352:1407–12.

70. Kim GP, Sargent DJ, Mahoney MR, et al. Phase III noninferiority trial comparing irinotecan with oxaliplatin, fluorouracil, and leucovorin in patients with advanced colorectal carcinoma previously treated with fluorouracil: N9841. J Clin Oncol. 2009;27:2848–54.

71. de Gramont A, Figer A, Seymour M, et al. Leucovorin and fluorouracil with or without oxaliplatin as first-line treatment in advanced colorectal cancer. J Clin Oncol. 2000;18:2938–47.

72. Giacchetti S, Perpoint B, Zidani R, et al. Phase III multicenter randomized trial of oxaliplatin added to chronomodulated fluorouracil-leucovorin as first-line treatment of metastatic colorectal cancer. J Clin Oncol. 2000;18:136–47.

73. Douillard JY, Cunningham D, Roth AD, et al. Irinotecan combined with fluorouracil compared with fluorouracil alone as first-line treatment for metastatic

colorectal cancer: a multicentre randomised trial. Lancet. 2000;355:1041–7.

74. Kohne CH, Van Cutsem E, Wils J, et al. Phase III study of weekly high-dose infusional fluorouracil plus folinic acid with or without irinotecan in patients with metastatic colorectal cancer: European Organisation for Research and Treatment of Cancer Gastrointestinal Group Study 40986. J Clin Oncol. 2005;23: 4856–65.

75. Saltz LB, Cox JV, Blanke C, et al. Irinotecan plus fluorouracil and leucovorin for metastatic colorectal cancer. N Engl J Med. 2000;343:905–14.

76. Lim DH, Park YS, Park BB, et al. Mitomycin-C and capecitabine as third-line chemotherapy in patients with advanced colorectal cancer: a phase II study. Cancer Chemother Pharmacol. 2005;56:10–4.

77. Rosati G, Rossi A, Germano D, et al. Raltitrexed and mitomycin-C as third-line chemotherapy for colorectal cancer after combination regimens including 5-fluorouracil, irinotecan and oxaliplatin: a phase II study. Anticancer Res. 2003;23:2981–5.

78. Glimelius B, Sorbye H, Balteskard L, et al. A randomized phase III multicenter trial comparing irinotecan in combination with the Nordic bolus 5-FU and folinic acid schedule or the bolus/infused de Gramont schedule (Lv5FU2) in patients with metastatic colorectal cancer. Ann Oncol. 2008;19:909–14.

79. Goldberg RM, Sargent DJ, Morton RF, et al. A randomized controlled trial of fluorouracil plus leucovorin, irinotecan, and oxaliplatin combinations in patients with previously untreated metastatic colorectal cancer. J Clin Oncol. 2004;22:23–30.

80. Tournigand C, Andre T, Achille E, et al. FOLFIRI followed by FOLFOX6 or the reverse sequence in advanced colorectal cancer: a randomized GERCOR study. J Clin Oncol. 2004;22:229–37.

81. Grothey A, Sargent D, Goldberg RM, et al. Survival of patients with advanced colorectal cancer improves with the availability of fluorouracil-leucovorin, irinotecan, and oxaliplatin in the course of treatment. J Clin Oncol. 2004;22:1209–14.

82. Koopman M, Antonini NF, Douma J, et al. Sequential versus combination chemotherapy with capecitabine, irinotecan, and oxaliplatin in advanced colorectal cancer (CAIRO): a phase III randomised controlled trial. The Lancet. 2007;370:135–42.

83. Seymour MT, Maughan TS, Ledermann JA, et al. Different strategies of sequential and combination chemotherapy for patients with poor prognosis advanced colorectal cancer (MRC FOCUS): a randomised controlled trial. Lancet. 2007;370:143–52.

84. Scheithauer W, Kornek GV, Raderer M, et al. Randomized multicenter phase II trial of two different schedules of capecitabine plus oxaliplatin as first-line treatment in advanced colorectal cancer. J Clin Oncol. 2003;21:1307–12.

85. Cassidy J, Clarke S, Diaz-Rubio E, et al. Randomized phase III study of capecitabine plus oxaliplatin compared with fluorouracil/folinic acid plus oxaliplatin as first-line therapy for metastatic colorectal cancer. J Clin Oncol. 2008;26:2006–12.

86. Diaz-Rubio E, Tabernero J, Gomez-Espana A, et al. Phase III study of capecitabine plus oxaliplatin compared with continuous-infusion fluorouracil plus oxaliplatin as first-line therapy in metastatic colorectal cancer: final report of the Spanish cooperative group for the treatment of digestive tumours trial. J Clin Oncol. 2007;25:4224–30.

87. Ducreux M, Bennouna J, Hebbar M, et al. Capecitabine plus oxaliplatin (XELOX) versus 5-fluorouracil/leucovorin plus oxaliplatin (FOLFOX-6) as first-line treatment for metastatic colorectal cancer. Int J Cancer 2011;128:682–90.

88. Porschen R, Arkenau HT, Kubicka S, et al. Phase III study of capecitabine plus oxaliplatin compared with fluorouracil and leucovorin plus oxaliplatin in metastatic colorectal cancer: a final report of the AIO Colorectal Study Group. J Clin Oncol. 2007;25:4217–23.

89. Arkenau HT, Arnold D, Cassidy J, et al. Efficacy of oxaliplatin plus capecitabine or infusional fluorouracil/leucovorin in patients with metastatic colorectal cancer: a pooled analysis of randomized trials. J Clin Oncol. 2008;26:5910–7.

90. Rothenberg ML, Cox JV, Butts C, et al. Capecitabine plus oxaliplatin (XELOX) versus 5-fluorouracil/folinic acid plus oxaliplatin (FOLFOX-4) as second-line therapy in metastatic colorectal cancer: a randomized phase III noninferiority study. Ann Oncol. 2008;19:1720–6.

91. Labianca R, Floriani I, Cortesi E, et al. Alternating versus continuous "FOLFIRI" in advanced colorectal cancer (ACC): a randomized "GISCAD" trial. ASCO 2006; abstract 3505.

92. Maughan TS, James RS, Kerr DJ, et al. Comparison of intermittent and continuous palliative chemotherapy for advanced colorectal cancer: a multicentre randomised trial. Lancet. 2003;361:457–64.

93. Tournigand C, Cervantes A, Figer A, et al. OPTIMOX1: a randomized study of FOLFOX4 or FOLFOX7 with oxaliplatin in a stop-and-go fashion in advanced colorectal cancer: a GERCOR study. J Clin Oncol. 2006;24:394–400.

94. Chibaudel B, Maindrault-Goebel F, Lledo G, et al. Can chemotherapy be discontinued in unresectable metastatic colorectal cancer? The GERCOR OPTIMOX2 study. J Clin Oncol. 2009;27:5727–33.

95. Hochster HS. Stop and go: yes or no? J Clin Oncol. 2009;27:5677–9.

96. Perez-Staub N, Chibaudel B, Figer A, et al. Who can benefit from chemotherapy holidays after first-line therapy for advanced colorectal cancer? A GERCOR study. ASCO 2008; abstract 4037.

97. Adams R, Wilson RH, Seymour MT, et al. Intermittent versus continuous oxaliplatin-fluoropyrimidine (Ox-Fp) chemotherapy (CT) in first-line treatment of patients (pts) with advanced colorectal cancer (aCRC): predictive factors (PF), quality of life (QL), and final efficacy results from the MRC COIN trial. ASCO 2010; abstract 3525.

98. Maughan T, Adams R, Wilson R, et al. Chemotherapy-free intervals for patients with metastatic colorectal cancer remain an option. J Clin Oncol. 2010;28:e275–6.

99. Tabernero J, Aranda E, Gomez A, et al. Phase III study of first-line XELOX plus bevacizumab (BEV) for 6 cycles followed by XELOX plus BEV or single-agent (s/a) BEV as maintenance therapy in patients (pts) with metastatic colorectal cancer (mCRC): The MACRO Trial (Spanish Cooperative Group for the Treatment of Digestive Tumours [TTD]). ASCO 2010; abstract 3501.
100. Pfeiffer P, Qvortrup C, Bjerregaard JK. Current status of treatment of metastatic colorectal cancer with special reference to cetuximab and elderly patients. Onco Targets and Therapy. 2009;2:17–27.
101. Sargent DJ, Goldberg RM, Jacobson SD, et al. A pooled analysis of adjuvant chemotherapy for resected colon cancer in elderly patients. N Engl J Med. 2001;345:1091–7.
102. Goldberg RM, Tabah-Fisch I, Bleiberg H, et al. Pooled analysis of safety and efficacy of oxaliplatin plus fluorouracil/leucovorin administered bimonthly in elderly patients with colorectal cancer. J Clin Oncol. 2006;24:4085–91.
103. Folprecht G, Seymour MT, Saltz L, et al. Irinotecan/ fluorouracil combination in first-line therapy of older and younger patients with metastatic colorectal cancer: combined analysis of 2,691 patients in randomized controlled trials. J Clin Oncol. 2008;26:1443–51.
104. Sanoff HK, Bleiberg H, Goldberg RM. Managing older patients with colorectal cancer. J Clin Oncol. 2007;25:1891–7.
105. McKibbin T, Frei CR, Greene RE, Kwan P, Simon J, Koeller JM. Disparities in the use of chemotherapy and monoclonal antibody therapy for elderly advanced colorectal cancer patients in the community oncology setting. Oncologist. 2008;13:876–85.
106. Tournigand C, Andre T, Bachet J, et al. FOLFOX4 as adjuvant therapy in elderly patients (pts) with colon cancer (CC): subgroup analysis of the MOSAIC trial. ASCO 2010; abstract 3522.
107. Haller DG, Cassidy J, Tabernero J, et al. Efficacy findings from a randomized phase III trial of capecitabine plus oxaliplatin versus bolus 5-FU/LV for stage III colon cancer (NO16968): impact of age on disease-free survival (DFS). ASCO 2010; abstract 3521.
108. Hurwitz H, Fehrenbacher L, Novotny W, et al. Bevacizumab plus irinotecan, fluorouracil, and leucovorin for metastatic colorectal cancer. N Engl J Med. 2004;350:2335–42.
109. Kabbinavar F, Hurwitz HI, Fehrenbacher L, et al. Phase II, randomized trial comparing bevacizumab plus fluorouracil (5-fluorouracil)/leucovorin (LV) with 5-fluorouracil/LV alone in patients with metastatic colorectal cancer. J Clin Oncol. 2003;21:60–5.
110. Kabbinavar F, Shulz J, McCleod M, et al. Addition of bevacizumab to bolus fluorouracil/leucovorin in first-line metastatic colorectal cancer: results of a randomized phase II trial. J Clin Oncol. 2005;23:3697–705.
111. Tebbutt NC, Wilson K, Gebski VJ, et al. Capecitabine, bevacizumab, and mitomycin in first-line treatment of metastatic colorectal cancer: results of the Australasian gastrointestinal trials group randomized phase III MAX study. J Clin Oncol. 2010;28:3191–8.
112. Saltz LB, Clarke S, Diaz-Rubio E, et al. Bevacizumab in combination with oxaliplatin-based chemotherapy as first-line therapy in metastatic colorectal cancer: a randomized phase III study. J Clin Oncol. 2008;26:2013–9.
113. Giantonio BJ, Catalano PJ, Meropol NJ, et al. Bevacizumab in combination with oxaliplatin, fluorouracil, and leucovorin (FOLFOX4) for previously treated metastatic colorectal cancer: results from the Eastern Cooperative Oncology Group study E3200. J Clin Oncol. 2007;25:1539–44.
114. Pfeiffer P, Qvortrup C, Eriksen JG. Current role of antibody therapy in patients with metastatic colorectal cancer. Oncogene. 2007;26:3661–78.
115. Cunningham D, Humblet Y, Siena S, et al. Cetuximab monotherapy and cetuximab plus irinotecan in irinotecan-refractory metastatic colorectal cancer. N Engl J Med. 2004;351(4):337–45.
116. Jonker DJ, O'Callaghan CJ, Karapetis CS, et al. Cetuximab for the treatment of colorectal cancer. N Engl J Med. 2007;357:2040–8.
117. Van Cutsem E, Peeters M, Siena S, et al. Open-label phase III trial of panitumumab plus best supportive care compared with best supportive care alone in patients with chemotherapy-refractory metastatic colorectal cancer. J Clin Oncol. 2007;25:1658–64.
118. Nielsen DL, Pfeiffer P, Jensen BV. Re-treatment with cetuximab in patients with severe hypersensitivity reactions to cetuximab. Two case reports. Acta Oncol. 2006;45(8):1137–8.
119. Nielsen DL, Pfeiffer P, Jensen BV. Six cases of treatment with panitumumab in patients with severe hypersensitivity reactions to cetuximab. Ann Oncol. 2009;20:798.
120. Sobrero AF, Maurel J, Fehrenbacher L, et al. EPIC: phase III trial of cetuximab plus irinotecan after fluoropyrimidine and oxaliplatin failure in patients with metastatic colorectal cancer. J Clin Oncol. 2008;26:2311–9.
121. Peeters M, Price TJ, Cervates A, et al. Randomized phase III study of panitumumab with fluorouracil, leucovorin, and irinotecan (FOLFIRI) compared with FOLFIRI alone as second-line treatment in patients with metastatic colorectal cancer. J Clin Oncol. 2010;28:4706–13.
122. Tabernero J, Pfeiffer P, Cervantes A. Two-weekly administration of cetuximab in the treatment of metastatic colorectal cancer: an effective, more convenient alternative to weekly administration? Oncologist. 2008;13:113–9.
123. Pfeiffer P, Nielsen D, Bjerregaard J, Qvortrup C, Yilmaz M, Jensen BV. Biweekly cetuximab and irinotecan as third line therapy in patients with advanced colorectal cancer after failure to irinotecan, oxaliplatin and 5-fluorouracil. Ann Oncol. 2008;2008(19):1141–5.
124. Jensen BV, Schou JV, Johannesen HH, et al. Cetuximab every second week with irinotecan in patients with metastatic colorectal cancer refractory to 5-FU, oxaliplatin, and irinotecan: KRAS mutation status and efficacy. ASCO 2010; abstract 3573.

125. Macarulla T, Ramos FJ, Elez E, Capdevila J, Peralta S, Tabernero J. Update on novel strategies to optimize cetuximab therapy in patients with metastatic colorectal cancer. Clin Colorectal Cancer. 2008;7:300–8.

126. Van Cutsem E, Kohne CH, Hitre E, et al. Cetuximab and chemotherapy as initial treatment for metastatic colorectal cancer. N Engl J Med. 2009;360:1408–17.

127. Bokemeyer C, Bondarenko I, Makhson A, et al. Fluorouracil, leucovorin, and oxaliplatin with and without cetuximab in the first-line treatment of metastatic colorectal cancer. J Clin Oncol. 2009;27:663–71.

128. Douillard JY, Siena S, Cassidy J, Tabernero J, et al. Randomized, phase III trial of panitumumab with infusional fluorouracil, leucovorin, and oxaliplatin (FOLFOX4) versus FOLFOX4 alone as first-line treatment in patients with previously untreated metastatic colorectal cancer: the PRIME study. J Clin Oncol. 2010;28:4697–705.

129. Maughan T, Adams RA, Smith CG, et al. Addition of cetuximab to oxaliplatin-based combination chemotherapy (CT) in patients with KRAS wild-type advanced colorectal cancer (ACRC): a randomised superiority trial (MRC COIN). ECCO 2009; abstract 6 LBA.

130. Lenz HJ, Chu E, Grothey A. KRAS mutation in metastatic colorectal cancer and its impact on the use of EGFR inhibitors. Clin Adv Hematol Oncol. 2008;6:1–13.

131. Amado RG, Wolf M, Peeters M, et al. Wild-type KRAS is required for panitumumab efficacy in patients with metastatic colorectal cancer. J Clin Oncol. 2008;26:1626–34.

132. Karapetis CS, Khambata-Ford S, Jonker DJ, et al. K-ras mutations and benefit from cetuximab in advanced colorectal cancer. N Engl J Med. 2008;359:1757–65.

133. Di Fiore F, Van Cutsem E, Laurent-Puig P, et al. Role of KRAS mutation in predicting response, progression-free survival, and overall survival in irinotecan-refractory patients treated with cetuximab plus irinotecan for a metastatic colorectal cancer: analysis of 281 individual data from published series. ASCO 2008; 4035.

134. Van Cutsem E, Lang I, Folprecht G, et al. Cetuximab plus FOLFIRI in the treatment of metastatic colorectal cancer (mCRC): the influence of KRAS and BRAF biomarkers on outcome: updated data from the CRYSTAL trial. ASCO GI 2010; abstract 281.

135. Saltz LB, Lenz HJ, Kindler HL, et al. Randomized phase II trial of cetuximab, bevacizumab, and irinotecan compared with cetuximab and bevacizumab alone in irinotecan-refractory colorectal cancer: the BOND-2 study. J Clin Oncol. 2007;25:4557–61.

136. Hecht JR, Mitchell E, Chidiac T, et al. A randomized phase IIIB trial of chemotherapy, bevacizumab, and panitumumab compared with chemotherapy and bevacizumab alone for metastatic colorectal cancer. J Clin Oncol. 2009;27:672–80.

137. Tol J, Koopman M, Cats A, et al. Chemotherapy, bevacizumab, and cetuximab in metastatic colorectal cancer. N Engl J Med. 2009;360:563–72.

138. Pfeiffer P, Rasmussen F. A multidisciplinary approach to the treatment of colorectal liver metastases is mandatory. Acta Radiol. 2009;50:707–8.

139. Adam R, Haller DG, Poston G. Toward optimized front-line therapeutic strategies in patients with metastatic colorectal cancer–an expert review from the International Congress on Anti-Cancer Treatment (ICACT) 2009. Ann Oncol. 2010;21:1579–84.

140. Nordlinger B, Sorbye H, Glimelius B, et al. Perioperative chemotherapy with FOLFOX4 and surgery versus surgery alone for resectable liver metastases from colorectal cancer (EORTC Intergroup trial 40983): a randomised controlled trial. Lancet. 2008;371:1007–16.

141. Sorbye H, Mauer M, Gruenberger T, et al. Predictive factors for the effect of perioperative FOLFOX for resectable liver metastasis in colorectal cancer patients (EORTC phase III study 40983). ASCO 2010; abstract 3544.

142. Mitry E, Fields A, Bleiberg H, et al. Adjuvant chemotherapy after potentially curative resection of metastases from colorectal cancer: a pooled analysis of Two randomized trials. J Clin Oncol. 2008;26:4906–11.

143. Folprecht G, Grothey A, Alberts S, et al. Neoadjuvant treatment of unresectable colorectal liver metastases: correlation between tumour response and resection rates. Ann Oncol. 2005;16:1311–9.

144. Mulier S, Ni Y, Jamart J, Michel L, Marchal G, Ruers T. Radiofrequency ablation versus resection for respectable colorectal liver metastases: time for a randomized trial? Ann Surg Oncol. 2008;15:144–57.

145. Curley SA. Radiofrequency ablation versus resection for resectable colorectal liver metastases: time for a randomized trial? Ann Surg Oncol. 2008;15:11–3.

146. Robinson PJA. The effects of cancer chemotherapy on liver imaging. Eur J Radiol. 2009;19:1752–62.

147. Poultsides GA, Servais EL, Saltz LB, et al. Outcome of primary tumour in patients with synchronous stage IV colorectal cancer receiving combination chemotherapy without surgery as initial treatment. J Clin Oncol. 2009;27:3379–84.

148. Kopetz S, Chang GJ, Overman MJ, et al. Improved survival in metastatic colorectal cancer is associated with adoption of hepatic resection and improved chemotherapy. J Clin Oncol. 2009;27:3677–83.

149. Dy GK, Hobday TJ, Nelson G, et al. Long-term survivors of metastatic colorectal cancer treated with systemic chemotherapy alone: a North Central Cancer Treatment Group review of 3811 patients, N0144. Clin Colorectal Cancer. 2009;8:88–93.

150. Sanoff HK, Sargent DJ, Campbell ME, et al. Five-year data and prognostic factor analysis of oxaliplatin and irinotecan combinations for advanced colorectal cancer: N9741. J Clin Oncol. 2008;26:5721–7.

151. Sorbye H, Pfeiffer P, Cavalli-Bjorkman N, et al. Clinical trial enrollment, patient characteristics, and survival differences in prospectively registered metastatic colorectal cancer patients. Cancer. 2009;115:4679–87.

Radiotherapy and Chemoradiation for Rectal Cancer: State of the Art in Europe, the USA and Asia

14

Bengt Glimelius

Abstract

In rectal cancer treatment, not only the local primary but also regional and systemic tumour deposits must be taken care of. The three major treatments, surgery, radiotherapy and drugs, each with their own advantages and limitations, must be combined to result in improved outcomes. Several large randomised trials, reviewed here, have proven that combinations of the three modalities have markedly improved the locoregional problem, but not yet had any major influence on the systemic problem, and thus overall survival. The best integration of the so far weakest modality, the drugs, is not known. The results of the trials are interpreted differently in the world. A new generation of trials exploring the best sequence of treatments, together with integration of the novel drugs, is required.

Introduction

Prognosis has traditionally been less favourable in rectal than in colon cancer, but this has recently changed [1, 2]. The most likely reasons for the presently slightly better 5-year survival rate in rectal cancer are the efforts to decrease rectal cancer local recurrence rates by better staging, improved surgery and incorporation of

B. Glimelius, MD, PhD
Department of Radiology, Oncology and Radiation Science, Uppsala University, Akademiska Sjukhuset, SE-751 85 Uppsala, Sweden

Department of Oncology and Pathology, Karolinska Institutet, SE-171 76, Stockholm, Sweden
e-mail: bengt.glimelius@onkologi.uu.se

radiotherapy [1, 2]. The local recurrence rates have also substantially decreased from 30–40 % a few decades ago down to 5–15 % in many recent studies, and this has had an impact on survival in certain Western populations. Survival has also improved with time for colon cancer, but proportionally not to the same extent as for rectal cancer [3].

When evaluating the impact of interventions in health care, it is important to look at the entire population and not only on a particular subgroup, like those with a successful surgical outcome (R0-resected or R0–1 resected) or included in a clinical trial. Lower local failure rates than the 5–15 % given above have been reported in literature, also from population-based registers, however only in subgroups. In order to best evaluate the collected efforts of the rectal cancer team, local recurrence rates in the population in which you intend to do a surgical resection or another locally curative approach, either upfront or after preoperative therapy, should be presented. Local failure rates give an estimate of the quality of parts of the team activities. It should then be calculated in the entire resected subgroup, irrespective of outcome, since only this gives a true reflection of the team activities. If only the R0-resected population is the denominator, the results can be biased. Local control, i.e. the sum of non-resected tumours and local failures, is the unbiased endpoint for the entire population reflecting the health-care system, but not directly the quality of the team since patients with very advanced tumours or those with severe comorbidities, both precluding active treatments, influence the results.

The Importance of Local Control: Overall Strategy of Rectal Cancer Care

Radical removal of the primary tumour and no local recurrence are prerequisites for cure although occasional local recurrences could be salvaged by secondary surgery and (chemo) radiotherapy ((C)RT). Avoidance of persistent or recurrent tumour in the pelvis is important, even if cure cannot be achieved, e.g. because of metastatic disease, since pelvic growth is usually associated with severe symptoms. Even if overall survival is not improved, improved local control is a legitimate outcome of different interventions in rectal cancer.

An important aim in rectal cancer is thus to treat so that the risk of residual disease in the pelvis is very low or preferably less than about 5 % in the population in whom curative treatment is intended. This should be possible in all but the few (≤ 10 %) cases presenting with a fixed tumour growing into a non-readily resectable organ (about half of those with clinical stage (c)T4). At the same time, however, as little acute and late morbidity as possible should be aimed at. Since surgery, particularly if extensive and additional

treatments, whether given pre- or postoperatively, add morbidity, these interventions should be used appropriately.

From a practical point of view, rectal cancers could be divided into four groups: very early (some cT1), early (cT1–T2, some cT3), intermediate (most cT3, some cT4) and locally advanced (some cT3, most cT4). Other factors than clinical T-stage like tumour height, closeness to the mesorectal fascia (mrf), potentially the circumferential margin (crm) (preoperatively, the term mrf is better to use than crm, since the crm cannot be defined until after surgery [4]), nodal (cN) stage and vascular and nerve invasion are also relevant. It is presently not possible to give a precise definition of which T and N substages belong to these groups, but this is discussed more below. The terms 'favourable or early or good', 'intermediate or bad' and 'locally advanced or ugly' can be used for categorising the rectal cancers into these clinical subgroups. In clinical practice and in many recent studies, the term 'locally advanced' has been commonly used for the 'intermediate/bad' group but is best reserved for the truly 'locally advanced/ugly' tumours [5–7]. Besides the variability in what is called locally advanced (there is a clear tendency in medicine to use terms that indicate advanced disease even if this is not present), there is unity about the need to subgroup along these lines. Subgrouping is an important step towards individualised medicine. Great discrepancies do however exist in many aspects of how treatment is delivered between centres and countries in these subgroups.

Differences Between Europe, the USA and Asia: An Overview

No doubts have the opinions about how to treat different risk groups varied between countries during the past decades. However, the differences should not be overemphasised, and they have tended to diminish with time. Europe has not been homogeneous in strategy, since some countries like Germany and many countries in Southern Europe have more resembled the

American traditions. An attempt to describe the differences and the development with time could be as follows, recognising that history depends upon who told it.

There has been and still is a clear difference in how the regional, subclinical tumour deposits frequently seen in advanced tumours below the peritoneal reflection are cared for between Asia, particularly Japan and the rest of the world. Should those areas be cleared surgically or using radiation? Surgical removal of the lateral nodes on one or both sides has been the preferred option in Asia, whereas the rest of the world has explored the value of radiation, in addition to surgery for the primary, to kill the tumour deposits. Since the radiation is not selectively irradiating the lateral nodes but also has included the primary tumour and the mesorectal nodes, the need for a meticulous surgical dissection technique did not develop as rapidly in the rest of the world as in Asia. Both extensive surgery and additional radiotherapy add morbidity. The questions are thus twofold: (1) which of the two alternatives are most efficient in eradicating all tumour cells, i.e. preventing a local failure, and (2) which alternative results in the least morbidity? There are no randomised studies comparing these two strategies. Comparisons between trials tell that the results are equally good at specialised centres, although patient selection precludes firm conclusions. Other evidence tells that it is more efficient to 'hunt' subclinical cancer deposits using radiation than using surgery. The morbidity is very different and thus hard to compare in different cultures.

In the Western world where the benefits of radiation therapy to surgery were studied, a preoperative approach was mainly explored in Europe, whereas a postoperative approach was explored in the USA. A few small studies indicated that postoperative CRT was better than postoperative radiotherapy (RT) in preventing local recurrence and that treatment was more effective than no additional treatment. Based upon this evidence, a NIH Consensus Conference and a subsequent NCI report stated that postoperative CRT should be standard treatment in rectal cancer stages II and III [8, 9]. A small Norwegian trial also found that postoperative CRT was better than no additional treatment, but the evidence for a clear benefit from postoperative CRT considering its toxicity over RT alone has been questioned [10]. This treatment strategy was however also adopted in several other countries like Canada and Germany and at many centres in Southern Europe.

In Europe, in contrast, several randomised trials compared surgery alone versus preoperative RT and surgery. These studies showed, particularly if a short-course RT, the Swedish 5×5 Gy schedule with immediate surgery was used [11], a relative reduction in local failure rates of 50–60 % in all trials including many hundreds to over thousand patients [12]. Based upon these experiences, preoperative RT was recommended as routine therapy in some countries.

For about two decades, two questions have dominated the arena: (1) should the RT be given before or after surgery, and (2) should it be long course or short course? A third question, (3) should the long-course RT be given alone or with chemotherapy, was also relevant and subject to trials in Europe where researchers were not convinced of the advantages of adding concomitant chemotherapy, as stated in the US documents. Further, (4) sphincter-saving surgery (SSS) and more recently organ preservation were considered important, and the chances for this could not be increased using short-course RT with immediate surgery.

Pre- or Postoperative?

A randomised trial early showed that preoperative short-course RT was more effective than postoperative long-course RT. Admittedly, this trial, the Uppsala trial [13, 14], compared two different radiation schedules, but a high-dose, optimised postoperative schedule was inferior to a brief preoperative schedule. Subsequently several trials comparing preoperative CRT with postoperative CRT were initiated. Only one of them completed patient accrual, the German trial [15, 16]. It showed that a preoperative approach was more efficient and less toxic. Since then, most of the world has more or less accepted that additional (C)RT in rectal cancer should be given before rather than after surgery. A collection of data from all randomised studies have also indicated that preoperative RT is more dose efficient than postoperative RT [17].

Short or Long Course?

The question of short-course (5×5 Gy) versus long-course conventional RT (1.8–2.0 Gy×25–28) is not yet settled although the efficacy appears similar in intertrial comparisons. A randomised study, the Stockholm III trial, has recently (Jan. 2013) closed patient entry when 840 patients have been randomised. Two trials including 316 and 326 patients, respectively, could not find a statistically significant difference in local recurrence rates, disease-free survival (DFS) and overall survival (OS) between the groups randomised to short-course RT alone or long-course CRT [18, 19]. A German trial from the Berlin area, again comparing these two treatments, has completed patient accrual.

The short-course schedule has gained much popularity in Northern European countries where the health-care system is rarely dependent upon private initiatives, whereas the long-course schedule is preferred in countries were hospital budgets are influenced by the number of treatments given. Reimbursement has thus likely influenced routines, although this has never officially been admitted. Much concerns have been expressed about the long-term consequences of hypofractionated RT. There is considerable evidence that the short-course schedule results in long-term morbidity, and the scale of that morbidity is presently well known [20] although even longer follow-up times with larger patient materials are still needed. The long-term morbidity of CRT whether given preoperatively or postoperatively has virtually not been studied why the extent of late morbidity is not known. Both options, short-course 5×5 Gy and long-course CRT, are considered valid in the intermediate group of rectal cancers [5, 7].

Without or with Chemotherapy?

The third question, whether the long-course RT should be combined with chemotherapy or not, got an answer after the completion of three randomised trials, two in the intermediate or bad group [21, 22] and one in the locally advanced or ugly group [23]. Local control was better in the combined treatment arm in all three studies, whereas a survival gain was only seen in the trial including locally advanced cancers [6, 23]. Whenever a patient with a locally advanced rectal cancer receives preoperative treatment, CRT should be used unless the patient cannot tolerate this treatment. This is today likely also the case worldwide.

Sphincter Preservation: Organ Preservation

Trials, again chiefly run in Europe, have explored whether long-course (C)RT with a delay before surgery could increase SSS rates, whereas other took it for granted that this was the case. The trials have later shown that this did not happen to any meaningful extent [24, 25]. The hopes about improved chances of SSS influenced routines in many countries, particularly in Southern Europe, Germany and the USA. Presently, the hopes about organ preservation (see below) influence treatment decision in different ways in different parts of the world.

Diagnosis and Staging

Appropriate diagnosis and staging are fundamental for adequate subgrouping. Thus, a few comments will be made in this chapter. Diagnosis is based on a digital rectal examination including rigid sigmoidoscopy with biopsy for histopathological examination. The purpose of the biopsy has so far been to obtain a cancer diagnosis prior to any treatment. The morphological pictures with the possible exception of poor differentiation and other cellular or molecular properties of the cancer have had very little impact on treatment decisions. It is hoped that reproducible characteristics with prognostic and/or predictive properties soon can be identified. Presently, the amount of cancer cells in the biopsy should be sufficient for analysis of kras mutation status since treatment with an epithelial growth factor receptor (EGFR) inhibitor could be an option in the future. Tumours with distal extension to 15 cm or less (as measured by rigid sigmoidoscopy) from the anal margin are classified as rectal and more proximal tumours as colonic. Whether this 15 cm limit is the best one for choosing a 'rectal cancer strategy' or a 'colon cancer strategy' could be discussed. Others prefer to separate colon and rectum cancer at the peritoneal reflection or about 9–12 cm from the anal verge. The localisation of the tumour in relation to other organs and structures and thus the distance from the anal verge are important for outcome and treatment. From a practical point of view, cancers between about 10 and 15 cm are best discussed as rectal cancers since RT is an important component of therapy, even if less frequently so than for lower rectal cancers (0–10 cm) [5].

Endoscopic ultrasound for the earliest tumours (cT1–T2) or rectal MRI for all tumours, including the earliest ones, is recommended in order to select patients for preoperative treatment and extent of surgery [26, 27]. The TNM staging system should be used. There is major controversy about which version to use. In this chapter, version 5 from 1997 is preferred over TNM versions 6 (2002) and 7 (2010) as the latter show marked interobserver variation in defining stage II and stage III [28, 29]. At the same time, there is a need for further subclassification, particularly of cT3 to individualise therapy every more, as indicated in Table 14.1.

Table 14.1 TNM classification (version 5, 1997) with subclassifications

TNM	Stage	Extension to	
Tis N0 M0	0	Carcinoma in situ: intraepithelial or invasion of lamina propria	
T1 N0 M0	I	Submucosa	
T2 N0 M0	I	Muscularis propria	
T3 N0 M0	IIA	Subserosa/perirectal tissue	
	Substaging[a]	T3a	Less than 1 mm
		T3b	1–5 mm
		T3c	5–15 mm
		T3d	15+ mm
T4 N0 M0	IIB	Perforation into visceral peritoneum (b) or invasion to other organs (a)[b]	
T1–2 N1 M0	IIIA	1–3 Regional nodes involved	
T3–4 N1 M0	IIIB	1–3 Regional nodes involved	
T1–4 N2 M0	IIIC	4 or more regional nodes involved	
T1–4 N1–2 M1	IV	Distant metastases	

[a]This subclassification based upon an evaluation using MRI prior to treatment decision is clinically valuable and used when describing the treatment strategy for primary rectal cancer. It can be used also in the histopathological classification but is not validated and not incorporated in any of the TNM versions (5–7)
[b]This is the subclassification in TNM 5. It has been reversed in TNM 6 and 7

Need for Quality Assurance and Control

Treatment of rectal cancer is demanding and requires great skill in the entire multidisciplinary team (MDT). Good surgery and good pathology as well as good radiation techniques and optimally given chemotherapy together with long-term complete follow-up, also including functional aspects, are important for quality control. Many countries have recently lounged quality assurance (QA) and quality control (QC) programmes in rectal cancer surgery. They have been beneficial for the outcome [30, 31]. Although other components than surgery have been dealt with within the clinical guidelines/care programmes, these, like RT and CRT, must also be fully integrated in the QA and QC programmes. Presently they are not [32].

Risk-Adapted Treatment

This description basically follows what is stated in the European Society of Medical Oncology (ESMO) guidelines [7, 33].

Very Favourable Rectal Cancer

In the earliest, most favourable cases, chiefly the malignant polyps (Haggitt 1–3, T1 sm 1 (–2?) N0), a local procedure, e.g. using the transanal endoscopic microsurgery (TEM) technique, is appropriate [34, 35]. The resection should be radical (R0) and no signs of vessel invasion or poor differentiation should be present. If this is not the case or if the tumour infiltrates deeper into the submucosa (Haggit 4, T1 sm (2?–)3) or a T2 tumour, the risk of recurrence because of remaining tumour cells or because of lymph node metastases is too high (≥10 %), and the patient should have postoperative CRT or, more safely, be recommended major (TME) surgery [36]. If the cancer diagnosis is verified in a biopsy, pre-surgical CRT is preferred if the intent is to perform a local procedure [34, 36]. As an alternative to local surgery, alone or with (preoperative) CRT, local RT (brachytherapy or contact therapy (Papillon technique)) can be used in the most favourable cases. The experiences of these treatments are limited outside specialised centres [37], and more prospective studies are required in order for these techniques to be part of clinical routines.

Favourable, 'Good' Rectal Cancers

In the early, favourable cases (cT1–T2, some early cT3, N0 [cT3a(–b) and clear mrf (mrf-) according to MRI], 'good' group) above the levators, surgery alone, meaning a sharp radical dissection using the total mesorectal excision (TME) technique, is appropriate, since the risk of local failure is very low [5]. A high cT3ab tumour with limited lymph node metastases (N1) according to MRI may also belong to the good group if mrf-. The role of TME in tumours situated in the upper third of the rectum has been much discussed. To avoid spillage of distal tumour cells, a margin of at least 5 cm distally to the tumour on an unfixed specimen is recommended. Although there are indications from the large randomised trials where short-course RT has been given that this treatment even further reduces local recurrence rates [11, 38, 39], surgery alone is recommended since the addition of preoperative RT results in overtreatment of too many individuals

[5, 12]. The balance between the reduction in local recurrence rates and long-term morbidity is intricate.

Intermediate, 'Bad' Rectal Cancers

In the intermediate or 'bad' group (most cT3 (cT3(b)c+ without threatened or involved mrf (mrf-) according to MRI), some cT4 (e.g. vaginal or peritoneal involvement only), N+), preoperative RT is recommended followed by TME, since this reduces local recurrence rates. Even in the absence of signs of extramural growth on ultrasound or MRI (cT2) in very low tumours (0–5 cm), preoperative RT may be indicated because the distance to the mesorectal fascia is very small. Twenty-five Gy during one week followed by immediate surgery (<10 days from the first radiation fraction) is a convenient, simple and low-toxic treatment [11, 38–40]. It has been used predominantly in Sweden, the Netherlands and the UK, where several clinical trials revealing its efficacy have been performed. The trials have shown that the risk of local failure in the randomised population selected for later resection, i.e. the intention to treat population, has been reduced by 50–70 % versus surgery alone. More demanding and not proven more effective alternatives are 46–50.4 Gy, 1.8–2 Gy/fraction without or preferably with 5-FU (bolus, continuous infusion or peroral) [18, 19, 21, 22]. The chemotherapy was added to the preoperative radiation primarily based upon extrapolations from the postoperative RT trials in rectal cancer (see below) and other GI cancer trials. As indicated above in the paragraph about different strategies in different parts of the world, two large European trials (FFCD 9203 and EORTC 22921 [21, 22]) however recently showed that the addition of 5-FU improves local control with reduced local failure rates after 5 years. These were 16–17 % in the preoperative RT arms alone and 8–10 % in the CRT arms. In the EORTC trial, the same reduction was seen whether the chemotherapy was given concomitantly or only postoperatively. Two trials (Polish, TROG 01.04) have randomised between preoperative 5×5 Gy and preoperative CRT (5-FU+50.4 Gy) without detecting any statistically significant difference in local recurrence rates, DFS and OS. In the Polish trial [18], local recurrence rates were 11 % in the 5×5 arm at 4 years and 16 % in the CRT arm ($p=0.2$). The corresponding figures were 7.5 and 4.4 % ($p=0.2$) in the Australasian trial [19]. In a third trial (MRC-CR07) [39], preoperative 5×5 Gy was randomly compared with postoperative CRT if crm was positive. Local recurrence rates favoured the preoperative arm (5 % vs. 17 %, $p<0.001$) [39]. In the MRC-CR07 trial including 1350 patients, DFS was superior in the preoperative arm (hazard ratio, HR, 0.76, $p=0.01$), whereas OS did not significantly differ (HR 0.91, $p=0.04$).

Whenever possible, preoperative treatment is preferred since it is more effective and less toxic than postoperative treatment [5, 15]. Postoperative chemotherapy has otherwise been extensively used in many countries, including Germany and the USA, since decades. The NIH consensus conference with the follow-up NCI statement in 1990 and 1991 stated that postoperative CRT should be standard treatment in stages II and III. The scientific support for these statements was considered strong and based upon several randomised clinical trials [8, 9]. Some of the trials were small (about 50 patients per treatment arm), the results were not entirely consistent, and it was difficult to firmly establish the role for local control and survival from the different treatment components (the RT, the concomitant chemotherapy with the radiation (CRT) or the chemotherapy given before or after the radiation). Taken together, these treatments during 6 months appear to reduce local recurrences in stages II and III with 50–60 % versus surgery alone [41].

Locally Advanced, 'Ugly' Rectal Cancers

In the most locally advanced, frequently non-resectable cases (cT3 crm+, cT4 with overgrowth to other organs [cT4a according to TNM5, cT4b according to TNM6 and 7, see Table 14.1]), preoperative CRT, 50.4 Gy, 1.8 Gy/fraction with concomitant 5-FU-based therapy should be used [5, 6, 23], followed by radical surgery 6–8 weeks later. In a Nordic randomised trial in locally advanced rectal cancers (cT4NXM0), local

control was significantly better after 5 years in the CRT arm (5-FU+50 Gy) than in the RT only arm (82 % vs. 67 %, $p=0.03$). Also, DFS and cancer-specific survival were significantly better in the combined modality arm, whereas OS did not significantly differ (66 % vs. 53 %, $p=0.09$) [23]. In very old patients (≥80–85 years) and in patients not fit for CRT, 5×5 Gy with a delay of approximately 8 weeks before surgery can be an alternative option [42–45].

Standard preoperative CRT means a dose of 46–50.4 Gy together with 5-FU given either as bolus injections with leucovorin at 6–10 times during the radiation (as in the trials proving that CRT provides better local control than the same RT alone) [6, 21–23], prolonged continuous infusion (likely better than bolus) or oral capecitabine or UFT. Extrapolations from other clinical situations and convenience tell that oral 5-FU is a valid treatment [46, 47]. Combinations of 5-FU or other antifolates with other cytostatics like oxaliplatin or irinotecan or targeted biologic drugs have been extensively explored in phase I–II trials, with claimed more favourable results (more downsizing, higher pathological complete response (pCR) rates) but also more acute toxicity. Several comparative randomised trials using oxaliplatin are ongoing. The initial results of these are not favourable [48–50], and these combinations are still experimental. Neither are the initial results of adding targeted drugs like cetuximab, panitumumab or bevacizumab favourable [51–55], although the first publications are, as usual, optimistic. When cetuximab was added to neoadjuvant oxaliplatin-capecitabine and preoperative CRT in the randomised phase II EXPERT-C trial, more radiological responses were seen in the cetuximab arm (89 % vs. 72 %, $p=0.003$) in the KRAS wild-type population ($n=90$) [56]. Overall survival was also improved (96 % vs. 81 % at 3 years, $p=0.04$).

Organ Preservation?

Besides the earliest tumours that can be treated with a local procedure or local RT, and described above, it has become increasingly popular to first give CRT, wait and restage the tumour with optimal multiple biopsies/excision biopsy of the previous tumour area in case good regression is seen [57–59]. If signs of no remaining tumour/no viable tumour cells, no further therapy is provided (organ preservation) and the patient is monitored closely for at least 5 years. It is then assumed that potential lymph node metastases have been eradicated parallel with the excellent response of the primary tumour. Although this undoubtedly may occur in some patients, this strategy has not been subject to properly controlled prospective studies. It is likely that this excellent response will not be frequently seen in the intermediate and locally advanced cases [60] but rather in the early cases. The advantages, no major surgery and no rectal excision if the tumour is very low, are apparent for certain individuals at very high risk for surgery or who cannot accept a stoma. However, the disadvantages for many others are seldom discussed. In most patients with an early 'good' rectal cancer, a low anterior resection alone is the preferred therapeutic option. Cure rates are high and morbidity is only a result of the surgery. If these patients are instead treated with the aim of organ preservation, all will receive CRT with its acute morbidity. Those clinically responding very well could then be cared for with a watch-and-wait policy. These are the patients potentially having a benefit of this approach, although they would all suffer from the long-term toxicity that can be seen after CRT. This is, as indicated above, not well studied. If the tumour is located low in rectum, at least part of the sphincters must be included in the irradiated volume, and poor anal function can be a result. For those not responding so well or those recurring during follow-up, major surgery is required. These patients will thus obtain the morbidity from both CRT and surgery. No study has so far had a prospective design so that it is possible to get an idea of the proportion of patients who do not need major surgery. With the CRT schedules available today, it is this author's opinion that the group of patients having a true advantage is much smaller than the group of patients who get extra morbidity.

Evaluation of Response After Preoperative (Chemo)radiotherapy

Since the response to preoperative therapy (5 × 5 Gy with a delay or prolonged CRT to 46–50.4 Gy) may influence prognosis [61–63] and thus subsequent therapy, both the extent of surgery and postoperative chemotherapy, attempts to clinically and pathologically restage the tumours have been made. There is an increasing experience in evaluating tumour response by repeat MRI or PET-CT. Using MRI, decrease in size can be seen as well as increase in fibrosis and mucous degeneration indicating response [64]. Using FDG-PET, decrease in uptake can be seen [65–68]. At present, the knowledge about the relevance of these changes is too uncertain to modify the extent of surgery.

Several systems for pathological tumour regression grading have been used (e.g. by [69–72]). The best (reproducibility, prognostic information, etc.) is not known. The tumours should at least be graded into three groups, complete response (pCR), some (potentially in the future good, moderate and poor) response and no response. The proportion of pCRs, meaning the absence of tumour cells after a given treatment for a certain substage, is influenced by intensity of dissection. A standardisation of the dissection is required if pCR rates should be used as a valid endpoint [73].

Postoperative Therapy

Postoperative CRT (e.g. about 50 Gy, 1.8–2.0 Gy/fraction) with concomitant 5-FU-based chemotherapy is as said above no longer recommended, but could be used in patients with positive crm and perforation in the tumour area or in other cases with high risk of local recurrence if preoperative RT has not been given. The strategy of giving postoperative CRT to crm+ tumours was, however, inferior to giving preoperative 5 × 5 Gy to all, according to the MRC-CR07-trial [39]. According to the NIH and NCI statements [8, 9], all patients with pT3–4 or N+ tumours were recommended postoperative CRT, but the routine use of this has been questioned for all pT3N0 tumours [74].

Similar to the situation in colon cancer stage III (and 'high-risk' stage II), adjuvant chemotherapy can be provided, even if the scientific support for sufficient effect is less than in colon cancer [75–78]. In the early, chiefly American trials, both chemotherapy and CRT were predominantly given, and thus it was difficult to ascertain which component was responsible for the survival gain [8, 9]. In a Hellenic trial [79], CRT with 4 additional cycles of chemotherapy was not more effective than CRT alone. In a Norwegian trial [80], CRT alone resulted in a survival gain compared to no postoperative therapy. It is possible that the efficacy of adjuvant chemotherapy is less if the tumour has not responded to the CRT, but this is based only upon a retrospective analysis of one trial [81].

Radiation Therapy Volumes and Doses

Whenever radiotherapy is indicated to lower the risk of local failure in the 'intermediate/bad' group or to cause downsizing to allow radical surgery in 'locally advanced/ugly' tumours, the primary tumour with the mesorectum and lymph nodes outside the mesorectum, at risk to contain tumour cells more than exceptionally, should be irradiated [82, 83]. In the 'early/good' group before or after a local procedure, only mesorectal nodes are considered at sufficient risk to be involved. The appropriate dose to subclinical disease is not precisely known, but should with 5-FU chemotherapy be at least 46 Gy in 1.8–2 Gy fractions. The relative reduction in local failure rates is then in the order of 50–60 %, why there is room for improvements. A boost of about 4–6 Gy in 2–4 fractions to the primary tumour is often given, limiting the radiation dose to the entire volume when long-course CRT is given. Elective para-aortic and liver radiotherapy did not improve survival in one trial [84].

The entire mesorectum is at great risk of having tumour deposits, often in the mesorectal lymph nodes, in all tumours except the very earliest (T1 sm1 (−2?)) and should be included in the clinical target volume (CTV). An exception is the high tumours where it is sufficient to include the 4–5 cm distal to the tumour. This means that in these tumours, the lower border of the beams can be about 5–6 cm distal to the tumour. Besides the mesorectal nodes, the presacral nodes along aa rectalis superior up to the level of S1–2 should be included. If presacral nodes are radiologically involved, the upper border of CTV should be even higher. Local recurrences above S1–2 are seldom seen [85–87]. The lateral nodes along aa rectalis inferior and aa obturatorii and the internal iliac nodes up to the bifurcation from aa iliac communis should be included in tumours below the peritoneal reflection, i.e. in tumours up to about 9–12 cm from the anal verge [88]. The risk of lateral node involvement in the Western world is not properly known, but studies from Asia show that these lymph nodes are seldom involved in low-mid rectal pT1–2 tumours and in high tumours irrespective of T-stage [89, 90]. External iliac nodes should only be included if an anterior organ like the urinary bladder, prostate or female sexual organs are involved to such an extent that there is a risk of involvement of these lymph node stations. The medial inguinal nodes need only to be prophylactically included when the tumour grows below the dentate line [91]. When lymph nodes are involved by metastatic disease so that this can be seen on imaging, there is always a risk of aberrant spread, and the CTV can be enlarged to include also other nodal stations than those described above.

Fossae ischiorectalis should only be included when the levator muscles and the internal and external sphincters are involved since the fascia inside the levators is considered to be a strong barrier to tumour cell penetration [92]. Other opinions have been expressed [82].

Treatment of Local Recurrences

Patients with recurrence (if radiotherapy was not given in the primary situation) should receive preoperative RT (about 50 Gy during 5–6 weeks) with concomitant chemotherapy similar to a locally advanced (ugly) rectal cancer. In patients previously irradiated, attempts at providing additional RT, externally, using intraoperative radiotherapy (IORT) or different brachytherapy techniques could be tried. It is often possible to re-irradiate many patients [93], although it is important to limit the dose to the small bowels as much as possible. Attempts of radical surgery should take place 6–10 weeks after RT. In patients with prior RT for whom salvage surgery is not an option, systemic chemotherapy should be considered.

Late Toxicity from Rectal Cancer Radiotherapy

It is extremely important to know the extent of late toxicity after rectal cancer RT if this is given pre- or postoperatively to diminish the risk of local recurrence. The prevention of a local failure with the severe morbidity it may have must be weighed against the morbidity from (C)RT that all treated patients can get. Studies have tried to estimate what minimal absolute gain should be present for patients to value RT. These studies are very difficult to interpret, although many patients accept an absolute 3 % difference for the risk of RT morbidity [94].

From the Swedish and Dutch randomised trials, we have good evidence of the morbidity that can be seen after 5×5 Gy RT (summarised in [20]). It is beyond the scope of this chapter to detail this toxicity, but increased risks of poor anal and sexual function, small bowel toxicity with obstruction and secondary malignancies have been reported. After having worked with rectal cancer patients for over 30 years, thus seeing many patients with a local recurrence during the first part of the period, and being actively involved in the research to estimate the risks of late toxicity up to 20 years after the RT, it is my opinion that an absolute risk reduction of in the order of 5 % unites motivates the recommendation to irradiate. Further and very important, the RT we give today, and the RT we can routinely give in only a few years, will mean less late toxicity than seen in the follow-up studies of the RT given during the 1980s–1990s [83].

A very important question not yet solved is the late toxicity from 5×5 Gy compared with the toxicity seen after 46–50 Gy in 25–28 fractions, usually with 5-FU. We know the long-term morbidity from 5×5 Gy up to at least 10 years' follow-up (with yesterday's techniques) from studies including thousands of patients. We do not have this knowledge from CRT to about 50 Gy. The Polish trial [18] and the MRC-CR07 trial [39] have reported late toxicity after 4 years of follow-up, without being able to detect any significant differences between 5×5 Gy and CRT to 46–50 Gy. The short-course schedule uses a high fraction size of 5 Gy, compared to 1.8–2.0 Gy, whereas the total dose is less (25 Gy compared to 46–50 Gy). Both the fraction size and the total dose are relevant. The relations between total dose, fraction size and toxicity are complex.

Another yet unresolved question is whether the addition of 5-FU, or in the future other drugs, increases late toxicity. Three randomised trials have been performed. Data from one of the two trials in the intermediate-risk group [21, 22] have shown that some dimensions of quality of life are less good in the CRT group [95]. Late toxicity has also been analysed in the smaller trial in the locally advanced/ugly group. More patients had a stoma or a poor anal function in the CRT group than in the RT group (89 % vs. 70 %, $p=0.046$) [96], but no differences in QoL were seen [97]. Whether this means that the chemotherapy addition results in more late toxicity or if this difference reflects survival of patients with more advanced tumours in the CRT group could not be deduced. Comparisons of population-based series where some have been irradiated and others not, reporting poorer long-term function among those irradiated, are extremely difficult to interpret due to the selection of more advanced cases for radiotherapy [98–100].

References

1. Birgisson H, Talback M, Gunnarsson U, Påhlman L, Glimelius B. Improved survival in cancer of the colon and rectum in Sweden. Eur J Surg Oncol. 2005;31:845–53.
2. den Dulk M, Krijnen P, Marijnen CA, Rutten HJ, van de Poll-Franse LV, Putter H, et al. Improved overall

survival for patients with rectal cancer since 1990: the effects of TME surgery and pre-operative radiotherapy. Eur J Cancer. 2008;44:1710–6.

3. Klint A, Engholm G, Storm HH, Tryggvadottir L, Gislum M, Hakulinen T, Bray F. Trends in survival of patients diagnosed with cancer of the digestive organs in the Nordic countries 1964–2003 followed up to the end of 2006. Acta Oncol. 2010;49:578–607.

4. Glimelius B, Beets-Tan R, Blomqvist L, Brown G, Nagtegaal I, Påhlman L, et al. Mesorectal fascia instead of circumferential resection margin in preoperative staging of rectal cancer. J Clin Oncol. 2011;29:2142–3.

5. Valentini V, Aristei C, Glimelius B, Minsky BD, Beets-Tan R, Borras JM, et al. Multidisciplinary rectal cancer management. Radiother Oncol. 2009;92:148–63.

6. Glimelius B, Holm T, Blomqvist L. Chemotherapy in addition to preoperative radiotherapy in locally advanced rectal cancer – a systematic overview. Rev Recent Clin Trials. 2008;3:204–11.

7. Schmoll HJ, Van Cutsem E, Stein A, Valentini V, Glimelius B, Haustermans K, et al. ESMO Consensus Guidelines for management of patients with colon and rectal cancer. A personalized approach to clinical decision making. Ann Oncol. 2012;23:2479–516.

8. NIH Consensus Conference. Adjuvant therapy for patients with colon and rectal cancer. JAMA. 1990;264:1444–50.

9. NCI. Clinical Announcement. Adjuvant therapy of rectal cancer, March 14. National Cancer Institute, Bethesda;1991.

10. Glimelius B. Chemoradiotherapy for rectal cancer – is there an optimal combination? Ann Oncol. 2001;12:1039–45.

11. Swedish Rectal Cancer Trial. Improved survival with preoperative radiotherapy in resectable rectal cancer. N Engl J Med. 1997;336:980–7.

12. Glimelius B. Multidisciplinary treatment of patients with rectal cancer: development during the past decades and plans for the future. Ups J Med Sci. 2012;117:225–36.

13. Påhlman L, Glimelius B, Graffman S. Pre- versus postoperative radiotherapy in rectal carcinoma: an interim report from a randomized multicentre trial. Br J Surg. 1985;72:961–6.

14. Påhlman L, Glimelius B. Pre- or postoperative radiotherapy in rectal carcinoma: a report from a randomized multicenter trial. Ann Surg. 1990;211:187–95.

15. Sauer R, Becker H, Hohenberger W, Rodel C, Wittekind C, Fietkau R, et al. Preoperative versus postoperative chemoradiotherapy for rectal cancer. N Engl J Med. 2004;351:1731–40.

16. Sauer R, Liersch T, Merkel S, Fietkau R, Hohenberger W, Hess C, et al. Preoperative versus postoperative chemoradiotherapy for locally advanced rectal cancer: results of the German CAO/ARO/AIO-94 randomized phase III trial after a median follow-up of 11 years. J Clin Oncol. 2012;30:1926–33.

17. Glimelius B, Isacsson U, Jung B, Påhlman L. Radiotherapy in addition to radical surgery in rectal cancer: evidence for a dose-response effect favouring preoperative treatment. Int J Radiat Oncol Biol Phys. 1997;37:281–7.

18. Bujko K, Nowacki MP, Nasierowska-Guttmejer A, Michalski W, Bebenek M, Kryj M, et al. Long-term results of a randomised trial comparing preoperative short-course radiotherapy vs preoperative conventionally fractionated chemoradiation for rectal cancer. Br J Surg. 2006;93:1215–23.

19. Ngan SY, Burmeister B, Fisher RJ, Solomon M, Goldstein D, Joseph D, et al. Randomized trial of short-course radiotherapy versus long-course chemoradiation comparing rates of local recurrence in patients with t3 rectal cancer: trans-tasman radiation oncology group trial 01.04. J Clin Oncol. 2012;30:3827–33.

20. Birgisson H, Påhlman L, Gunnarsson U, Glimelius B. Late adverse effects of radiation therapy for rectal cancer – a systematic overview. Acta Oncol. 2007;46:504–16.

21. Gerard JP, Conroy T, Bonnetain F, Bouche O, Chapet O, Closon-Dejardin MT, et al. Preoperative radiotherapy with or without concurrent fluorouracil and leucovorin in T3-4 rectal cancers: results of FFCD 9203. J Clin Oncol. 2006;24:4620–5.

22. Bosset JF, Collette L, Calais G, Mineur L, Maingon P, Radosevic-Jelic L, et al. Chemotherapy with preoperative radiotherapy in rectal cancer. N Engl J Med. 2006;355:1114–23.

23. Braendengen M, Tveit KM, Berglund Å, Birkemeyer E, Frykholm G, Påhlman L, et al. A randomized phase III study (LARCS) comparing preoperative radiotherapy alone versus chemoradiotherapy in non-resectable rectal cancer. J Clin Oncol. 2008;26:3687–94.

24. Bujko K, Kepka L, Michalski W, Nowacki MP. Does rectal cancer shrinkage induced by preoperative radio(chemo)therapy increase the likelihood of anterior resection? A systematic review of randomised trials. Radiother Oncol. 2006;80:4–12.

25. Gerard JP, Rostom Y, Gal J, Benchimol D, Ortholan C, Aschele C, Levi JM. Can we increase the chance of sphincter saving surgery in rectal cancer with neoadjuvant treatments: lessons from a systematic review of recent randomized trials. Crit Rev Oncol Hematol. 2012;81:21–8.

26. Bipat S, Glas AS, Slors FJ, Zwinderman AH, Bossuyt PM, Stoker J. Rectal cancer: local staging and assessment of lymph node involvement with endoluminal US, CT, and MR imaging–a meta-analysis. Radiology. 2004;232:773–83.

27. Smith N, Brown G. Preoperative staging in rectal cancer. Acta Oncol. 2008;47:20–31.

28. Quirke P, Williams GT, Ectors N, Ensari A, Piard F, Nagtegaal I. The future of the TNM staging system in colorectal cancer: time for a debate? Lancet Oncol. 2007;8:651–7.

29. Quirke P, Cuvelier C, Ensari A, Glimelius B, Laurberg S, Ortiz H, et al. Evidence-based medicine: the time has come to set standards for staging. J Pathol. 2010;221:357–60.

30. Pahlman L, Bohe M, Cedermark B, Dahlberg M, Lindmark G, Sjodahl R, et al. The Swedish rectal cancer registry. Br J Surg. 2007;94:1285–92.

31. Wibe A, Moller B, Norstein J, Carlsen E, Wiig JN, Heald RJ, et al. A national strategic change in treatment policy for rectal cancer–implementation of total mesorectal excision as routine treatment in Norway. A national audit. Dis Colon Rectum. 2002;45:857–66.

32. Valentini V, Glimelius B, Frascino V. Quality assurance and quality control for radiotherapy/medical oncology in Europe: guideline development and implementation. Eur J Surg Oncol. 2013;39: 938–44.

33. Glimelius B, Tiret E, Cervantes A, Arnold D. Rectal cancer: ESMO Clinical Practice Guidelines for diagnosis, treatment and follow-up. Ann Oncol. 2013;24 Suppl 6:vi81–8.

34. Doornebosch PG, Tollenaar RA, De Graaf EJ. Is the increasing role of Transanal Endoscopic Microsurgery in curation for T1 rectal cancer justified? A systematic review. Acta Oncol. 2009;48:343–53.

35. Baatrup G, Endreseth BH, Isaksen V, Kjellmo A, Tveit KM, Nesbakken A. Preoperative staging and treatment options in T1 rectal adenocarcinoma. Acta Oncol. 2009;48:328–42.

36. Stamos MJ, Murrell Z. Management of early rectal T1 and T2 cancers. Clin Cancer Res. 2007;13:6885s–99.

37. Gerard JP, Ortholan C, Benezery K, Ginot A, Hannoun-Levi JM, Chamorey E, et al. Contact X-ray therapy for rectal cancer: experience in Centre Antoine-Lacassagne, Nice, 2002–2006. Int J Radiat Oncol Biol Phys. 2008;72:665–70.

38. Kapiteijn E, Marijnen CAM, Nagtegaal ID, Putter H, Steup WH, Wiggers T, et al. Preoperative radiotherapy in combination with total mesorectal excision improves local control in resectable rectal cancer. Report from a multicenter randomized trial. New Engl J Med. 2001;345:638–46.

39. Sebag-Montefiore D, Stephens RJ, Steele R, Monson J, Grieve R, Khanna S, et al. Preoperative radiotherapy versus selective postoperative chemoradiotherapy in patients with rectal cancer (MRC CR07 and NCIC-CTG C016): a multicentre, randomised trial. Lancet. 2009;373:811–20.

40. Folkesson J, Birgisson H, Påhlman L, Cedermark B, Glimelius B, Gunnarsson U. Swedish Rectal Cancer Trial: long lasting benefits from radiotherapy on survival and local recurrence rate. J Clin Oncol. 2005;23:5644–50.

41. Colorectal Cancer Collaborative Group. Adjuvant therapy for rectal cancer: a systematic overview of 8507 patients from 22 randomised trials. Lancet. 2001;358:1291–304.

42. Radu C, Berglund Å, Påhlman L, Glimelius B. Short course preoperative radiotherapy with delayed surgery in rectal cancer – a retrospective study. Radiother Oncol. 2008;87:343–9.

43. Valentini V, Glimelius B. Rectal cancer radiotherapy: towards European consensus. Acta Oncol. 2010;49: 1206–16.

44. Hatfield P, Hingorani M, Radhakrishna G, Cooper R, Melcher A, Crellin A, et al. Short-course radiotherapy, with elective delay prior to surgery, in patients with unresectable rectal cancer who have poor performance status or significant co-morbidity. Radiother Oncol. 2009;92:210–4.

45. Pettersson D, Holm T, Iversen H, Blomqvist L, Glimelius B, Martling A. Preoperative short-course radiotherapy with delayed surgery in primary rectal cancer. Br J Surg. 2012;99:577–83.

46. Hofheinz RD, Wenz F, Post S, Matzdorff A, Laechelt S, Hartmann JT, et al. Chemoradiotherapy with capecitabine versus fluorouracil for locally advanced rectal cancer: a randomised, multicentre, non-inferiority, phase 3 trial. Lancet Oncol. 2012;13:579–88.

47. Crane CH, Sargent DJ. Substitution of oral fluoropyrimidines for infusional fluorouracil with radiotherapy: how much data do we need? J Clin Oncol. 2004;22:2978–81.

48. Gerard JP, Azria D, Gourgou-Bourgade S, Martel-Laffay I, Hennequin C, Etienne PL, et al. Comparison of two neoadjuvant chemoradiotherapy regimens for locally advanced rectal cancer: results of the phase III trial ACCORD 12/0405-Prodige 2. J Clin Oncol. 2010;28:1638–44.

49. Aschele C, Cionini L, Lonardi S, Pinto C, Cordio S, Rosati G, et al. Primary tumor response to preoperative chemoradiation with or without oxaliplatin in locally advanced rectal cancer: pathologic results of the STAR-01 randomized phase III trial. J Clin Oncol. 2011;29:2773–80.

50. Rodel C, Liersch T, Becker H, Fietkau R, Hohenberger W, Hothorn T, et al. Preoperative chemoradiotherapy and postoperative chemotherapy with fluorouracil and oxaliplatin versus fluorouracil alone in locally advanced rectal cancer: initial results of the German CAO/ARO/AIO-04 randomised phase 3 trial. Lancet Oncol. 2012;13:679–87.

51. Horisberger K, Treschl A, Mai S, Barreto-Miranda M, Kienle P, Strobel P, et al. Cetuximab in combination with capecitabine, irinotecan, and radiotherapy for patients with locally advanced rectal cancer: results of a Phase II MARGIT trial. Int J Radiat Oncol Biol Phys. 2009;74:1487–93.

52. Glynne-Jones R, Mawdsley S, Harrison M. Cetuximab and chemoradiation for rectal cancer–is the water getting muddy? Acta Oncol. 2010;49:278–86.

53. Pinto C, Di Fabio F, Maiello E, Pini S, Latiano T, Aschele C, et al. Phase II study of panitumumab, oxaliplatin, 5-fluorouracil, and concurrent radiotherapy as preoperative treatment in high-risk locally advanced rectal cancer patients (StarPan/STAR-02 Study). Ann Oncol. 2011;22(11):2424–30.

54. Resch G, De Vries A, Ofner D, Eisterer W, Rabl H, Jagoditsch M, et al. Preoperative treatment with capecitabine, bevacizumab and radiotherapy for primary locally advanced rectal cancer–a two stage phase II clinical trial. Radiother Oncol. 2012;102:10–3.

55. Nogue M, Salud A, Vicente P, Arrivi A, Roca JM, Losa F, et al. Addition of bevacizumab to XELOX induction therapy plus concomitant capecitabine-based chemoradiotherapy in magnetic resonance imaging-defined poor-prognosis locally advanced

rectal cancer: the AVACROSS study. Oncologist. 2011;16:614–20.

56. Dewdney A, Cunningham D, Tabernero J, Capdevila J, Glimelius B, Cervantes A, et al. Multicenter randomized phase II clinical trial comparing neoadjuvant oxaliplatin, capecitabine, and preoperative radiotherapy with or without cetuximab followed by total mesorectal excision in patients with high-risk rectal cancer (EXPERT-C). J Clin Oncol. 2012;30:1620–7.

57. Habr-Gama A, Perez RO, Nadalin W, Sabbaga J, Ribeiro Jr U, Silva e Sousa Jr AH, et al. Operative versus nonoperative treatment for stage 0 distal rectal cancer following chemoradiation therapy: long-term results. Ann Surg. 2004;240:711–7.

58. Baxter NN, Garcia-Aguilar J. Organ preservation for rectal cancer. J Clin Oncol. 2007;25:1014–20.

59. Maas M, Beets-Tan RG, Lambregts DM, Lammering G, Nelemans PJ, Engelen SM, et al. Wait-and-see policy for clinical complete responders after chemoradiation for rectal cancer. J Clin Oncol. 2011;29: 4633–40.

60. Hughes R, Harrison M, Glynne-Jones R. Could a wait and see policy be justified in T3/4 rectal cancers after chemo-radiotherapy? Acta Oncol. 2010;49:378–81.

61. Glynne-Jones R, Mawdsley S, Pearce T, Buyse M. Alternative clinical end points in rectal cancer–are we getting closer? Ann Oncol. 2006;17:1239–48.

62. Bujko K, Kolodziejczyk M, Nasierowska-Guttmejer A, Michalski W, Kepka L, Chmielik E, et al. Tumour regression grading in patients with residual rectal cancer after preoperative chemoradiation. Radiother Oncol. 2010;95:298–302.

63. Park IJ, You YN, Agarwal A, Skibber JM, Rodriguez-Bigas MA, Eng C, et al. Neoadjuvant treatment response as an early response indicator for patients with rectal cancer. J Clin Oncol. 2012;30:1770–6.

64. Barbaro B, Fiorucci C, Tebala C, Valentini V, Gambacorta MA, Vecchio FM, et al. Locally advanced rectal cancer: MR imaging in prediction of response after preoperative chemotherapy and radiation therapy. Radiology. 2009;250:730–9.

65. Calvo FA, Domper M, Matute R, Martinez-Lazaro R, Arranz JA, Desco M, et al. 18F-FDG positron emission tomography staging and restaging in rectal cancer treated with preoperative chemoradiation. Int J Radiat Oncol Biol Phys. 2004;58:528–35.

66. Lambrecht M, Deroose C, Roels S, Vandecaveye V, Penninckx F, Sagaert X, et al. The use of FDG-PET/CT and diffusion-weighted magnetic resonance imaging for response prediction before, during and after preoperative chemoradiotherapy for rectal cancer. Acta Oncol. 2010;49:956–63.

67. Martoni AA, Di Fabio F, Pinto C, Castellucci P, Pini S, Ceccarelli C, et al. Prospective study on the FDG-PET/CT predictive and prognostic values in patients treated with neoadjuvant chemoradiation therapy and radical surgery for locally advanced rectal cancer. Ann Oncol. 2011;22:650–6.

68. Yoon MS, Ahn SJ, Nah BS, Chung WK, Song JY, Jeong JU, Nam TK. The metabolic response using 18F-fluorodeoxyglucose-positron emission tomography/computed tomography and the change in the carcinoembryonic antigen level for predicting response to pre-operative chemoradiotherapy in patients with rectal cancer. Radiother Oncol. 2011;98: 134–8.

69. Mandard AM, Dalibard F, Mandard JC, et al. Pathologic assessment of tumor regression after preoperative chemoradiotherapy of esophageal carcinoma. Clinicopathologic correlations. Cancer. 1994;73: 2680–6.

70. Dworak O, Keilholz L, Hoffmann A. Pathological features of rectal cancer after preoperative radiochemotherapy. Int J Colorectal Dis. 1997;12:19–23.

71. Wheeler JM, Warren BF, Mortensen NJ, et al. Quantification of histologic regression of rectal cancer after irradiation: A proposal for a modified staging system. Dis Colon Rectum. 2002;45:1051–6.

72. Rödel CL, Martus P, Papadoupolos T, et al. Prognostic significance of tumor regression after preoperative chemoradiotherapy for rectal cancer. J Clin Oncol. 2005;23:8688–96.

73. Quirke P, Morris E. Reporting colorectal cancer. Histopathology. 2007;50:103–12.

74. Gunderson LL, Sargent DJ, Tepper JE, O'Connell MJ, Allmer C, Smalley SR, et al. Impact of T and N substage on survival and disease relapse in adjuvant rectal cancer: a pooled analysis. Int J Radiat Oncol Biol Phys. 2002;54:386–96.

75. Quasar Collaborative Group, Gray R, Barnwell J, McConkey C, Hills RK, Williams NS, Kerr DJ. Adjuvant chemotherapy versus observation in patients with colorectal cancer: a randomised study. Lancet. 2007;370:2020–9.

76. Sakamoto J, Hamada C, Yoshida S, Kodaira S, Yasutomi M, Kato T, et al. An individual patient data meta-analysis of adjuvant therapy with uracil-tegafur (UFT) in patients with curatively resected rectal cancer. Br J Cancer. 2007;96:1170–7.

77. Glimelius B. Adjuvant chemotherapy in rectal cancer – an issue or a non-issue? Ann Oncol. 2010;21: 1739–41.

78. Bujko K, Glynne-Jones R, Bujko M. Does adjuvant fluoropyrimidine-based chemotherapy provide a benefit for patients with resected rectal cancer who have already received neoadjuvant radio(chemo)therapy? A systematic review of randomized trials. Ann Oncol. 2010;21:1743–50.

79. Fountzilas G, Zisiadis A, Dafni U, Konstantaras C, Hatzitheoharis G, Liaros A, et al. Postoperative radiation and concomitant bolus fluorouracil with or without additional chemotherapy with fluorouracil and high-dose leucovorin in patients with high-risk rectal cancer: a randomized phase III study conducted by the Hellenic Cooperative Oncology Group. Ann Oncol. 1999;10:671–6.

80. Tveit KM, Guldvog I, Hagen S, Trondsen E, Harbitz T, Nygaard K, et al. Randomized controlled trial of postoperative radiotherapy and short-term time-scheduled 5-fluorouracil against surgery alone in the

treatment of Dukes B and C rectal cancer. Br J Surg. 1997;84:1130–5.

81. Collette L, Bosset JF, den Dulk M, Nguyen F, Mineur L, Maingon P, et al. Patients with curative resection of cT3-4 rectal cancer after preoperative radiotherapy or radiochemotherapy: does anybody benefit from adjuvant fluorouracil-based chemotherapy? J Clin Oncol. 2007;25:4379–86.

82. Roels S, Duthoy W, Haustermans K, Penninckx F, Vandecaveye V, Boterberg T, De Neve W. Definition and delineation of the clinical target volume for rectal cancer. Int J Radiat Oncol Biol Phys. 2006;65: 1129–42.

83. Ippolito E, Mertens I, Haustermans K, Gambacorta MA, Pasini D, Valentini V. IGRT in rectal cancer. Acta Oncol. 2008;47:1317–24.

84. Bosset JF, Horiot JC, Hamers HP, Cionini L, Bartelink H, Caspers R, et al. Postoperative pelvic radiotherapy with or without elective irradiation of para-aortic nodes and liver in rectal cancer patients. A controlled clinical trial of the EORTC Radiotherapy Group. Radiother Oncol. 2001;61:7–13.

85. Syk E, Torkzad MR, Blomqvist L, Ljungqvist O, Glimelius B. Radiological findings do not support lateral residual tumour as a major cause of local recurrence of rectal cancer. Br J Surg. 2006;93:113–9.

86. Syk E, Torkzad MR, Blomqvist L, Nilsson PJ, Glimelius B. Local recurrence in rectal cancer: anatomic localization and effect on radiation target. Int J Radiat Oncol Biol Phys. 2008;72:658–64.

87. Nijkamp J, Kusters M, Beets-Tan RG, Martijn H, Beets GL, van de Velde CJ, Marijnen CA. Three-dimensional analysis of recurrence patterns in rectal cancer: the cranial border in hypofractionated preoperative radiotherapy can be lowered. Int J Radiat Oncol Biol Phys. 2011;80:103–10.

88. Kusters M, Wallner C, Lange MM, Deruiter MC, van de Velde CJ, Moriya Y, Rutten HJ. Origin of presacral local recurrence after rectal cancer treatment. Br J Surg. 2010;97:1582–7.

89. Wang C, Zhou ZG, Yu YY, Li Y, Lei WZ, Cheng Z, Chen ZX. Patterns of lateral pelvic lymph node metastases and micrometastases for patients with lower rectal cancer. Eur J Surg Oncol. 2007;33:463–7.

90. Yano H, Moran BJ. The incidence of lateral pelvic side-wall nodal involvement in low rectal cancer may be similar in Japan and the West. Br J Surg. 2008;95: 33–49.

91. Taylor N, Crane C, Skibber J, Feig B, Ellis L, Vauthey JN, et al. Elective groin irradiation is not indicated for patients with adenocarcinoma of the rectum extending to the anal canal. Int J Radiat Oncol Biol Phys. 2001;51:741–7.

92. West NP, Finan PJ, Anderin C, Lindholm J, Holm T, Quirke P. Evidence of the oncologic superiority of cylindrical abdominoperineal excision for low rectal cancer. J Clin Oncol. 2008;26:3517–22.

93. Das P, Delclos ME, Skibber JM, Rodriguez-Bigas MA, Feig BW, Chang GJ, et al. Hyperfractionated accelerated radiotherapy for rectal cancer in patients with prior pelvic irradiation. Int J Radiat Oncol Biol Phys. 2010;77:60–5.

94. Bakx R, Emous M, Legemate DA, Zoetmulder FA, van Tienhoven G, Bemelman WA, van Lanschot JJ. Harm and benefits of short-term pre-operative radiotherapy in patients with resectable rectal carcinomas. Eur J Surg Oncol. 2006;32:520–6.

95. Tiv M, Puyraveau M, Mineur L, Calais G, Maingon P, Bardet E, et al. Long-term quality of life in patients with rectal cancer treated with preoperative (chemo)-radiotherapy within a randomized trial. Cancer Radiother. 2010;14:530–4.

96. Braendengen M, Tveit KM, Bruheim K, Cvancarova M, Berglund Å, Glimelius B. Late patient-reported toxicity after preoperative radiotherapy or chemoradiotherapy in nonresectable rectal cancer: results from a randomized phase III study. Int J Radiat Oncol Biol Phys. 2011;81:1017–24.

97. Braendengen M, Tveit KM, Hjermstad MJ, Johansson H, Berglund K, Brandberg Y, Glimelius B. Health-related quality of life (HRQoL) after multimodal treatment for primarily non-resectable rectal cancer. Long-term results from a phase III study. Eur J Cancer. 2012;48:813–9.

98. Bruheim K, Guren MG, Dahl AA, Skovlund E, Balteskard L, Carlsen E, et al. Sexual function in males after radiotherapy for rectal cancer. Int J Radiat Oncol Biol Phys. 2010;76:1012–7.

99. Bruheim K, Guren MG, Skovlund E, Hjermstad MJ, Dahl O, Frykholm G, et al. Late side effects and quality of life after radiotherapy for rectal cancer. Int J Radiat Oncol Biol Phys. 2010;76:1005–11.

100. Bruheim K, Tveit KM, Skovlund E, Balteskard L, Carlsen E, Fossa SD, Guren MG. Sexual function in females after radiotherapy for rectal cancer. Acta Oncol. 2010;49:826–32.

Short- and Long-Term Side Effects from Adjuvant and Neoadjuvant Treatment of Rectal Cancer

15

Rune Sjödahl

Abstract

Adjuvant therapy in rectal cancer patients involves most often chemotherapy or in rare cases radiotherapy after the tumour has been removed surgically without any signs of remnant macroscopic or microscopic disease. Neoadjuvant treatment means radiotherapy, chemotherapy, or chemoradiation before the tumour has been removed surgically. As chemotherapy inhibits and kills cancer cells as well as normal cells, some side effects are often unavoidable. Ideally benefits and side effects should be balanced, but at present, it is not possible to individualise the treatment with respect to differences in pharmacodynamics and pharmacokinetics. Not only the frequency but also the severity of the side effects must be evaluated, and scoring systems like the Common Toxicity Criteria can be used. Nausea and vomiting may be prevented to some extent by various measures. Both early and late side effects of radiotherapy are dependent on irradiated volume, total dose, fractionation, and total time for treatment. Early toxicity is more frequent after chemoradiation than after radiotherapy alone. Ageing involves a reduction of physiologic reserves, absorption, metabolism, and elimination which may be associated with increased toxicity. However, performance status and functional status should be more important than age alone for recommending adjuvant or neoadjuvant therapy.

Adjuvant therapy in rectal cancer patients involves chemotherapy or radiotherapy after the tumour has been removed surgically without any signs of remnant macroscopic or microscopic disease. The rationale for adjuvant therapy is that in spite of an R0 resection, there may be residual clusters of tumour cells with metastatic potential in the tumour area or in distant locations. This, however, does not occur in the majority of patients, and it must be remembered that although chemotherapy has made great progress, the response rates are still limited to around 50 %. Consequently, a substantial amount of patients are overtreated when

R. Sjödahl
Department of Surgery, Linköping University,
SE-585 81 Linköping, Sweden
e-mail: rune.sjodahl@lio.se

"number to treat" is calculated. The documentation of the benefit of adjuvant treatment regarding reduced local recurrence rate and particularly improved survival is limited in rectal cancer patients. Therefore, significant and permanent side effects should not be accepted.

Neoadjuvant treatment in rectal cancer means radiotherapy, chemotherapy, or a combination of them before the tumour has been removed surgically. This preoperative treatment is offered selected patients with a resectable rectal cancer as it may destroy cancer cells in the periphery of the tumour area but also more distantly. More seldom neoadjuvant treatment is given when the tumour is so advanced that it is uncertain whether it can be completely removed with surgery. Then there is a need to downsize or even downgrade the tumour before surgery and improve the possibility to perform a radical operation. Obviously more side effects should be accepted in this situation.

Cytotoxic chemotherapy inhibits and kills cancer cells as well as normal cells, and some side effects are thus unavoidable. It is therefore crucial to balance benefits against complications to the treatment. But this is difficult as the effects of chemotherapy are still unpredictable in the individual patient. At present our knowledge is insufficient to individualise the treatment with respect to differences in pharmacodynamics and pharmacokinetics. Genetic differences in drug handling are probably important both for some of the variations in the response and for some side effects of chemotherapy [1].

Radiotherapy

Neoadjuvant or adjuvant radiotherapy before or after surgery with curative intent is for many patients an overtreatment, as local recurrence rate is reduced from merely 10–15 % after surgery alone to 5–8 %. Therefore, it is of great importance to avoid serious side effects.

The side effects of radiotherapy are dependent on the following:
- Irradiated volume
- Total dose
- Fractionation
- Total time for treatment

Early side effects after radiation are well known with fatigue, pain, and other symptoms from the gastrointestinal tract, loss of weight, and sometimes dermatological manifestations. In a recent interim analysis [2], there was a trend towards less complications after long-term irradiation compared with 5 Gy given for 5 days. Moreover, the rate of complications and the mortality in elderly patients was increased when surgery was performed 11–17 days after the start of short-term irradiation. To reduce the side effects of 5×5 Gy, the recommendation was to perform the operation either within 5 days or after 4–8 weeks after the start of irradiation. After abdominoperineal resection, septic complications of the perineal wound are doubled from about 10 % to about 20 % [3, 4]. Other surgical complications as anastomotic leakage have not been increased in randomised studies, but this is in contrast to population-based studies where postoperative complications have been increased in irradiated patient groups. Such a difference between various patient materials may be due to differences in comorbidity of the included patients. Early studies with a big radiation volume reported an increased postoperative mortality but with modern technique using four fields, and smaller irradiated volumes the mortality is not increased [5]. A rare complication reported after short-course radiation has been acute neuropathy with pain in the buttocks and the thighs. There is a slight increase in side effects after postoperative radiotherapy compared with preoperative radiotherapy.

Late side effects. In studies where the anal sphincters were included in the irradiated field, the anal function was impaired twice as often after preoperative radiation and surgery compared to surgery alone with low anterior resection. The discomfort seems, however, tolerable as it does not influence on the quality of life [6, 7]. There is also a slight decrease in sexual function after irradiation and resectional surgery. It has been reported that 2 years after treatment, 67 % of males were sexually active after irradiation combined with surgery and 76 % after surgery alone. Corresponding figures for females were 72 % versus 90 % [8]. In the early studies, intestinal obstruction and pathological fractures of the pelvic region were seen, but those findings have not been confirmed in later studies with modern radiation techniques [6]. However, secondary tumours are more common in the pelvic area among irradiated patients. A systematic overview of 22 randomised trials showed that fewer patients who had preoperative radiotherapy died from rectal cancer than did those who had surgery alone (45 % versus 50 %), but overall, deaths within 1 year after treatment were increased in irradiated patients (8 % versus 4 %) [9].

Chemotherapy

In rectal cancer patients, chemotherapy is used postoperatively in selected patients with stage III tumours or in T3–T4 tumours. In addition chemotherapy is considered when the resectional margin is narrow or after an R1–2 resection in patients irradiated before surgery. Usually the adjuvant treatment will continue for about 6 months, and during that time more or less awkward side effects may appear. They comprise both subjective feelings and objective effects which can influence on the management of chemotherapeutic agents and sometimes even be life threatening. It is generally accepted that certain factors may increase the risk for side effects such as pharmacodynamic characteristics, inappropriate dosage, interactions with other drugs, variations of metabolic inactivation, changes of metabolism or elimination, or malnutrition. When various chemotherapeutic agents are combined, the side effects are not reduced, but their panorama may get wider. Side effects are extremely common, and it is important that they are described not only regarding their frequency but also regarding their severity.

In general, the various side effects can be managed quite successfully with prevention, symptomatic treatment, and changes of dosage of the chemotherapeutic agents.

Organ-Related Side Effects

Nausea and vomiting are the biggest problems of chemotherapy for cancer, and in rare cases the treatment must be interrupted. The degree of these symptoms differs from patient to patient but is also depending on type of drug, dose, way of administration, combination with other drugs, and duration of the treatment. It is not clear whether nausea is caused by mucosal irritation, disordered motility in the gastrointestinal tract, or a direct effect on the central nervous system. The consequence of nausea and vomiting is not only discomfort, but they are also negative factors for energy intake, nutritional status, and fluid/electrolyte balance. The vomiting can appear within 24 h or later but usually during the first 1–2 h after treatment. Vomiting can also be conditioned which is experienced in 20–60 % of patients when they merely think of their treatment or even when they see the hospital building.

Muscle and nerve symptoms. Weakness, fatigue, or tenderness of muscles may occur. Other symptoms are burning sensations in hands and feet, spasms, disordered fine motility, and disordered body balance.

Alopecia. Many patients worry about this, but nowadays it is uncommon in patients treated with adjuvant or neoadjuvant chemotherapy for rectal cancer.

Dermatological problems. These are not common among chemotherapeutic regimens used for rectal cancer. Palmar and plantar erythema or pathological changes of the nails are reported to occur in 1/100–1/1,000 of treated patients but may be more frequent.

Stomatitis. The cells comprising the mucous membranes are highly proliferating and thus sensitive to chemotherapy. Consequently, symptoms from the mouth or the pharynx are very common overall (30–60 %) in connection with chemotherapy but are uncommon in patients treated for rectal cancer

Diarrhoea. This is a common symptom in patients on chemotherapy for rectal cancer but can also be caused by irradiation. Treatment with fluorouracil is often associated with diarrhoea. It can be treated effectively with drugs containing diphenoxylate.

Bone marrow toxicity. The myelosuppressive effect is a major risk factor for septic manifestations and may be life threatening, but fortunately it occurs very seldom. Laboratory tests reveal granulocytopenia, thrombocytopenia, and anaemia. As the life time of granulocytes is limited to hours/days and thrombocytes to days/week, the granulocytopenia is noted before the thrombocytopenia (9–14 days versus 7–17 days) and the anaemia. Colony-stimulating factors are the current treatment of severe granulocytopenia.

Thromboembolic disease. There is an increased risk for pulmonary embolism by both fluorouracil and oxaliplatin (1/10–1/100 of treated patients).

Other manifestations. Complications from the heart, lung, blood vessels, kidneys, and liver are not often seen in connection with chemotherapy for rectal cancer.

Severity of Side Effects

The National Cancer Institute of Canada (NCIC) has published a detailed Common Toxicity Criteria in order to score side effects from 0 to 4, where grades 3 and 4 are associated with a substantial symptomatic load [10]. Some examples relevant for chemotherapy in rectal cancer are shown in Table 15.1.

According to another classification, neurological side effects are graded as 1–2 for sensory and grades 3–4 for motor manifestations.

Measures to Prevent or Treat Nausea/Vomiting and Stomatitis

Nausea and vomiting shall be prevented. Most effective prevention and treatment is obtained by various modifications of 5-HT$_3$ receptor blockers. Sometimes merely changes of eating habits are of great value. Relaxing measures can reduce nausea and vomiting particularly in patients where the symptoms are conditioned. Acupressure and acupuncture have also been reported to be beneficial. Careful hygiene of the oral cavity, e.g. by regular rinsing, is of value to prevent stomatitis. Cryotherapy during 30 min before chemotherapy is reported to decrease the mucositis.

Table 15.1 Grading of severity of side effects associated with chemotherapy according to NCIC 2.0

Fatigue

0 None
1 Increased but not altering normal activities
2 Moderate, difficulty performing some activities
3 Severe, cannot perform some activities
4 Bedridden or disabling

Nausea

0 None
1 Able to eat
2 Oral intake significantly decreased
3 No significant intake, intravenous nutrition
4 –

Vomiting

0 None
1 1/day
2 2–5/day
3 ≥6/day
4 Requiring parenteral nutrition or intensive care

Stomatitis

0 None
1 Painless erythema
2 Painful erythema or ulcers but can eat
3 Requiring intravenous hydration
4 Requiring parenteral or enteral nutrition

Diarrhoea

0 None
1 1–3/day
2 4–6/day
3 >6/day
4 Requiring intensive care

Constipation

0 None
1 Requiring stool softener
2 Requiring laxatives
3 Requiring enema
4 Obstruction or toxic megacolon

Dermatological manifestations

0 None
1 Redness
2 Ulcerations/blisters, pain
3 Extensive ulcerations/blisters
4 Generalised exfoliative or ulcerative dermatitis

Neuropathy, sensory

0 None
1 Paraesthesia or loss of tendon reflexes
2 Objective sensory loss or paraesthesia interfering with function

(continued)

Table 15.1   (continued)

3	Sensory loss or paraesthesia interfering with daily living
4	Permanent sensory loss interfering with function
Neuropathy, motor	
0	Normal
1	Subjective weakness
2	Mild objective weakness
3	Objective weakness interfering with daily living
4	Paralysis

Adjuvant and Chemotherapeutic Agents in Rectal Cancer

Fluorouracil. Fluorouracil is a common cause of nausea and vomiting (1/10–1/100 of treated patients). This drug can also cause cerebral ataxia (1/10–1/100), confusion or nystagmus (1/1,000–1/10,000). It is stated that alopecia occurs after treatment with fluorouracil in 1/10–1/100 patients. Fluorouracil causes stomatitis in 40–60 % (1/10–1/100) which often is the first sign of toxicity, and it will cause leucopenia quite often (1/10–1/100). It is sometimes associated with changes in ECG (1/10–1/100) but more seldom with arrhythmia and coronary angina (1/100–1/1,000) or heart failure/myocardial infarction (1/1,000–1/10,000). Increased secretion of tears, pathological visual changes, or hypersensitivity for light is reported after treatment with fluorouracil (1/1,000–1/10,000).

Fluorouracil has been used extensively for adjuvant chemotherapy, but the treatment-associated mortality is less than 1 %.

Capecitabine

Capecitabine is converted into the active drug in tumours containing thymidine phosphorylase and should therefore be less toxic than 5-FU. Consequently, the safety profile is improved compared with 5-FU regimens. Most common side effects are gastrointestinal symptoms, fatigue, and hand-foot syndrome, but they are significantly less than for 5-FU. Very rare side effects are stenosis of the lacrimal duct and liver failure (1/1,000–1/10,000).

Oxaliplatin. The most frequent side effects associated with oxaliplatin are symptoms from the gastrointestinal tract, but also haematologic and neurological side effects are common. Oxaliplatin is often associated with nausea and vomiting (>1/10). Neurological side effects have been reported in up to 95 % of the patients. The complications include sensory perineuritis characterised by dysaesthesia/paraesthesia with or without muscle spasm triggered by cold. The neurological manifestations are most important as they are restricting the dose. After the treatment is completed, about 90 % of the patients are free from neurological symptoms, and after 3 years only about 3 % have moderate or severe paraesthesia. Treatment with oxaliplatin is very often associated with fatigue, peripheral sensory neuropathy, hypoaesthesia, disordered sense of taste, headache, and back pain (>1/10). Other common symptoms are neuritis in motoric nerves, dizziness, insomnia, dysuria, and conjunctivitis (1/10–1/100). Oxaliplatin treatment often causes exfoliation (hand-foot syndrome). A less common side effect is intestinal obstruction (1/100–1/1,000). Oxaliplatin is rarely associated with colitis or diarrhoea caused by *Clostridium difficile* (1/1,000–10,000). It is a common cause of disturbed electrolyte concentrations in plasma and of allergic reactions (>1/10). Sometimes it is associated with arthralgia (1/10–1/100).

Various side effects caused by oxaliplatin are not severe. All grades of nausea have been reported to occur in 73.7 % of the patients, but only 5.1 % are grades 3–4. Vomiting occurs in 47.2 % of the patients, but only 5.8 % are grades 3–4. Stomatitis is seen in 42.1 and 2.9 %, respectively. Sepsis in connection with neutropenia occurs in 1.1 and 1.0 %, respectively.

Oxaliplatin is used extensively for adjuvant/neoadjuvant chemotherapy, but like fluorouracil the treatment-associated mortality is less than 1 %.

Chemoradiation

This is most often used preoperatively in selected patients when the imaging shows a suspected T3–T4 cancer or a suspected stage III cancer.

Chemotherapeutic agents serve as radiosensitisers to enhance the radiation therapy but also to target any occult metastases.

Side effects are more common after chemoradiation than after radiotherapy alone, both in the neoadjuvant/preoperative and in the adjuvant/postoperative setting. The morbidity in the gastrointestinal tract is increased from 5–10 % to 20–50 % [11]. Chronic proctitis is more common after chemoradiation than after radiotherapy. A recent study reported that perineal wound complications after abdominoperineal resection were diagnosed in 16.2 % without chemoradiation and in 20.6 % in patients who received neoadjuvant chemoradiation. That difference did, however, not reach statistical significance. Partly contradictory results have been reported regarding the effect of chemoradiation on anorectal function, but the addition of chemotherapeutic agents does not seem to increase the morbidity caused by radiotherapy and surgery. Preoperative chemoradiation is better tolerated than postoperative chemoradiation – grade 3–4 toxicity is about 25 % against 40 % [12].

There are still only few reports of late side effects after chemoradiation, but as the irradiation doses are about 50 Gy and chemotherapeutic agents are added, one can expect an increased frequency in comparison with radiotherapy alone. In a recent study, the early toxicity was higher in the chemoradiation group than in the group having only radiotherapy before surgery (18.2 % versus 3.2 %). However, toxicity after a median follow-up of 48 months was not increased – 28.3 and 27.0 %, respectively [13]. Several studies have shown that postoperative mortality is not increased in modern series of chemoradiation.

Elderly Patients

The current median age is about 72 years when the diagnosis of rectal cancer is made. Ageing involves a gradual reduction of physiologic reserves, absorption, metabolism, and elimination, which may lead to impaired pharmacological effects and increased toxicity. Furthermore, there is often an increase in comorbidity among elderly patients.

A serious concern is, however, that most trials have not included elderly patients; the majority has been below 65 years. Therefore, meta-analyses and pooled analyses have been done in an attempt to address the effectiveness and toxicity of neoadjuvant and adjuvant therapy in elderly patients. Adjuvant therapy with fluorouracil-based regimens has been compared with no adjuvant chemotherapy in over 3,000 patients operated on for colon cancer. The side effects were the same in younger and elderly patients, but there was a trend towards a higher incidence of leucopenia among the elderly. However, only 0.7 % of the patients who participated in the seven randomised trials were over the age of 80 [14]. Other studies have confirmed that elderly people who are fit enough for participation in the studies are as likely to tolerate and benefit from adjuvant chemotherapy as younger patients.

Studies have also shown that capecitabine is as least as effective as 5-FU in patients older than 70 years without any increase in toxicity [15]. But it should be used with caution in elderly patients with renal insufficiency and in those using anticoagulants because of the risk for bleeding.

Oxaliplatin is more toxic in elderly than in younger patients regarding haematologic toxicity, but there has been no difference between elderly and younger patients in treatment-associated mortality or neuropathy. Age per se is therefore not a limiting factor for using oxaliplatin and fluorouracil/capecitabine as adjuvant therapy. But as with fluorouracil/capecitabine, the documentation is weak for treating patients older than 80 years with oxaliplatin.

Fifty percent of the patients are older than 72 years when a rectal cancer is diagnosed. Scientific studies reported until now do not support that there is an increased toxicity or lack of benefit in the elderly, but to be included in those trials, the patients had to be in good condition both physically and mentally. Furthermore, as mentioned before, the documentation is weak for patients older than 80 years. Performance and functional status as well as comorbidity – compensated or not – should be more important for the decision of offering adjuvant chemotherapy than age alone.

References

1. Sanoff HK, McLeod HL. Predictive factors for response and toxicity in chemotherapy: pharmacogenomics. Semin Colon Rectal Surg. 2008;19:226–30.
2. Pettersson D, Cedermark B, Holm T, Radu C, Påhlman L, Glimelius B, Martling A. Interim analysis of the Stockholm III trial of preoperative radiotherapy regimens for rectal cancer. Br J Surg. 2010;97:580–7.
3. Swedish Rectal Cancer Trial. Preoperative irradiation followed by surgery vs surgery alone in resectable rectal carcinoma – postoperative morbidity and mortality in a Swedish multicenter trial. Br J Surg. 1993;80:1333–6.
4. Marijnen CAM, Kapiteijn E, van de Velde CJ, Martijn H, Steup WH, Wiggers T, Kranenberg EK, Leer JW. Acute side effects and complications after short-term preoperative radiotherapy combined with total mesorectal excision in primary rectal cancer: report of a multicenter randomized trial. J Clin Oncol. 2002;3:817–25.
5. Lim YK, Law WL, Liu R, Poon JTC, Fan JFM, Lo SH. Impact of neoadjuvant treatment on total mesorectal excision for ultra-low rectal cancers. World J Surg Oncol. 2010;8:23.
6. Pollack J, Holm T, Cedermark B, Altman D, Holmström B, Glimelius B, Mellgren A. Late adverse effects of short-course preoperative radiotherapy in rectal cancer. Br J Surg. 2006;93:1519–25.
7. Birgisson H, Påhlman L, Gunnarsson U, Glimelius B. Adverse effects of preoperative radiation therapy for rectal cancer: long-term follow-up of the Swedish rectal cancer trial. J Clin Oncol. 2005;23:8697–705.
8. Marijnen CA, van de Velde CJ, Putter H, van den Brink M, Maas CP, Martijn H, Rutten HJ, Wiggers T, Kranenberg EK, Leer JW, Stiggelbout AM. Impact of short-term preoperative radiotherapy on health-related quality of life and sexual functioning in primary rectal cancer: report of a multicenter randomized trial. J Clin Oncol. 2005;23:1847–58.
9. Colorectal Cancer Collaborative Group. Adjuvant radiotherapy for rectal cancer: a systematic overview of 8507 patients from 22 randomised trials. Lancet. 2001;358:1291–304.
10. Cancer Therapy Evaluation Program. Common toxicity criteria, version 2.0. DCTD, NCI, NIH, DHHS, March 1998. http://www.redjournal.org/article/S0360-3016(99)00559-3/abstract.
11. Krook JE, Moertel CG, Gunderson LL, Wieand HS, Collins RT, Beart DL, Collins RT, Beart RW, Kubista TP, Poon MA, Meyers WC, Maillard JA. Effective surgical adjuvant therapy for high-risk rectal cancer. N Engl J Med. 1991;324:709–15.
12. Sauer R, Becker H, Hohenberger W, Rödel C, Wittekind C, Fietkau R, Martus P, Tschmelitsch J, Hager E, Hess C, Karstens J, Liersch T, Schmidberger H, Raab R, German Rectal Cancer Study Group. Preoperative versus postoperative chemoradiotherapy for rectal cancer. N Engl J Med. 2004;351:1731–40.
13. Bujko K, Nowacki MP, Nasierowska-Guttmejer A, Michalski W, Bebenek M, Kryj M, Polish Colorectal Study Group. Long-term results of a randomized trial comparing preoperative short-course radiotherapy with preoperative conventionally fractionated chemoradiation for rectal cancer. Br J Surg. 2006;93:1215–23.
14. Goldberg RM, Tabah-Fisch I, Bleiberg H, de Gramont A, Tournigand C, Andre T, Rothenberg ML, Green E, Sargent DJ. Pooled analysis of safety and efficacy of oxaliplatin plus fluorouracil/leucovorin administered bimonthly in elderly patients with colorectal cancer. J Clin Oncol. 2008;26:1443–51.
15. Power DG, Lichtman SM. Adjuvant and palliative chemotherapy for colon cancer in the elderly patient. Semin Colon Rectal Surg. 2008;19:239–46.

Chemo-Radiotherapy for Locally Advanced T3/T4 Rectal Cancer: What Should We Do with Complete Responders?

16

Robert Glynne-Jones and Rob Hughes

Abstract

A proportion of patients, who receive preoperative chemoradiation (CRT) for locally advanced (cT3, cT4, NX) rectal cancer, achieve a pathological complete response (pCR). Less frequently a complete clinical response (cCR) is observed prior to surgery. So support is growing for the concept of 'waiting to see' and *not* proceeding to radical surgery if a cCR is observed – particularly when a permanent stoma is planned. We aimed to evaluate how often cCR is achieved following CRT, the concordance with pCR and the outcome, if patients who achieve cCR are observed rather than proceed to radical surgery. The rationale and outcome of non-radical surgical approaches are discussed.

It remains uncertain whether the degree of response to chemoradiation in terms of cCR or pCR is a useful clinical endpoint. cCR is inconsistently defined and insufficiently robust with only partial concordance with pCR. Studies, which include T3 rectal cancer, are associated with high local recurrence rates after nonsurgical treatment. Few studies report long-term outcome after achievement of a cCR.

The rationale of a 'wait-and-see policy' relies on retrospective observations which do not support this policy as routine except in patients who are recognised to be unfit for or refuse radical surgery. The strategy of examining the histology of a local excision merits further investigation. We would therefore encourage careful observational studies in this setting.

R. Glynne-Jones, FRCR (✉) • R. Hughes, FRCR
Department of Radiotherapy, Centre for Cancer
Treatment, Mount Vernon Hospital,
Northwood, Middlesex, UK
e-mail: rob.glynnejones@nhs.net;
robert.hughes@nhs.net

G. Baatrup (ed.), *Multidisciplinary Treatment of Colorectal Cancer*,
DOI 10.1007/978-3-319-06142-9_16, © Springer International Publishing Switzerland 2015

Introduction

Rectal cancer is a common malignancy. The combination of preoperative radiotherapy and surgery in the form of total mesorectal excision (TME) has reduced the risk of local recurrence to less than 10 % [1, 2]. The ability to control local disease with radiotherapy and surgery comes at a considerable risk of long-term complications in terms of bowel, urinary and sexual function [3, 4]. Furthermore treatment is associated with an overall mortality of 2 %. The risk is especially high in the elderly, where the mortality following major surgery has been demonstrated in the Dutch TME study to be almost one third of those over 80 years, within 6 months [5]. There is also a high psychological morbidity and dissatisfaction with a permanent stoma, when this is required – particularly in southern Europe.

The improvements in local disease control do not seem to have led to improvements in overall survival, with the development of metastases appearing to be relatively independent of local treatment, as recent clinical trials demonstrate that 25–40 % of patients with resectable disease develop metastases despite increasingly low rates of local recurrence.

Pathological complete response (pCR) – i.e. where no residual viable tumour cells are found in the resected specimen – is a not infrequent observation following chemoradiation. Rates of 13–30 % pCR have been reported in phase II and phase III trials following 5FU-based preoperative CRT. A review of 3157 patients from 77 phase II and phase III trials showed an overall pCR rate in these studies was 13.5 % [6]. It is questionable whether these patients receive any benefit from surgical resection. So, when a surgeon performs an APER for low rectal cancer after CRT, and the pathologist tells us in our multidisciplinary meeting that there is no tumour in the specimen, a sense of failure prevails – why could we not have recognised this excellent response and avoided the mutilating surgery? The paradigm of squamous cell cancer of the anus is often cited, where chemoradiation has become the prime modality.

Over 35 years ago, Rider questioned the need in all cases of rectal cancer for surgery [7].

Hence, others previously have called for a nonoperative approach in patients who have a complete clinical response – particularly in early tumours [8, 9]. This strategy is supported by nonoperative series from Canada [10] and has been recently examined in a detailed review [11].

Patients, who obtain excellent symptomatic benefit during CRT, also often question the need to proceed with surgical resection.

The unease engendered by the above thoughts has been focussed by the results of Angelita Habr-Gama in Brazil, who showed that about a third of patients treated with chemoradiation, who achieved a clinical complete response, if appropriately assessed and watched carefully, could avoid major surgery and have the same long-term outcome as a similar group treated with surgery, who had achieved a pathological complete response [12]. Subsequent data from the same authors confirmed that patients, who recurred relapse endoluminally and could be surgically salvaged [13]. For these reasons, interest in nonsurgical management as an alternative to an abdominoperineal resection (APER) is rising, and many countries in Europe including Denmark and the United Kingdom have sponsored 'wait-and-see' registries and clinical studies to define the possibilities more carefully. However, in the United Kingdom, a recent questionnaire sent to members of the Association of Coloproctology could not obtain a consensus on how to define a complete response, and there was a marked resistance and anxiety in offering nonoperative treatment to patients fit for curative surgery [14].

Many remain sceptical of the watch-and-wait approach [15–17]. They argue that many in these series are selected early cases and not locally advanced T3/T4 defined by MRI. The difficulties of accurate prediction of complete pathological response also limit the use of clinical response alone as an end point for determining future management. In addition, several small observational studies show that complete pathological response (ypT0) in the primary tumour only partially correlates with sterilisation of microscopic disease within the pelvic lymph nodes [18–23]; therefore, 15–25 % of patients may still have positive lymph nodes leading to the potential of regional local or pelvic relapse. Other shortcomings of these series include opaque methods of selection of suitable patients and poorly defined follow-up programmes.

The aim of this short chapter is to examine the current evidence for a 'wait-and-see' nonsurgical approach and examine future possibilities.

The Evidence

What Is the Evidence for a Watch-and-wait approach?

A 'watch-and-wait approach' is not a laissez-faire strategy but represents a positive decision to delay or avoid a potentially curative resection. The original Habr-Gama series [24] reported 118 patients with potentially resectable low rectal cancer, who received preoperative chemoradiation (50.4 Gy combined with 5FU and folinic acid for three consecutive days on the first and last 3 days of radiotherapy). In this retrospective study, a total of 36/118 (30 %) achieved a clinical complete response. When 6 of these proceeded to surgery, there was no residual tumour found in the surgical specimen. This complete clinical response was confirmed in the remaining 30 patients by clinical examination, pelvic CT, transrectal ultrasound and finally by a negative biopsy. These 30 patients did not proceed to radical surgery. In this series 8/30 (27 %) eventually failed locally and proceeded to a salvage resection within 3–14 months of the completion of radiation. The outcome in terms of local recurrence and survival was found to be similar for those achieving cCR and entering into surveillance compared to patients found at surgery to have achieved a pCR. In an abstract updating this preliminary data [25] with a total of 201 patients, 64 (32 %) achieved a cCR. Of these, 11 proceeded to have a pCR at surgery, and 10 patients who were initially considered as complete responders relapsed locally 3–14 months later.

In a subsequent paper [12], 71/265 patients (27 %) with a complete clinical response at 8 weeks are described. All these patients were observed rather than proceeding to radical sur-gery. With a mean follow-up of 57.3 months, only three patients (2.8 %) are reported to have suffered an endoluminal recurrence and three had developed systemic metastases. Unfortunately, there is no description in this report of patients requiring surgery between 8 weeks and 14 months.

Habr-Gama's next updated experience with longer follow-up relates to these 71 selected patients who continued to maintain complete clinical response after 14 months [13]. The paper describes a meticulous follow-up protocol where patients were followed on a monthly basis and closely observed without submitting them to radical surgery. The presence of an obvious clinical tumour, a significant ulcer or a positive biopsy following chemoradiation was considered an incomplete response. The paper specifically states that only patients with a sustained complete tumour response at 12 months were considered as complete clinical responders and were managed by observation and not surgery. In the 71 patients who maintained a complete clinical response at 14 months, with a median follow-up of almost 5 years, there are no deaths due to rectal cancer, and only three patients have relapsed locally.

A further paper [26] discusses a total of 360 clinically staged T2–T4 patients treated with chemoradiation of whom 99 (27.5 %) achieved a cCR (patients again had to sustain a cCR for a year). Overall recurrence rates were similar for complete and incomplete responders (11 % for cCR and 12.5 % for incomplete responders): 5-year survival rates were lower for the resected patients ($p = 0.42$) – but not significantly so. Only six local recurrences were reported in the surveillance arm. The authors comment that local recurrences in this series were always endoluminal and hence amenable to surgical salvage. The fact that all the recurrences were endoluminal suggests that the initial tumours in the cCR group were node negative and potentially lower stage and of smaller size. This hypothesis would also account for the slightly better survival in the cCR group.

Finally, a further paper [27] describes 361 patients of whom 122 were considered to have a cCR at the first assessment, but only 99 sustained cCR at 12 months (27.4 %). The 23 patients who recurred early are excluded from the study. In patients with sustained cCR, all recurrences were endoluminal and surgically salvageable – there were no pelvic recurrences.

The outcome of the 23 patients who did not achieve a sustained clinical response to 12 months has been reported [28]. These patients had an interval to surgery of 48 weeks (±0.4 weeks). Disease recurred in 8/23 (35 %), with a 5-year DFS of 51.6 % and overall survival of 84.9 %. Compared to patients who proceeded to surgery within 12 weeks of CRT, those with delayed surgery had significantly earlier pathological disease and less lymph node metastases. Without being able to compare the original clinical staging in this group, it's difficult to assess whether the 23 patients were disadvantaged by a watch-and-wait approach.

Defining Pathological Complete Response

Pathological complete response (pCR) after chemoradiation is defined as ypT0N0. A recent long-term analysis of data in 566 patients achieving a pCR [29, 30] showed that patients with pCR have a favourable prognosis with 5-year rates of disease-free and overall survival of 85 and 92 %. This study did not compare outcome with a control group of patients who had residual disease after chemoradiation. A more recent pooled analysis showed prognosis is significantly better for those achieving pCR than in a control group of 2,621 patients without pCR. This study demonstrated a pCR prevalence of 16 % [30]. Patients with pCR had clinically smaller T1 and T2 tumours significantly more often than patients with residual disease post-chemoradiation ((10 % vs. 4 %), $p < 0.0001$). Additionally only 0.88 % of patients with complete pathological response within the primary had positive involved nodes at pathological examination. In contrast in smaller single-centre studies, regional nodes have been found in 7–17 % of patients who achieve pCR in the primary tumour, i.e. ypT0N1 [23, 31]. This

observation may represent differences in initial tumour staging or potential differences in radiotherapy field sizes.

Defining Complete Clinical Response

The definition of cCR is poorly described and inconsistent. Studies have evaluated clinical response according to World Health Organisation (WHO) criteria [32–36] using the same diagnostic tool, which categorised initial clinical stage prior to CRT [37] or CT-based assessment alone [38]. Most studies categorised cCR as patients with no detectable tumour present on clinical examination [39] or clinical examination and endoscopy [40]. Only one group used an independent radiologist who was blinded to subsequent outcome [35, 41]. Some authors required both a clinical absence of tumour and a negative biopsy [12, 42]. Yet, digital rectal examination (DRE) is only able to identify a small proportion of patients who actually achieve a pCR [43], and only about 25–50 % of patients achieving a cCR are confirmed as a pCR at subsequent surgery [44]. In a pooled analysis, clinical complete response was associated with pCR in only 30 % of cases [45]. Some studies [46, 47], which describe a high rate of cCR, are misleading in that they define cCR as cases where no histological residual disease or only microscopic foci could be found in the resected specimen.

Can We Predict Pathological Complete Response?

Many biological factors have been evaluated as potential predictors of pCR and long-term outcome, including p53, epidermal growth factor receptor (EGFR), Ki-67, p21 and Bax/bcl-2, VEGF and apoptotic index. Microarray studies of genetic profiles and gene signatures [48] have been compared between responding and nonresponding tumours. Although these studies are hypothesis generating, their results are derived from small sample sizes, and the results need to be interpreted with caution. To date, there are no robust methods of predicting pCR prior to treatment.

How Could cCR Be Confirmed as a pCR?

Non-invasive functional imaging can assess response without increasing the morbidity for the patient prior to surgery and might identify patients where surgery can be omitted or to allow minimally invasive surgery. Change in 18FDG uptake, using the standardised uptake value (SUV), appears to predict outcome [29, 49], and one study showed that change in SUV max at 2 weeks into treatment could predict ultimate response [50]. An alternative method is diffusion-weighted MRI (DW-MRI) [51], which detects molecular diffusion, i.e. Brownian motion of water molecules [52]. However, the sensitivity and specificity to differentiate between persistent disease in the primary tumour and posttreatment tissue fibrosis or inflammation remain uncertain. It seems more likely that these techniques will identify nonresponding patients early on during treatment more easily than complete responders.

Radiotherapy as Definitive Treatment

The use of radiotherapy as a definitive treatment is not novel and was used extensively in the 1920s. The evidence for this approach is based on observational series of endocavitry, local contact therapy or brachytherapy either alone or in combination with external beam radiotherapy in selected patients with early cancers [53]. External beam radiotherapy alone has been successfully used in patients unsuitable for radical surgery [10], but the dose is limited by the tolerance of structures such as the bladder and small bowel. The curative use of radiotherapy as a sole modality of treatment has been usually confined to specialists with considerable expertise [54].

The unique data from Habr-Gama is not entirely consistent between the three reports as regards the time points (e.g. 8 weeks, 12 months or 14 months) for assessment and the number of patients subsequently failing. In addition, these excellent results have not been duplicated in any other unit. The data is consistent in that approximately 27 % of each series achieve a cCR. The strength of the Habr-Gama data lies in the rigorous initial selection of patients suitable for a watch-and-wait approach – i.e. low tumours which would require APER; the meticulous methods of defining cCR by clinical, endoscopic, radiological and metabolic imaging confirmed histologically with a local excision of residual thickening; and the painstaking intensive follow-up over the first year in order to confirm a sustained cCR. The latter in particular may explain the finding that all local recurrences were endoluminal and amenable to surgical salvage.

Only 7 other studies were found in which patients with clinically staged tumours were treated with radiotherapy/chemoradiation alone and did not routinely proceed to surgery. In contrast to Habr-Gama, these studies treated unselected patients who were usually unfit for or refused surgery. The results of these studies are shown in Table 16.1. These studies in general used lower doses of radiotherapy, often represent more advanced cases and had less rigorous follow-up. The studies, which included cT1 and T2 patients, fare much better in terms of local control (Table 16.1).

The shortcomings of these series are that patients in the Habr-Gama series were clinically staged without MRI and often without TRUS. It is stated that 20 % were clinically staged as T2N0. Many others are likely to have been small tumours as the median size of the patients who failed to achieve cCR was only 4 cm. One could speculate that this approach is more suitable for small cT2 tumours – as in the recent ACCORD study where pCR was common in cT2 patients (Table 16.2). In addition, most published studies have up to 10 % of patients lost to follow-up. The Habr-Gama series does not appear to have any patients lost to follow-up. Also the original denominator – i.e. how many patients after completion of chemoradiation at 6 weeks achieve a complete clinical response – remains unclear.

Table 16.1 Patients with clinically staged T2/T3 tumours treated with radiotherapy/chemoradiation who did not proceed to surgery – long-term outcome of a wait-and-see policy

Authors	No. of pts	RT dose Gy/fractions/ days	T2	Chemo	Procedure	cCR	No failing	Local failure
Habr-Gama et al. [24]	118	50.4/28/38	Yes	Bolus FUFA	No surgery	32 %	8/30 27 %	Not fully stated
Rossi et al. [55]	16	50.4/28/38 + 30Gy b	Not stated	FUFA	No surgery	6/16 38 %	5/6 83 %	5/6 83 %
Birnbaum et al. [56]	72	45/25/33 + 30Gy brachy	Yes	No chemo	No surgery	Not stated	26/72 36 %	26/72 36 %
Nagakawa et al. [57]	52	45–50.4/28/38	No	FUFA	No surgery	19 %	Not stated	Not fully stated
Gerard et al. [58]	29	70 contact + 39/13/17 EBRT	Yes T1–3	No chemo	No surgery	Not stated	8/29 28 %	8/29 28 %
Gerard et al. [54]	63	80 contact + 39/13/17 EBRT	Yes T2/3	No chemo	No surgery	58/63 92 %	17/63 16 %	37 %
Habr-Gama et al. [13]	260	50.4/28/38	Yes 20 %	FUFA	No surgery	71/260 28 %	5/70 7 %	4.2 %
Wang et al. [10]	271	40–52/20	Yes	No chemo	No surgery	80/271 30 %	Not stated	78 %
Lim et al. [59]	48	Variable, mean 50Gy/25 fractions	Yes T1 and T2 (33 %)	PVI 5FU 92 %	No surgery	56 %	18/48 37 %	11/48 23 %
Hughes et al. [15]	58	45Gy/25/33	No 50 % T4	FUFA	No surgery	10/58 17 %	6/10 60 %	6/10 60 %

Table 16.2 ACCORD-12 PRODIGE trial: percentage of ypCR according to clinical T stage in both arms [60]

	T2 (%)	T3 (%)	T4 (%)
CAPOX 50Gy	47	18	13
CAP 45Gy	33	13	7

The use of a delayed time point, for assessing response, loses important information on those patients, who relapse within the first year. Unless we have definitive information on the downside of this approach in terms of those patients who have an initial complete clinical response, who then recur locally within the first year or subsequently develop metastatic disease, it is not possible to assess the validity of the watch-and-wait approach.

What Are the Risks to Wait and See?

Recurrent rectal cancer is often a diffuse pelvic process, particularly following radiotherapy, and is often associated with metastatic disease. For these reasons, local recurrence is rarely surgically salvaged and is associated with poor outcomes particularly after preoperative radiotherapy [61]. Patients risk being left with very difficult to manage pelvic symptoms, which can be very challenging to palliate adequately.

In the Habr-Gama series [28], patients with apparent cCR where a delay in surgery was instituted did not appear to experience a negative impact regarding survival. In the original Habr-Gama data, only 2 patients developed a local pelvic relapse. When further updated in 2005 and 2006 with an additional 28 patients (i.e. 99 patients) being identified as having had a cCR (99/360), only 3 more local relapses were identified. However, this finding is not necessarily extrapolated to locally advanced T3/T4 tumours where up to 70 % are node positive.

Sterilisation of Pelvic Lymph Nodes

The second major concern regarding chemoradiotherapy as a definitive treatment especially in locally advanced disease is the ability of chemoradiotherapy to adequately sterilise the pelvic lymph nodes. Residual viable disease within the lymph nodes leaves a potential source of pelvic relapse. Chemoradiotherapy does result in the downstaging of pelvic lymph node disease in locally advanced disease; however, the concordance between the eradication of disease within the primary and within the lymph nodes is not absolute with some patients appearing to have obtained pathological complete responses within the primary but not in the lymph nodes. Pelvic residual disease is obviously more likely in advanced lesions where CRT is administered for a bulky tumour which threatens the CRM than a small T1/T2 tumour [62]. Tumours which are clinically and radiologically node negative are more likely to achieve a pCR [63].

The difficulty in predicting the status of pelvic lymph nodes remains a major issue. To date imaging has proved insufficiently accurate. We have 'a chicken or an egg' situation because to date the best method of predicting lymph node status is the clinical and pathological response to radiotherapy and chemoradiation. For this reason, it may be possible to predict retrospectively the initial status of the lymph nodes by the pathological response to chemoradiation in the primary tumour.

Long-Term Follow-up Is Required

Data on long-term outcome of 271 patients with rectal cancer suggest radical external beam radiotherapy is a reasonable management option in rectal carcinoma for patients who are not fit surgical candidates or refuse surgery [10]. However, despite achieving a cCR, the majority of patients in this series eventually failed locally. Habr-Gama's data show recurrences occur late, and this observation is supported by other small series [15]. Hence, small studies with short follow-up do not add to our knowledge of the risks of this approach [64]. Current prospective studies will require a costly long-term follow-up programme of sequential MRIs and PET scans.

Increasing the Rate of Pathological Complete Response

Can we increase the likelihood of patients with rectal cancer achieving a pCR with more aggressive neoadjuvant treatment, such as neoadjuvant chemotherapy, biological agents, higher local radiation doses, more potent cytotoxic radiosensitisers or brachytherapy boosts on the primary tumour? To date these strategies have not been very effective [60, 65, 66]. A different option to increase pCR may be to lengthen the interval between chemoradiation and surgery. Other strategies are to increase the radiation dose to the primary with brachytherapy boost [67]. Habr-Gama recently reported that by extending the duration of the chemotherapy post-chemoradiation, a cCR of 48 % and an overall complete response (i.e. including cCR and pCR) could be increased to an astonishing 65 % [68].

This strategy could potentially be extrapolated to a full course of post-chemoradiation adjuvant chemotherapy using 5FU and oxaliplatin to consolidate the local response and address the potential for distant metastases. However, we are not aware of any randomised studies in this setting.

Retrospective studies reporting a 'watch-and-wait' approach have limitations because they are hampered by the landmark method, which omits important data on outcome for patients who fail in the first year. Habr-Gama attempts to provide information on this group [28]. In 23 such patients failing in the first year, the recurrence rate was 34 %. The authors suggest the outcomes of 5-year OS and DFS rates were 84 and 51.6 %, respectively, and not significantly different to the remaining patients who did not achieve a cCR and proceeded directly to radical surgery. Yet this is a flawed comparison, because the downstaging required to achieve a cCR (even if not sustained for 12 months) should select out a group with a more favourable prognosis.

The Role of Local Excision After Chemoradiation

Local excision and transanal endoscopic microsurgical resection (TEMS) are attractive alternative techniques to radical surgery because of the low morbidity and mortality and better functional outcome. However, the primary curative goal of surgery cannot always be achieved through these techniques, as the pelvic lymph nodes are not resected [69]. The stumbling block for accepting that in fit patients local excision is curative therapy is the challenge of developing and validating selection criteria that identify those patients where local excision alone is safe and does not compromise cure. Surgical series [70] suggest that the likelihood of having microscopic perirectal or mesorectal nodal involvement would be rare in T1 tumours but 10–30 % for T2 tumours and as high as 60 % risk in T3 tumours. For this reason, most surgeons would not accept that T3 tumours can be treated by local excision alone.

Retrospective studies demonstrate that tumours <3 cm in size, which are limited to superficial layers of the muscularis propria and are well or moderately well differentiated (as opposed to poorly differentiated), without lymphovascular invasion or extramural vascular invasion are the most reliable clinical and pathological features whereby the risk of lymph node involvement is predicted to be small and a local excision alone may prove sufficient treatment. Tumours with these characteristics are associated with a low risk of microscopic lymph node involvement and a late local recurrence rate of <10 % provided adequate surgical margins can be achieved. In principle chemoradiotherapy is likely to be more effective and pCR more frequent in such smaller earlier T stage tumours.

Hence, local excision might be a viable treatment option in more advanced tumours if patients are selected for avoidance of radical surgery by their response to preoperative CRT [18]. Following chemoradiation, patients who achieved a clinical good response had the residual tumour resected. With a mean follow-up at 24 months, there were no recurrences in patients who had a complete pathological response. In a similar study but using radiotherapy alone, an Italian group performed transanal endoscopic microsurgery (TEM) on the residual [71]. The local recurrence rate was only 2.85 % with a median follow-up of 38 months (range 24–96). However, few studies accurately document the rate of subsequent local recurrences that are amenable to salvage by AP excision of the rectum [72]. In summary, the advantage of preoperative chemoradiation is that the subsequent histopathology and regression can categorise patients between very high and very low risk.

In a study of 272 patients receiving preoperative chemoradiation [73], there were positive nodes in 1.6 % of ypT0, 6.3 % of ypT1 and 24 % of patients achieving tumour regression grade 2 (TRG2). A pooled analysis showed that after CRT, the local recurrence for patients achieving pCR was only 1 %, for ypT1 8 % and for ypT2 11 %, respectively [74].

The same author has reported an early analysis of a prospective study using short-course radiation in small rectal cancers prior to local excision. The rate of pCR was 41 %, and the strategy appears feasible [75]. A further small randomised study of chemoradiation prior to radical surgery or TEM in a highly selected group of small early tumours suggests that the results of conservative and radical surgery are equivalent if the tumour is downstaged to pCR or ypT1 [76].

Taking the assumption that the characteristics of patients in large randomised studies are likely to be the same in both arms, and that the populations of these studies reflect mainly patients with cT3/T4 stage, there were 33.3 % node-positive patients in the preoperative arm of the NSABP R03 compared with 47.5 % in the postoperative control arm [77]. This nodal sterilisation is almost identical in the POLISH study with 32 % in the preoperative chemoradiation arm versus 48 % in the SCPRT (where the histology will not have changed because insufficient time has elapsed for downstaging), respectively. In the German AIO trial [78], the node positivity was 25 % versus 40 % for the preoperative and postoperative arms. Data from these three trials of preoperative chemoradiation consistently suggest that if patients with cT3/T4 stage are selected, only approximately one third of involved lymph nodes will be sterilised by chemoradiation.

However, clinical nodal status may also impact on the chance of achieving a pCR. In a small retrospective study [63], clinically N0 tumours had a rate high rate of pCR – ($p = 0.02$); in contrast, only 3/33 (9 %) cN1–N2 patients responded with a pCR. So, node-negative patients may be more likely to achieve a pCR.

The most convincing evidence that patients with early stage presumed cN0 can be safely selected for a neoadjuvant, and local excision approach comes from the preliminary results of the ACOSOG Z6041 trial [79]. Patients with ultrasound-defined uT2N0 were treated with capecitabine and oxaliplatin and radiotherapy and local excision. In all, 36/90 achieved a pCR. Only six patients (6 %) had ypT3 tumours, and of the five local excision specimens, which contained lymph nodes, only one (a ypT3 tumour) had a positive node. The exciting results of this highly selected study demonstrated concordance between cCR and pCR in 31 of 36 patients.

So Where Do We Go from Here?

Some have tried to use the available data to develop a decision-analytic model examining the relative benefits of surgery versus observation in rectal cancer patients who achieve clinical complete response after neoadjuvant chemoradiation [80]. It seems unlikely that we can enhance the algorithm by achieving a well-designed noninferiority randomised controlled trial on this question. Randomisation would probably be unacceptable to patients, and the numbers required would prove enormous.

We would therefore encourage careful observational studies in this setting. We are aware of several such studies. There is ongoing observational study at the Royal Marsden 'Avoiding Surgery in Rectal Cancer After Pre-Operative Therapy' (NCT01047969). The primary outcome measures are to estimate the percentage of patients who can safely omit surgery, defined as the percentage of patients at 2 years after end of CRT who have not had surgery and who are in CR (no detectable local disease), and also to prove the safety of deferred surgery, as measured by the percentage of patients who have local failure at 2 years, where local failure is defined as positive margin status of resected tumour or surgically unsalvageable disease. Many including the authors of this chapter feel that 2 years is a very short time frame for accepting the safety of this strategy.

There is also a Danish Colorectal Cancer Group Protocol (clinical trials gov. identification NCT00952926), which is a prospective observational study of patients with rectal cancer after concomitant radiation and chemotherapy. The objectives are to examine frequency of local recurrence at 1, 3 and 5 years after radiation and concomitant chemotherapy without subsequent operation patients with low rectal cancer. The first phase requires 30 patients. This study uses PET/CT as part of the follow-up evaluation.

A third study in the Netherlands (NCT00939666) follows complete responders, and some good responders are treated with a TEM. The United Kingdom in the North of England also has a registration programme run by surgeons. Finally in addition a formal European registry, the European Network for Watchful waiting (ENWW), has been initiated in Denmark – kfe.onk@slb.regionsyddanmark.dk

Conclusion

Controversial management options following CRT – such as a watch-and-wait approach (i.e. the omission of surgery) in case of a complete response, or local excision of the residual – remain experimental. These less invasive treatments have some obvious advantages, such as fewer potential surgical deaths, less morbidity in terms of urinary and faecal incontinence, sexual problems and fewer colostomies than after standard radical total mesorectal excision.

Yet the present limitations in assessing complete response still undermine our confidence in a watch-and-wait approach. Hence, methods to define pCR without resorting to radical surgery warrant further investigation and have been prioritised by the American College of Surgeons. Currently a local excision following chemoradiation is the most promising strategy. A local excision with complete or almost complete histopathological regression in the primary tumour may render radical pelvic surgery unnecessary. Selection of patients with cT2N0 tumours

for this approach is more likely to demonstrate concordance between cCR and pCR than serendipitously observing more locally advanced tumours particularly cT3/T4 with an initial threatened circumferential margin. In addition, the role of additional 'adjuvant' chemotherapy needs to be defined.

However, current and future studies will have to provide definitive evidence about the long-term (at least 7 years) oncological safety and late effects. We may be able to use a smaller scalpel, but it seems unlikely we can throw it away.

References

1. Peeters KC, Marijnen CA, Nagtegaal ID, Dutch Colorectal Cancer Group, et al. The TME Trial after a Median Follow-up of 6 Years: increased local control but no survival benefit in irradiated patients with resectable rectal Carcinoma. Ann Surg. 2007;246(5): 693–701.
2. Sebag-Montefiore D, Stephens RJ, Steele R, et al. Preoperative radiotherapy versus selective postoperative chemoradiotherapy in patients with rectal cancer (MRC CR07 and NCIC-CTG C016): a multicentre, randomised trial. Lancet. 2009;373(9666):811–20.
3. Gervaz PA, Wexner SD, Pemberton JH. Pelvic radiation and anorectal function: introducing the concept of sphincter-preserving radiation therapy. J Am Coll Surg. 2002;195:387–94.
4. Bujko K, Nowacki MP, Nasierowska-Guttmejer A, Polish Colorectal Study Group. Long-term results of a randomized trial comparing preoperative short-course radiotherapy with preoperative conventionally fractionated chemoradiation for rectal cancer. Br J Surg. 2006;93(10):1215–23.
5. Rutten HJ, den Dulk M, Lemmens VE, et al. Controversies of total mesorectal excision for rectal cancer in elderly patients. Lancet Oncol. 2008;9(5): 494–501.
6. Hartley A, Ho K, McConkey C, et al. Pathological complete response following pre-operative chemoradiotherapy in rectal cancer: analysis of phase II/III trials. Br J Radiol. 2005;78:934–8.
7. Rider WD. The 1975 Gordon Richards Memorial Lecture: Is the Miles operation really necessary for the treatment of rectal cancer? J Can Assoc Radiol. 1975;26:167–75.
8. Rich TA. Infusional chemoradiation for operable rectal cancer: post-, pre-, or nonoperative management? Oncology (Williston Park). 1997;11(3):295–300, 305; discussion 306 passim. Review.
9. Rich TA, Gunderson LL. Radical nonoperative management of early rectal cancer. Int J Radiat Oncol Biol Phys. 1995;31(3):677–8.

10. Wang Y, Cummings B, Catton P, et al. Primary radical external beam radiotherapy of rectal adenocarcinoma: long term outcome of 271 patients. Radiother Oncol. 2005;77(2):126–32.

11. Higgins KA, Willett CG, Czito BG. Nonoperative management of rectal cancer: current perspectives. Clin Colorectal Cancer. 2010;9(2):83–8.

12. Habr-Gama A, Perez RO, Nadalin W, et al. Operative versus nonoperative treatment for stage 0 distal rectal cancer following chemoradiation therapy: long term results. Ann Surg. 2004;240:711–71.

13. Habr Gama A, Perez RO, Nadalin W, et al. Long term results of preoperative chemoradiation for distal rectal cancer: correlation between final stage and survival. J Gastrointest Surg. 2005;9:90–101.

14. Wynn GR, Bhasin N, Macklin CP, George ML. Complete clinical response to neoadjuvant chemoradiotherapy in patients with rectal cancer: opinions of British and Irish specialists. Colorectal Dis. 2010; 12(4):327–33.

15. Hughes R, Harrison M, Glynne-Jones R. Could a wait and see policy be justified in T3/4 rectal cancers after chemo-radiotherapy? Acta Oncol. 2010;49(3):378–81.

16. Nyasavajjala SM, Shaw AG, Khan AQ, Brown SR, Lund JN. Neoadjuvant chemo-radiotherapy and rectal cancer: can the UK watch and wait with Brazil? Colorectal Dis. 2010;12(1):33–6. Epub.

17. Dos Santos LV, dos Anjos Jacome AA, Carcano FM, et al. Watch and wait policy remains experimental for the management of rectal cancer. Colorectal Dis. 2010;12:833.

18. Kim CJ, Yeatman TJ, Coppula D, Trotti A, Williams B, Barthel JS, et al. Local excision of T2 and T3 rectal cancers after downstaging chemoradiation. Ann Surg. 2001;234:352–8.

19. Mohiuddin M, Marks G, Bannon J. High dose preoperative radiation full thickness local excision – a new option for selective T3 distal rectal cancer. Int J Radiat Oncol Biol Phys. 1994;30:845–9.

20. Onaitis MW, Noone RB, Fields R, Hurwitz H, Morse M, Jowell P, et al. Complete response to neoadjuvant chemoradiation for rectal cancer does not influence survival. Ann Surg Oncol. 2001;8:801–6.

21. Schell SR, Zlotecki RA, Mendenhall WM, et al. Transanal excision of locally advanced rectal cancers downstaged using neoadjuvant chemoradiotherapy. J Am Coll Surg. 2002;194:584–90.

22. Bonnen M, Crane C, Vauthey JN, et al. Long term results using local excision after preoperative chemoradiation among selected T3 rectal cancer patients. Int J Radiat Oncol Biol Phys. 2004;60:1098–105.

23. Hughes R, Glynne-Jones R, Grainger J, et al. Can pathological complete response in the primary tumour following pre-operative pelvic chemoradiotherapy for T3-T4 rectal cancer predict for sterilisation of pelvic lymph nodes, a low risk of local recurrence and the appropriateness of local excision? Int J Colorectal Dis. 2006;21(1):11–723.

24. Habr-Gama A, de Souza PM, Ribeiro U, et al. Low rectal cancer: impact of radiation and chemotherapy on surgical treatment. Dis Colon Rectum. 1998;41: 1087–96.

25. Habr-Gama A, de Souza PM, Ribeiro U, et al. Multimodality therapy in low rectal cancer: long-term outcome of complete responders. Dis Colon Rectum. 2001;44:A18.

26. Habr-Gama A, Perez RO, Proscurshim I, et al. Patterns of failure and survival for non-operative treatment of stage C0 distal rectal cancer following neoadjuvant chemoradiation therapy. J Gastrointest Surg. 2006;10:1319–29.

27. Habr-Gama A. Assessment and management of the complete clinical response of rectal cancer to chemoradiotherapy. Colorectal Dis. 2006;8 suppl 3:21–4.

28. Habr-Gama A, Perez RO, Proscurshim I, et al. Interval between surgery and neoadjuvant chemoradiation therapy for distal rectal cancer: does delayed surgery have an impact on outcome? Int J Radiat Oncol Biol Phys. 2008;71(4):1181–8.

29. Capirci C, Rubello D, Pasini F, et al. The role of dual-time combined 18-fluorodeoxyglucose positron emission tomography and computed tomography in the staging and restaging workup of locally advanced rectal cancer, treated with preoperative chemoradiation therapy and radical surgery. Int J Radiat Oncol Biol Phys. 2009;74(5):1461–9.

30. Maas M, Nelemans PJ, Valentini V, et al. Long-term outcome in patients with a pathological complete response after chemoradiation for rectal cancer. Lancet Oncol. 2010;11(9):835–44.

31. Stipa F, Zernecke A, Moore HG, et al. Residual mesorectal lymph node involvement following neoadjuvant combined-modality therapy: rationale for radical resection? Ann Surg Oncol. 2004;11(2):187–91.

32. De la Torre A, Ramos S, Valcarcel VJ, et al. Phase II study of radiochemotherapy with UFT and low dose oral leucovorin in patients with unresectable rectal cancer. Int J Radiat Oncol Biol Phys. 1999;45:629–34.

33. Uzcudun AE, Batlle JF, Velasco JF, et al. Efficacy of preoperative radiation therapy for respectable rectal adenocarcinoma when combined with oral tegafururacil modulated with leucovorin. Dis Colon Rectum. 2002;45:1349–58.

34. Ratto C, Valentini V, Morganti AG, et al. Combined modality therapy in locally advanced primary rectal cancer. Dis Colon Rectum. 2003;46:59–67.

35. Chau I, Allen M, Cunningham D, et al. Neoadjuvant systemic fluorouracil and mitomycin C prior to synchronous chemoradiation is an effective strategy in locally advanced rectal cancer. Br J Cancer. 2003;88:1017–24.

36. Gambacorta MA, Valentini V, Morganti AG, et al. Chemoradiation with raltitrexed (tomudex) in preoperative treatment of stage II –III resectable rectal cancer: a phase II study. Int J Radiat Oncol Biol Phys. 2004;60:130–8.

37. De Paoli A, Chiara S, Luppi G, et al. Capecitabine in combination with preoperative radiation therapy in locally advanced, resectable, rectal cancer: a multicentre phase II study. Ann Oncol. 2006;17:246–51.

38. Burke SJ, Percapio BA, Knight DC, Kwasnik EM. Combined preoperative radiation and mitomycin/5-fluorouracil treatment for locally advanced rectal adenocarcinoma. J Am Coll Surg. 1998;187:164–70.
39. Benzoni E, Cerato F, Cojutti A, et al. The predictive value of clinical evaluation of response to neoadjuvant chemoradiation therapy for rectal cancer. Tumori. 2005;91(5):401–5.
40. Zmora O, Dasilva GM, Gurland B, et al. Does rectal wall tumor eradication with preoperative chemoradiation permit a change in the operative strategy? Dis Colon Rectum. 2004;47(10):1607–12.
41. Chau I, Brown G, Cunningham D, et al. Neoadjuvant capecitabine and oxaliplatin followed by synchronous chemoradiation and total mesorectal excision in magnetic resonance imaging –defined poor-risk rectal cancer. J Clin Oncol. 2006;24:668–74.
42. Chari RS, Tyler DS, Anscher MS, et al. Preoperative radiotherapy and chemotherapy in the treatment of adenocarcinoma of the rectum. Ann Surg. 1995;221: 778–87.
43. Guillem J, Chessin D, Shia J, et al. Clinical examination following preoperative chemoradiation for rectal cancer is not a reliable surrogate end point. J Clin Oncol. 2005;23(15):3475–9.
44. Tulchinsky H, Rabau M, Shacham-Shemueli E, et al. Can rectal cancers with pathological T0 after neoadjuvant chemoradiation (ypT0) be treated by transanal excision alone? Ann Surg Oncol. 2005;13:347–52.
45. Glynne-Jones R, Wallace M, Livingstone JL, Meyrick–Thomas J. Complete clinical response after preoperative chemoradiation in rectal cancer: is a "wait and see" policy justified? Dis Colon Rectum. 2008;51(1):10–9.
46. Grann A, Feng C, Wong D, et al. Preoperative combined modality for clinically resectable uT3 rectal adenocarcinoma. Int J Radiat Oncol Biol Phys. 2001;49:987–95.
47. Crane CH, Skibber JM, Birnbaum EH, et al. The addition of continuous infusion 5-FU to preoperative radiation therapy increases tumor response, leading to increased sphincter preservation in locally advanced low rectal cancer. Int J Radiat Oncol Biol Phys. 2003;57:84–9.
48. Kim IL, Lim SB, Kang HC. Microarray gene expression profiling for predicting complete response to preoperative chemoradiotherapy in patients with advanced rectal cancer. Dis Colon Rectum. 2007;50:1342–53.
49. Mak D, Joon DL, Chao M, Wada M, Joon ML, See A, Feigen M, Jenkins P, Mercuri A, McNamara J, Poon A, Khoo V. The use of PET in assessing tumor response after neoadjuvant chemoradiation for rectal cancer. Radiother Oncol. 2010;97(2):205–11.
50. Janssen MH, Ollers MC, van Stiphout RG, et al. Evaluation of early metabolic responses in rectal cancer during combined radiochemotherapy or radiotherapy alone: sequential FDG-PET-CT findings. Radiother Oncol. 2010;94(2):151–5.
51. Patterson DM, Padhani AR, Collins DJ. Technology insight: water diffusion MRI–a potential new biomarker of response to cancer therapy. Nat Clin Pract Oncol. 2008;5(4):220–33.
52. Sun YS, Zhang XP, Tang L, et al. Locally advanced rectal carcinoma treated with preoperative chemotherapy and radiation therapy: preliminary analysis of diffusion-weighted MR imaging for early detection of tumor histopathologic downstaging. Radiology. 2010; 254(1):170–8.
53. Papillon J. Present status of radiation therapy in the conservative management of rectal cancer. Radiother Oncol. 1990;17(4):275–83.
54. Gerard JP, Chapet O, Ramailoli A, et al. Long term control of T2-T3 rectal adenocarcinoma with radiotherapy alone. Int J Radiat Oncol Phys. 2002;54: 142–9.
55. Rossi B, Nakagawa W, Novaes P, et al. Radiation and chemotherapy instead of surgery for low infiltrative rectal adenocarcinoma: a prospective trial. Ann Surg Oncol. 1998;5(2):113–8.
56. Birnbaum EH, Ogunbiyi OA, Gagliardi G, et al. Selection criteria for treatment of rectal cancer with combined external beam and endocavitary radiation. Dis Colon Rectum. 1999;42:727–33.
57. Nakagawa W, Rossi B, de O Ferreira F, Ferrigno R, Filho P, Nishimoto I, Vieira R, Lopes A. Chemoradiation instead of surgery to treat mid and low rectal tumours: is it safe? Ann Surg Oncol. 2002;9(6):568–73.
58. Gerard JP, Ayzac L, Coquard R, et al. Endocavitry irradiation for early rectal carcinomas T1 (T2). A series of 101 patients treated with Papillon's technique. Int J Radiat Biol Phys. 1996;34:775–83.
59. Lim L, Chao M, Shapiro J, et al. Long term outcomes of patients with localized rectal cancer treated with chemoradiation or radiotherapy alone because of medical inoperability or patient refusal. Dis Colon Rectum. 2007;50(12):2032–9.
60. Gérard JP, Azria D, Gourgou-Bourgade S, et al. Comparison of two neoadjuvant chemoradiotherapy regimens for locally advanced rectal cancer: results of the phase III trial ACCORD 12/0405-Prodige 2. J Clin Oncol. 2010;28(10):1638–44.
61. Van den Brink M, Stiggelbout A, van den Hout W, et al. Clinical nature and prognosis of locally recurrent rectal cancer after total mesorectal excision with or without preoperative radiotherapy. J Clin Oncol. 2004;22:3958–64.
62. Steup WH, Moriya Y, van de Velde CJH. Patterns of lymphatic spread in rectal cancer. A topographical analysis on lymph node metastases. Eur J Cancer. 2002;38:911–8.
63. Negri FV, Campanini N, Camisa R, et al. Biological predictive factors in rectal cancer treated with preoperative radiotherapy or radiochemotherapy. Br J Cancer. 2008;98(1):143–7.
64. O'Neill B, Brown G, Heald R, et al. Non-operative treatment after neoadjuvant chemoradiotherapy for rectal cancer. Lancet Oncol. 2007;8:625–33.

65. Aschele C, Pinto C, Rosati G, Luppi G, Bonetti A, Miraglia S, et al. Preoperative (FU)-based chemoradiation with and without weekly oxaliplatin in locally advanced rectal cancer; pathologic response analysis of the Studio Terapia Adjuvante Retto (STAR)-01 randomized phase III trial. J Clin Oncol. 2009;27:18S (part II of II) : 804s (Abstract CRA 4008).

66. Glynne-Jones R, Sebag Montefiore D. Are we ready to use an early alternative end point as the primary end point of a phase III study in rectal cancer? J Clin Oncol. 2010;28(29): e581–2.

67. Gerard JP, Chapet O, Nemoz C, et al. Improved sphincter preservation in low rectal cancer with high-dose preoperative radiotherapy: the lyon R96-02 randomized trial. J Clin Oncol. 2004;22(12):2404–9.

68. Habr-Gama A, Perez RO, Sabbaga J, et al. Increasing the rates of complete response to neoadjuvant chemoradiotherapy for distal rectal cancer: results of a prospective study using additional chemotherapy during the resting period. Dis Colon Rectum. 2009;52(12):1927–34.

69. Garcia-Aguilar J, Mellgren A, Sirivongs P, et al. Local excision of rectal cancer without adjuvant therapy. Ann Surg. 2000;231:345–51.

70. Paty PB, Nash GM, Baron P, et al. Long-term results for the excision of rectal cancer. Ann Surg. 2002; 236:522–30.

71. Lezoche E, Guerrieri M, Paganini M, et al. Long term results of pT2 rectal cancer treated with radiotherapy and transanal endoscopic microsurgical excision. World J Surg. 2002;26:1170–4.

72. Friel C, Cromwell J, Marra C, et al. Salvage radical surgery after failed local excision for early rectal cancer. Dis Colon Rectum. 2002;45:875–9.

73. Coco C, Manno A, Mattana C, et al. The role of local excision in rectal cancer after complete response to neoadjuvant treatment. Surg Oncol. 2007;16 Suppl 1:S101–4.

74. Bujko K, Sopylo R, Kepka L. Local excision after radio(chemo)therapy for rectal cancer: is it safe? Clin Oncol (R Coll Radiol). 2007;19(9):693–700.

75. Bujko K, Richter P, Kołodziejczyk M, Polish Colorectal Study Group, et al. Preoperative radiotherapy and local excision of rectal cancer with immediate radical re-operation for poor responders. Radiother Oncol. 2009;92(2):195–201.

76. Lezoche G, Baldarelli M, Guerrieri M, et al. A prospective randomized study with a 5-year minimum follow-up evaluation of transanal endoscopic microsurgery versus laparoscopic total mesorectal excision after neoadjuvant therapy. Surg Endosc. 2008;22(2): 352–8.

77. Roh MS, Colangelo LH, O'Connell MJ, et al. Preoperative multimodality therapy improves disease-free survival in patients with carcinoma of the rectum: NSABP-R03. J Clin Oncol. 2009;27:5124–30.

78. Sauer R, Becker H, Hohenberger W, German Rectal Cancer Study Group, et al. Preoperative versus postoperative chemoradiotherapy for rectal cancer. N Engl J Med. 2004;351:1731–40.

79. Garcia-Aguilar J, Shi Q, Thomas CR Jr, et al. Pathologic complete response (pCR) to neoadjuvant chemoradiation (CRT) of uT2N0 rectal cancer (RC) treated by local excision (LE): results of the ACOSOG Z6041 trial. J Clin Oncol. 2010;28(15S):part I of II:263s (abstract 3510).

80. Neuman HB, Elkin EB, Guillem JG, Paty PB, Weiser MR, Wong WD, Temple LK. Treatment for patients with rectal cancer and a clinical complete response to neoadjuvant therapy: a decision analysis. Dis Colon Rectum. 2009;52(5):863–71.

Part IV

Imaging and Staging

Introduction: Preoperative Staging by Imaging

17

Regina G.H. Beets-Tan

Abstract

In the recent decade, the role of imaging in local staging of rectal cancer has evolved. Whereas in the past its role has been restricted mainly to endorectal ultrasound, it has recently extended to modern imaging such as CT and MRI. This chapter "imaging and staging" will address the two most frequently used imaging methods in rectal cancer management: endorectal ultrasound (ERUS) and magnetic resonance imaging (MRI). For each, experts in the field will elaborate on how these methods can identify the relevant risk factors for local recurrence and which protocol should be used to ensure a high-quality performance. In this introduction section, a helicopter view is given on the role of each method, ERUS and MRI, in the context of clinical decision making and its role put in perspective of one another. The introduction finalizes with recommendations for use in clinical practice.

The local recurrence rate after rectal cancer surgery has significantly decreased in the past two decades. This is mainly due to the introduction of a total mesorectal excision (TME) surgery. In addition preoperative radiotherapy is now given instead of a postoperative course because trials have shown that preoperative radiotherapy is more effective in reducing the local recurrence rate than postoperative. Therefore, the role of imaging in the staging of these tumors has changed. Whereas previously most decisions on whether or not to give adjuvant treatment were based on the risk assessment for recurrence through histological evaluation of the tumor and the lymph nodes, the decisions on neoadjuvant treatment are now based on risk assessment through imaging. Although modern CT techniques are improving and to some extent able to provide information for locoregional staging, endorectal ultrasonography (ERUS) and MRI are considered as the two best locoregional staging methods for rectal cancer. When comparing ERUS with MRI, there are several issues that require consideration. In addition to the accuracy in predicting certain risk factors for local recurrence, there is the treatment strategy that dictates

R.G.H. Beets-Tan, MD, PhD
Department of Radiology, Maastricht University
Medical Center, Maastricht, The Netherlands
e-mail: r.beets.tan@mumc.nl

what information will have a clinical consequence. Besides, issues of cost, availability, and expertise may influence the local treatment strategy and thus the choice of the imaging method.

The risk factors associated with local recurrence are the T stage, N stage, distance of the tumor to the mesorectal fascia, extramural vascular invasion, perineural invasion, lymph vessel invasion, and histological grade [1, 2]. Of these risk factors, the T and N stages are commonly used for (neo)adjuvant treatment decisions (NCCN guidelines) [3] and recently the distance of the tumor to the mesorectal fascia [4]. The TNM classification system has reproducible and straightforward histological cutoff values, such as the distinction between a T2 and T3 tumor. It does however not always easily transfer to staging through imaging. All imaging methods are good in showing the bulk of the tumor but will have difficulty in predicting the exact microscopical tumor extension to a histological interface. It is therefore unrealistic to expect a 100 % accuracy from imaging technology in predicting a histological classification.

The accuracy of the T stage assessment with ERUS in the smaller series is generally higher than in larger and more recent data [5–8]. ERUS is reliable to stage rectal cancer for the degree of invasion in the rectal wall, but high accuracies are only obtained in expert centers. The agreement between the uT stage and pT stage in larger studies is 65–70 %, with 10–15 % understaging and 20 % overstaging [9–11]. In uT1 there is understaging in 15–20 % and in uT2 stage 15–30 %. Overstaging in uT3 occurred in 25–30 %. Some series address the specific question of distinguishing mucosal T0 lesions from T1 tumors, showing a risk of understaging with uT0 of only 5–15 % [12–15]. It is therefore generally considered that ERUS is good in imaging the smaller tumors and in selecting the eligible patients for a local excision. An overview of the ERUS technique and its role including the drawbacks is provided by Nonner and coauthors in Chap. 19 of this section. For the larger T3 and T4 lesions, ERUS can perfectly identify ingrowth in surrounding structures that are within the field of view such as the vagina, prostate, and seminal

vesicles. The difficulties arise when tumors are located high in the rectum. It then provides insufficient anatomical information in specific on the extent to the dorsal and lateral pelvic wall.

The importance of the involvement of the mesorectal fascia as a prognostic factor and as a parameter of surgical quality has been recognized and confirmed in the last 20 years [2]. The ideal plane of resection in a total mesorectal excision is just outside the mesorectal fascia, and a positive circumferential resection margin can be the result of inadequate TME surgery. An involved mesorectal fascia is defined as a closest distance of ≤1 mm between the tumor and the mesorectal fascia, as this represents the optimal prognostic cutoff point. Preoperative assessment of the mesorectal fascia involvement is important whenever a short preoperative course of 5×5 Gy is considered in patients without a threatened or involved margin. Although it has been shown that 5×5 Gy is a very efficient and cost-effective way to prevent local recurrences in many patients, it is much less effective when the tumor comes close to or invades the mesorectal fascia [16]. These tumors should be identified and treated with a preoperative long course of chemoradiation to provide downsizing. For centers that only use a long course of chemoradiation as a neoadjuvant treatment, the distance of the tumor to the mesorectal fascia is usually not very important in the preoperative decision process, as all tumors that extend beyond the muscular wall are considered candidates for a long course of chemoradiation, providing an opportunity for downsizing. Regardless of the neoadjuvant treatment strategies, it is however important for the surgeon to know the exact anatomical relation of the tumor to the mesorectal fascia and the surrounding structures in order to obtain a complete resection. Therefore, when it comes to staging the large rectal tumors, MRI is recommended as the preferred staging method [17–20]. For MRI of rectal cancer, it is important to obtain good standard high-resolution images. In Chap. 18 of this section, Hunter et al. elaborate on the state-of-the-art imaging protocol, on the strength but also the weaknesses for staging rectal tumors with modern planar imaging techniques, MRI and CT.

Nodal disease is one of the most important risk factors for both local and distant recurrence and is generally considered an indication for neoadjuvant therapy. Identifying nodal disease with imaging remains difficult because size criteria used on its own result in only a moderate accuracy. Lymph nodes with a diameter of ≥ 10 mm are invariably malignant, but the majority of involved nodes are smaller than 5 mm [21, 22]. In addition to size, morphological criteria such as shape, texture, and border of the nodes can be assessed in the larger nodes and improve the identification of the true node positives. But overall, the assessment of the smaller nodes remains difficult also because these criteria cannot always be applied. The difficulties in nodal staging with the standard imaging methods are illustrated by a recent multicentre report in which T3N0 tumors, staged with ERUS and/or MRI, were found to be node positive at histology in 22 %, despite preoperative chemoradiation [23].

How does one work in practice with a suboptimal accuracy of preoperative lymph node imaging? One approach is only to rely on imaging information on nodal status when the tumor is associated with round large nodes (>5 mm) that are irregular in border and/or heterogeneous in signal or echogenecity. Whenever these criteria for node positivity are absent on ERUS or MRI for any of the visualized nodes, information on nodal status is not reliable. An extreme approach is to disregard the imaging data on nodal status and to give neoadjuvant treatment in most patients, accepting overtreatment rather then undertreatment. This strategy exposes all patients to the side effects while only a few patients benefit of the improved local control. A third approach is to take into account the prevalence of nodal metastases according to the T stage and to give neoadjuvant therapy for T3 lesions, regardless of nodal imaging results, but not for T2N0 lesions [23]. This strategy of selective use of neoadjuvant radiotherapy only for patients most at risk for local recurrence is further supported by evidence from two large European trials of the lack of survival benefit of radiotherapy when good TME surgery is performed [18, 24].

Future Perspectives

Currently, there is also a trend to study alternative treatment options after a good response to treatment, such as a local excision or even a nonoperative wait and see approach. Given the increasing use of preoperative (chemo)radiation in rectal cancer, selection of the candidates for these alternative treatments by imaging should be a topic for further studies, because imaging technologies such as ERUS, CT, MRI, and PET are continuously improving. With modern more powerful machines, functional data can be generated and combined with morphological data. 3D-ERUS, diffusion MR imaging, perfusion MRI, perfusion CT, or perfusion PET/CT could all be of help in monitoring treatment response. New lymph node-specific MR contrast agents are on the way that may finally move us one step forward in our search for better identification of patients with nodal metastases. This new role of imaging to detect small volumes of residual disease in fibrotic scar tissue in the rectal wall and in the lymph nodes is now still work in progress, but it is clear that imaging in future will play an important role in the selection and follow-up of patients after neoadjuvant treatment.

Recommendations

ERUS and MRI should be seen more as complementary rather than competitive techniques. Each has its own strengths and weaknesses. ERUS has the advantage over MRI that the equipment is less costly and that it can be readily used in the office, immediately providing information that is important for further treatment planning. MRI on the other hand has the advantage over ERUS that the images can be more easily interpreted and read by other radiologists and clinicians. The images can also be used by radiotherapists for planning the radiotherapy fields and by surgeons to guide the resection in advanced cases. ERUS is without doubt the best imaging method for the selection of the candidates for local excision, whereas MRI is recommended for the larger more advanced tumors. MRI is accurate in identifying the different risk groups and in stratifying these patients into their treatment according to their risk. In the absence of easy access to MRI, MDCT is a good alternative for the high tumors, but it lacks accuracy in the low tumors. For lymph node imaging, all techniques are at present only moderately accurate. The most practical strategy seems to use the information on lymph node staging in the preoperative decision making, keeping in mind the suboptimal accuracy. In addition to the standard treatment with TME, there is a small group of patients with a superficial tumor where the surgeon is considering a local excision with a small risk of leaving behind involved lymph nodes in the mesorectum. Accurate selection of node-negative disease would be of help in the selection for this procedure, and future research should focus on developing imaging techniques that can better identify nodal disease.

References

1. Gunderson LL, Sargent DJ, Tepper JE, et al. Impact of T and N substage on survival and disease relapse in adjuvant rectal cancer: a pooled analysis. Int J Radiat Oncol Biol Phys. 2002;54(2):386–96.
2. Nagtegaal ID, Quirke P. What is the role for the circumferential margin in the modern treatment of rectal cancer? J Clin Oncol. 2008;26(2):303–12.
3. NIH Consensus Conference. Adjuvant therapy for patients with colon and rectal cancer. JAMA. 1990;264(11):1444–50.
4. Marijnen CA, Nagtegaal ID, Kapiteijn E, et al. Radiotherapy does not compensate for positive resection margins in rectal cancer patients: report of a multicenter randomized trial. Int J Radiat Oncol Biol Phys. 2003;55(5):1311–20.
5. Edelman BR, Weiser MR. Endorectal ultrasound: its role in the diagnosis and treatment of rectal cancer. Clin Colon Rectal Surg. 2008;21(3):167–77.
6. Schaffzin DM, Wong WD. Endorectal ultrasound in the preoperative evaluation of rectal cancer. Clin Colorectal Cancer. 2004;4(2):124–32.
7. Harewood GC. Assessment of publication bias in the reporting of EUS performance in staging rectal cancer. Am J Gastroenterol. 2005;100(4):808–16.
8. Bipat S, Glas AS, Slors FJ, Zwinderman AH, Bossuyt PM, Stoker J. Rectal cancer: local staging and assessment of lymph node involvement with endoluminal US, CT, and MR imaging–a meta-analysis. Radiology. 2004;232(3):773–83.
9. Marusch F, Koch A, Schmidt U, et al. Routine use of transrectal ultrasound in rectal carcinoma: results of a prospective multicenter study. Endoscopy. 2002;34(5):385–90.
10. Ptok H, Marusch F, Meyer F, et al. Feasibility and accuracy of TRUS in the pre-treatment staging for rectal carcinoma in general practice. Eur J Surg Oncol. 2006;32(4):420–5.
11. Garcia-Aguilar J, Pollack J, Lee SH, et al. Accuracy of endorectal ultrasonography in preoperative staging of rectal tumors. Dis Colon Rectum. 2002;45(1):10–5.
12. Adams WJ, Wong WD. Endorectal ultrasonic detection of malignancy within rectal villous lesions. Dis Colon Rectum. 1995;38(10):1093–6.
13. Kim JC, Yu CS, Jung HY, et al. Source of errors in the evaluation of early rectal cancer by endoluminal ultrasonography. Dis Colon Rectum. 2001;44(9):1302–9.
14. Staib L, Schirrmeister H, Reske SN, Beger HG. Is (18)F-fluorodeoxyglucose positron emission tomography in recurrent colorectal cancer a contribution to surgical decision making? Am J Surg. 2000;180(1):1–5.
15. Starck M, Bohe M, Simanaitis M, Valentin L. Rectal endosonography can distinguish benign rectal lesions from invasive early rectal cancers. Colorectal Dis. 2003;5(3):246–50.
16. Peeters KC, Marijnen CA, Nagtegaal ID, et al. The TME trial after a median follow-up of 6 years: increased local control but no survival benefit in irradiated patients with resectable rectal carcinoma. Ann Surg. 2007;246(5):693–701.
17. Beets-Tan RG, Beets GL, Vliegen RF, et al. Accuracy of magnetic resonance imaging in prediction of tumour-free resection margin in rectal cancer surgery. Lancet. 2001;357(9255):497–504.
18. MERCURY Study Group. Extramural depth of tumor invasion at thin-section MR in patients with rectal cancer: results of the MERCURY study. Radiology. 2007;243(1):132–9.
19. Bissett IP, Fernando CC, Hough DM, et al. Identification of the fascia propria by magnetic resonance imaging and its relevance to preoperative assessment of rectal cancer. Dis Colon Rectum. 2001;44(2):259–65.
20. Blomqvist L, Machado M, Rubio C, et al. Rectal tumour staging: MR imaging using pelvic phased-array and endorectal coils vs endoscopic ultrasonography. Eur Radiol. 2000;10(4):653–60.

21. Lahaye MJ, Engelen SM, Nelemans PJ, et al. Imaging for predicting the risk factors–the circumferential resection margin and nodal disease–of local recurrence in rectal cancer: a meta-analysis. Semin Ultrasound CT MR. 2005;26(4):259–68.

22. Wang C, Zhou Z, Wang Z, et al. Patterns of neoplastic foci and lymph node micrometastasis within the mesorectum. Langenbecks Arch Surg. 2005;390(4):312–8.

23. Guillem JG, Diaz-Gonzalez JA, Minsky BD, et al. cT3N0 rectal cancer: potential overtreatment with preoperative chemoradiotherapy is warranted. J Clin Oncol. 2008;26(3):368–73.

24. Sebag-Montefiore D, Stephens RJ, Steele R, et al. Preoperative radiotherapy versus selective post-operative chemoradiotherapy in patients with rectal cancer (MRC CR07 and NCIC-CTG C016): a multicentre, randomised trial. Lancet. 2009; 373(9666):811–20.

MRI and CT for the Preoperative T and N Staging of Rectal Cancer

Chris Hunter and Gina Brown

Abstract
Local staging of rectal cancer is becoming increasingly important as more treatment options become available. A number of modalities are used for this purpose, including endoscopic ultrasound, CT and MRI. Endoscopic ultrasound may be useful for distinguishing early T-stage tumours. CT has a wider field of view but is limited by poor soft tissue contrast. MRI is able to very accurately assess the relationship of rectal tumours to the mesorectal fascia and so determine whether the circumferential resection margin will be involved following total mesorectal excision. It is therefore the preferred modality for assessing whether patients require downstaging preoperative chemoradiotherapy.

The preoperative staging of rectal tumours requires consideration of certain specific features. Colon and rectal tumours probably share similar pathogenesis, as suggested by their common premalignant conditions, histopathological appearances and modes of spread. However, the anatomical location of the rectum within the limited confines of the bony pelvis and close relations with the other pelvic organs plays a significant role in disease progression and recurrence. Preoperative staging and neoadjuvant and surgical treatment of rectal cancer are therefore quite different to colon cancer, and for these reasons, it should be considered as a separate disease entity.

The Importance of Local Staging

There is a general consensus of opinion that the primary rectal cancer should be resected in most patients, even in the presence of metastatic disease. This is because growth of the primary rectal cancer within the limited space of the pelvis is often associated with severe pain, which can be difficult to palliate. Local effects, such as faecal frequency, tenesmus and rectal bleeding [1], can also severely impact on the patients' quality of life.

C. Hunter • G. Brown (✉)
Department of Radiology, Royal Marsden Hospital, Downs Road, Sutton, Surrey SM2 5PT, UK
e-mail: chris_j_hunter@hotmail.com; gina.brown@rmh.nhs.uk

G. Baatrup (ed.), *Multidisciplinary Treatment of Colorectal Cancer*,
DOI 10.1007/978-3-319-06142-9_18, © Springer International Publishing Switzerland 2015

However, the lateral resection margins are limited within the pelvis, both by the restricted space and adjacent organs. High-quality surgical resection, paying close attention to anatomical planes and removing the rectum in an intact mesorectal envelope (total mesorectal excision, TME), results in low local recurrence rates of 4–5 % with tumour more than 1 mm from the circumferential margin [2–4]. However, if clear circumferential margins are not achieved, local recurrence rates are high. In the absence of adjuvant therapy, involved circumferential resection margins are associated with local recurrence of around 22 % with TME surgery [3].

Three large prospective trials have shown lower recurrence rates in preoperative radiotherapy than in selective postoperative radiotherapy or chemoradiotherapy (12 % vs. 21 %, 6 % vs. 13 %, 4.4 % vs. 10.6 %), as well as a lower incidence of side effects [5–7]. However, radiotherapy is not without problems, which include perineal wound breakdown if APR is performed, diarrhoea, rectal bleeding and small bowel obstruction. It is therefore desirable to preoperatively identify those patients who are at high risk of local recurrence following TME surgery and will derive most benefit from radiotherapy.

Conversely, in tumours confined to the submucosa (T1 tumours), local excision with transanal excision (TAE) or transendoscopic microsurgery (TEMS) may be considered [8]. This is an alternative to anterior resection or abdominoperineal resection (APR) which avoids the morbidity associated with major surgery, although local recurrence rates are higher [9] and careful postoperative surveillance is required.

Accurate preoperative staging of rectal cancer allows tailoring of therapy for individual patients. Those with very early-stage disease and no adverse features can consider local excision, with associated lower operative morbidity than radical surgery. Patients with T1 tumours choosing radical surgery, T2 tumours or T3 tumours with a clear circumferential margin, may proceed directly to high-quality TME surgery with a low local recurrence rate and good overall 5-year survival. Those with poor prognosis T3 tumours or T4 tumours will benefit from neoadjuvant therapy.

Modalities Available for Local Staging

Endoscopic Ultrasound

Endoscopic ultrasound is most useful in distinguishing the T stage of early (T1 and T2) rectal cancers. It is discussed in detail later in this chapter and so will not be discussed in detail here.

Computed Tomography (CT)

CT offers potential advantages over other imaging modalities for the local staging of rectal cancer. It is widely available, well tolerated, relatively inexpensive and rapidly acquired and has few contraindications, particularly if intravenous contrast agents are not required. It is also widely used for the assessment of metastatic disease in rectal cancer. A number of early small-scale trials reported promising results for local staging of rectal cancers [10, 11]. Unfortunately, these early encouraging results were not confirmed in larger trials [12]. More recently, technological advances have seen some renewed interest in local staging with CT. These include multi-detector CT scanners, which allow a spatial resolution of around 1 mm to be achieved, and multiplanar reconstruction which allow images to be viewed perpendicular or parallel to the tumour, rather than solely in the axial acquisition plane. These technical advances have improved T staging, with accuracies of up to 87 % being reported, compared with an accuracy of 73 % reported in the same trial using axial images alone [13]. However, in a recent large prospective multicentre study of 250 patients, the sensitivity of CT in predicting an involved circumferential resection margin was only 75 % [14]. This limits its usefulness in determining the need for neoadjuvant therapy, and so CT should still be reserved for those who have contraindications to MR imaging.

Magnetic Resonance Imaging (MRI)

The staging of rectal cancers with MRI has gone through considerable development over the 20 years since its first assessment. Early studies tended to involve small numbers of patients and focus on the use of an endorectal coil and the assessment of T and N staging [15]. Although the use of an endorectal coil helps to identify the inner layers of the bowel wall which is helpful for distinguishing the T stage of early tumours [16], the volume of sensitivity using these coils is limited. Technical problems are also common, with stenosis, patient discomfort, coil migration and difficulty in reaching upper rectal tumours all limiting its usefulness. Reported accuracy in these early studies varied between 31 and 80 % in determining T stage and between 57 and 70 % for identifying lymph node metastases, with higher accuracy reported for correctly identifying T3 tumours than distinguishing T1 from T2 tumours [15, 17, 18].

However, during the same period, the acceptance of TME surgery and the recognition of the importance of CRM involvement resulted in a shift in the focus in preoperative assessment of rectal cancer from T and N staging to the assessment of the CRM and depth of tumour invasion. A number of larger studies, using a phased-array pelvic surface coil, subsequently demonstrated that MRI could reliably identify the mesorectal fascia and predict its involvement [19, 20]. In a subsequent multicentre study where the depth of extramural tumour invasion was compared between preoperative MRI and histology in 311 patients undergoing primary surgery, accuracy to within 0.5 mm was achieved in 95 % of cases [21]. Further studies have failed to show benefit for gadolinium-enhanced T1-weighted sequences in addition to T2-weighted TSE sequences [22, 23] or 3D volume acquisition T2-weighted sequences over 2D T2-weighted sequences [24]. In fact intravenous contrast enhancement may cause overstaging due to peritumoural vessel enhancement [25]. It is now widely accepted within Europe that high-resolution T2-weighted MRI with a phased-array pelvic coil provides the most accurate imaging for determining an involved or threatened CRM and so determining the need for neoadjuvant therapy prior to TME for rectal cancer.

Nodal staging of rectal cancer remains comparatively poor. In a meta-analysis of 19 studies, performed in 2004, Bipat found that MRI had a sensitivity of 66 % and a specificity of 76 % for predicting lymph node metastases [26]. Most of these studies used size criteria to determine whether lymph nodes should be considered to contain metastases, although cutoff values varied. More recent studies have used alternative criteria to size to identify lymph node metastases, including border irregularity or signal heterogeneity. These have resulted in moderate improvement in the accuracy of staging mesorectal lymph nodes, with a sensitivity of 85 % and a specificity of 96 % in a study of 42 patients where 281 lymph nodes identified on MRI were correlated with histological findings [27].

Staging of pelvic side wall lymph nodes may be slightly more accurate than staging of mesorectal lymph nodes. Akasu recently demonstrated a sensitivity of 87 % and a specificity of 87 % for identifying pelvic sidewall lymph node metastases, compared to a sensitivity of 83 % and a specificity of 64 % for identifying mesorectal lymph node metastases in the same study [28]. This may be related to a lower prevalence of reactive lymph nodes in this area.

Technical Aspects of Rectal Cancer Imaging

Computed Tomography

Recent years have seen continuing technological developments both in CT hardware and image reconstruction software, which are likely to continue. Multi-detector CT scanners are now routinely found in clinical practice, and 64-slice scanners not uncommon. There continues to be a trade-off between signal to noise ratio, spatial resolution, scan time and radiation dose. However, these technological advances have allowed higher resolutions to be achieved while keeping the signal to noise ratio high and the radiation dose acceptable. We currently use MDCT with the following parameters: acquisition of the abdomen and pelvis from the diaphragm to the pubic symphysis, collimation 2–3 mm and slice reconstruction 3 mm. This can be acquired in a single breath hold of around 25 s. However, the aim is to obtain images with the maximum spatial resolution and signal to noise ratio which can be acquired in a single breath hold with an acceptable radiation dose, and so these parameters should be adjusted according to the available scanner hardware.

All scans should be acquired with iodinated intravenous contrast infused at a rate of 3–4 ml/s unless there are contraindications to its use. Oral contrast, such as 1.5 L of water or 1 L of 2.1 % barium sulphate solution administered 40 min to 1 h prior to scanning, is also helpful. An alternative to this is rectal insufflation with air following cathartic bowel preparation. This allows CT colonography to be performed to assess the colon for synchronous polyps or tumours simultaneously with staging the rectal tumour and may also allow accurate staging of colorectal cancers [29].

Images should be viewed on a dedicated workstation which allows multiplanar reconstruction (MPR). This allows images to be viewed in planes other than the axial acquisition plane, overcoming one of the limitations of CT compared to MR. Modern software will allow reconstruction of images in oblique planes, so that the tumour can be visualised at 90° to its long axis. Image interpretation using MPR has been demonstrated to increase staging accuracy over viewing solely in the acquisition plane in CT [13].

Magnetic Resonance Imaging

The referring team should provide basic information relevant to the staging of the rectal cancer when referring the patient, particularly tumour location (described in terms of height above the anal verge), details of any previous pelvic surgery and any known coincident pelvic pathology. The patient should be assessed for any contraindications to MRI scanning, including cardiac pacemaker, shrapnel in sensitive biological areas, ferromagnetic aneurysm clips and cochlear implants [30]. The removal of shrapnel is occasionally required to facilitate optimal preoperative staging. The patient should be pain-free, positioned comfortably on the MRI scanner and fully informed about the scan duration and experience; this will improve patient compliance and reduce the likelihood of nondiagnostic scans due to patient movement [31].

The patient is positioned supine on the MRI table, with a pillow under the head and knees. A multielement flexible pelvic phased-array coil is placed firmly over the pelvis, ensuring the entire imaging volume is covered. This requires the lower edge of the coil to be at least 10 cm below the pubic symphysis. A full bladder is not necessary and may increase patient discomfort when the surface coil is strapped tightly over the pelvis. Although small bowel movement and associated movement artefact is not generally a major problem in pelvic imaging, antiperistaltic medication may slightly improve the image quality and is generally well tolerated [32].

The patient may be imaged with a 1.0 T or 1.5 T MRI system, for which the accuracy of MRI in staging has been demonstrated. Although there are not yet large-scale trials of the accuracy of rectal cancer staging at 3.0 T, some small trials have shown that similar accuracy can be achieved at this field strength [24, 33]. Increasing field strength offers the potential benefit of increased signal to noise ratio or shorter scanning time.

Three to five sequences are required for adequate MRI staging of rectal cancer dependent on the location of the tumour:

Sequence 1: Sagittal T2-weighted fast spin echo (T2W-FSE, 5 mm slices). This allows identification of the primary tumour and planning of the subsequent sequences.

Sequence 2: Large field of view axial sections (T2W-FSE, 5 mm slices). These should include the whole volume of the pelvis, from the pubic symphysis to the iliac crest.

Sequences 1 and 2 allow visualisation of the whole pelvis to identify any possible sites of lymph node metastases. While the second sequence is being acquired, the first sequence can be used to plan the high-resolution images through the tumour.

Sequence 3: High-resolution oblique axial sections through the tumour and peritumoural tissues (T2W-FSE, 16 cm FOV, 3 mm slices). It is essential that these sequences are obtained perpendicular to the long axis of the tumour so that the depth of tumour invasion can be accurately assessed.

Sequence 4: For lower 1/3rd rectal tumours. High-resolution coronal sections through the sphincter complex (T2W-FSE, 16 cm FOV, 3 mm slices). These demonstrate the levator ani muscles, sphincter complex and inter-sphincteric plane and allow the rectal wall to be clearly differentiated from the levator. If these sequences are omitted, low rectal tumours may be overstaged.

Sequence 5: For low anterior wall rectal tumours. High resolution, small field of view sagittal sections (T2W-FSE, 16 cm, 3 mm slices). These help to delineate the exact relationship between the edge of the tumour and anterior structures (prostate or posterior vaginal wall).

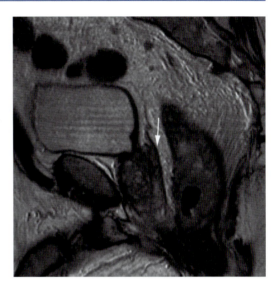

Fig. 18.1 Urogenital septum. Sagittal view demonstrating the urogenital septum (*white arrow*)

Radiological Anatomy

Bill Heald has described the anatomy of the rectum and important features in relation to rectal cancer in Chap. 4. In this section we will demonstrate the radiological appearance of this anatomy, so as to describe its relationship to the rectal tumour.

The Urogenital Septum

The urogenital septum is an avascular layer of connective tissue, which arises from the pelvic floor during embryological development. This layer of connective tissue separates the hindgut (posteriorly, containing the rectum and perirectal tissues) from the urogenital organs (anteriorly). This layer has been demonstrated to be present in both men, where it is called Denonvilliers' fascia, and women, where it is described as the recto-vaginal septum [34]. This layer can be easily visualised in both sexes on MRI as a layer of low signal intensity, which continues superiorly as far as the peritoneal reflection (Fig. 18.1).

Pelvic Nerve Plexuses

The autonomic nerve supply in the pelvis is important for sexual and urological function and is potentially at risk during rectal cancer surgery.

The nerve plexuses can be readily identified on MRI, which allows the relationship to the tumour to be appreciated preoperatively to aid in surgical or neoadjuvant treatment planning. The inferior hypogastric plexus lies sagittally; in the male, the tip of the seminal vesicle marks the midpoint of the plexus, whereas in the female the anterior half of the plexus lies against the upper third of the vagina. The hypogastric plexus lies in a plane just medial to the vessels of the pelvic sidewall and forms a meshwork of interconnecting nerves which can be identified on the coronal (Fig. 18.2) and sagittal (Fig. 18.3) views on MRI.

Peritoneum

The peritoneum extends from the superior aspect of the bladder posteriorly to the side walls of the pelvis and the anterior surface of the rectum. The peritoneum forms an acute angle in the recess between the bladder in the male and the uterus in female (the rectovesical or recto-uterine pouch). This peritoneal reflection is best seen on sagittal MR images, where it can be recognised as a low signal intensity layer extending over the surface of the bladder and continuing to

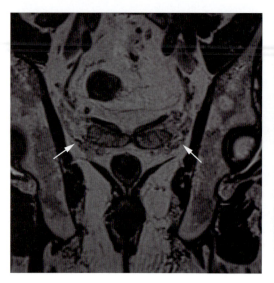

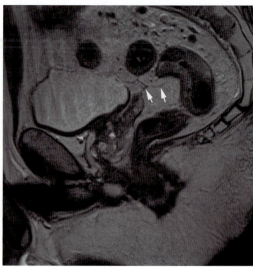

Fig. 18.2 Pelvic nerve plexuses, coronal. Coronal view demonstrating the pelvic nerve plexuses (*white arrows*)

Fig. 18.4 Peritoneal reflection. Sagittal view showing the peritoneal reflection (*white arrows*)

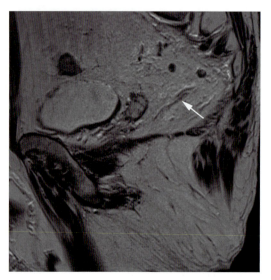

Fig. 18.3 Pelvic nerve plexuses; sagittal. Sagittal view showing the pelvic nerves (*white arrow*) extending towards the neurovascular bundle of the prostate

its attachment on the anterior surface of the rectum (Fig. 18.4).

Mesorectum and the Mesorectal Fascia

As described previously, the mesorectum is a distinct structure which derives embryologically

from the hindgut. This contains the rectum, its associated vessels and draining lymphatics in a package of fatty connective tissue. This package is contained within a fascial layer, the mesorectal fascia, which is derived from the visceral peritoneum. The importance of this fascia in terms of surgical technique and outcome is now well understood [35]. The great strength of MRI compared to other imaging techniques for staging rectal cancer is that this layer can be readily identified on high-resolution T2-weighted images. It is most easily appreciated on axial sequences as a band of low signal intensity surrounding the mesorectum (Fig. 18.5).

The Bowel Wall

Histologically, the bowel wall can be divided into four layers; the innermost mucosal layer, the muscularis mucosa, the submucosa and the muscularis propria. The muscularis propria can be further subdivided into inner circular and outer longitudinal layers, separated by a thin layer of connective tissue. On MRI, the mucosal layer can be identified as a thin line of low signal intensity overlying the thicker higher signal intensity submucosa. The muscularis mucosa cannot usually be identified as a distinct layer on MRI. The two layers of the muscularis propria can sometimes be identified as two distinct layers (Fig. 18.6); otherwise, it appears as one layer of low signal intensity surrounded by the perirectal tissues which are of high signal intensity due to their high fat content.

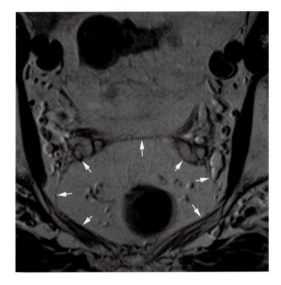

Fig. 18.5 Mesorectal fascia. Transaxial view demonstrating the mesorectal fascia (*white arrows*)

Image Interpretation for MRI Staging of Rectal Cancer

Tumour Morphology

An appreciation of the morphological appearance of rectal cancers, typical patterns of development and spread and common variations is very helpful for understanding the appearances of imaging. Rectal cancers are usually adenocarcinomas, which are thought to arise from adenomas in most cases. These adenomas can be either polypoid or sessile in nature.

Some tumours maintain an exophytic appearance similar to the polypoid adenomas from which they arise. These lesions are often low-grade malignancies even when they form large masses projecting into the bowel lumen [36]. On MRI, these tumours can be seen projecting into the bowel lumen. A preserved layer of high signal intensity representing the submucosal layer is frequently evident, as these are often early-stage tumours. The surface of these tumours often has clefts containing mucous fluid which is high signal on MRI (Fig. 18.7).

The most common appearance of adenocarcinomas is annular or semiannular. This appearance can be recognised on MRI as an elevated plaque of intermediate signal intensity projecting

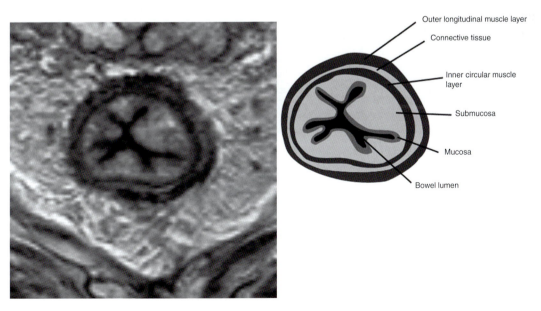

Fig. 18.6 Layers of the bowel wall. Transaxial view demonstrating the layers of the bowel wall. This image was acquired following radiotherapy, so the layers of the bowel wall are exaggerated due to tissue oedema

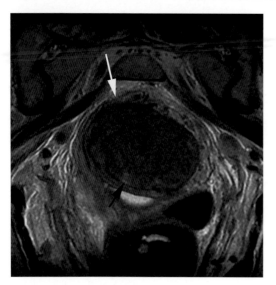

Fig. 18.7 Polypoidal tumour. Transaxial view demonstrating a polypoidal tumour entirely filling the rectal lumen. There is invasion through the base of the stalk (*white arrow*). The surface of the tumour has clefts containing mucin secretion (*black arrow*)

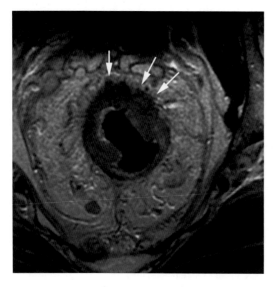

Fig. 18.8 Semiannular early T3 tumour. Transaxial view showing a semiannular tumour extending around the anterior three quarters of the bowel wall. There is early invasion into the mesorectal tissues (*white arrows*), making this an early T3 tumour

into the bowel lumen and extending around the bowel lumen in a U-shape (Fig. 18.8).

As the tumour advances and increases in size, the central portion frequently begins to ulcerate.

This area of ulceration overlies the area of deepest invasion through the bowel wall. These features can often be identified on MR imaging.

If the tumour advances further, then it invades through the wall of the bowel into the perirectal tissues. Rectal tumours usually do this with a well-circumscribed border. However, around 25 % of tumours do so with poorly defined borders. In these cases, the malignant cells invade between normal structures, so there is not a distinct leading edge to the tumour. This pattern of spread is associated with a worse prognosis [37]. The former pattern of spread is recognised on MRI as intermediate signal intensity with a broad pushing margin (Fig. 18.8). The latter type is indicated by the presence of fingerlike projections of intermediate signal intensity extending into the perirectal tissues.

Some tumours have preponderance for ulceration at a relatively small size. These tumours may cause diffuse thinning of the bowel wall which can make identification of the layers of the rectum more difficult. This can also make determining the degree of extramural spread more difficult than in other morphological types.

Mucinous tumours are defined as tumours containing more than 75 % mucin [38]. Although this morphological subtype accounts for only 10 % of tumours, they are important because they are associated with a poorer prognosis. This is thought to be due to the fact that they have a poorly defined margin and are often advanced at the time of presentation. They may also spread intramurally which is rare in other morphological subtypes of rectal tumours, unlike upper gastrointestinal tumours. This form of tumour can be recognised on MRI by their very high signal intensity on T2-weighted imaging. As these tumours are often diffusely infiltrating, anatomical layers may be preserved by expanded by high signal intensity (Fig. 18.9).

T Stage

In histological terms, T1 tumours have invaded into, but not through, the submucosa. On MRI, part of the high signal intensity submucosa is

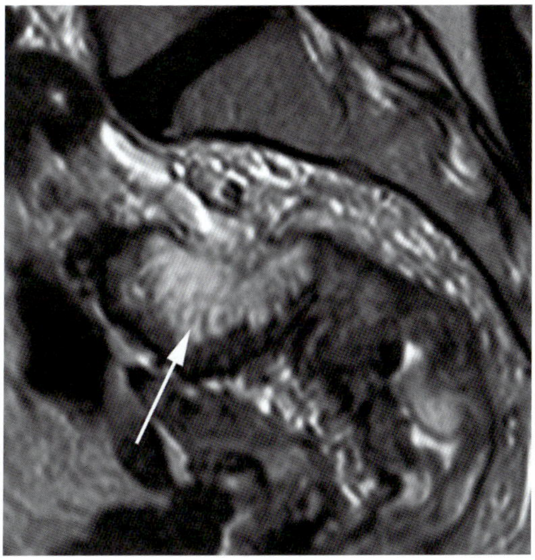

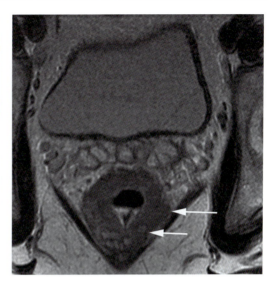

Fig. 18.9 Mucinous tumour. Sagittal view showing a mucinous tumour (*white arrow*). The invasive border (posteriorly) is diffusely infiltrating

Fig. 18.10 Poor prognosis T3 tumour. Transaxial view showing a poor prognosis T3 tumour. The mesorectal fascia is threatened posterolaterally on the left side (*white arrows*)

sometimes still preserved. In this case, it has a high positive predictive value for a T1 tumour.

Unfortunately, loss of the high signal submucosal layer does not necessarily allow differentiation between T1 and T2 tumours. This is because microscopic infiltration of the tumour into the muscular layer (T2) is indistinguishable on MRI from complete replacement of the submucosa without infiltration into the muscular layer (T1). Similarly, it is difficult to differentiate between a tumour occupying the whole thickness of the bowel wall without invasion through the wall (T2) from a tumour with very early invasion into the perirectal tissues (T3). The distinction between of T2 and early T3 tumours (T3a <1 mm invasion into perirectal fat or T3b 1–5 mm invasion into perirectal fat) is of less prognostic significance than the distinction between early and advanced T3 tumours (T3c 5–15 mm extramural invasion, T3d >15 mm extramural invasion).

T3 tumours show invasion into the perirectal tissues. This can be identified on MRI as a broad-based pushing or nodular margin of intermediate signal intensity moving beyond the bowel wall into the perirectal fat (Figs. 18.8 and 18.10).

T4 tumours are defined as invading into an adjacent organ or having perforated the perito-

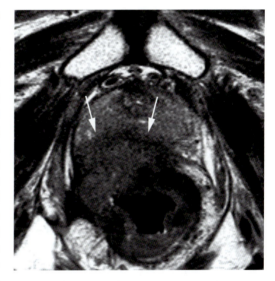

Fig. 18.11 T4 tumour. Transaxial view showing a T4 tumour with invasion into the prostate anteriorly (*white arrows*)

neum (Fig. 18.11). It is important to look carefully for evidence of these features in advanced tumours. Structures at risk will be dependent on the site of the tumour and the direction of the leading margin of the tumour. In the upper and mid rectum, in the anterior direction the uterus or

Table 18.1 T-staging rectal tumours using MRI

T stage	Definition	MRI appearances
Tx	Primary tumour cannot be assessed	
T0	No evidence of primary tumour	
T1	Tumour invades submucosa	Tumour signal intensity within submucosal layer **or** replacement of submucosal layer by tumour signal intensity but not extending into muscularis propria
T2	Tumour invades but confined to muscularis propria	Tumour signal intensity within muscularis propria **or** tumour signal intensity replaces muscularis propria but does not extend into mesorectal fat
T3	Tumour invades through muscularis propria into subserosa (mesorectum)	Broad-based bulge or nodular projection (but not fine speculation) of tumour signal intensity beyond outer muscular layer
T3a	Tumour extends <1 mm beyond muscularis propria	
T3b	Tumour extends 1–5 mm beyond muscularis propria	
T3c	Tumour extends 5–15 mm beyond muscularis propria	
T3d	Tumour extends >15 mm beyond muscularis propria	
T4	Tumour invades other organs or penetrates peritoneum	Extension of tumour signal intensity into adjacent organ OR extension of tumour signal intensity through peritoneal reflection

Adapted from Taylor et al. [39], with permission

Tumour signal intensity is intermediate, lower than submucosa and mesorectum, and higher than muscle

bladder is at risk, as well as the peritoneal surface. Laterally, the tumour may invade into the pelvic sidewall, and in the posterior direction, the sacrum may be involved by an advanced tumour. Tumours in the lower third of the rectum place will invade the structures of the pelvic floor if they become locally advanced. The prostate, seminal vesicles or vagina may be involved anterior to the rectum, the levator muscles laterally, and the sacrum or coccyx in the posterior direction. The MRI T-staging system for rectal tumours is summarised in Table 18.1.

Circumferential Resection Margin

The circumferential resection margin (CRM) involvement is the most important factor in determining local recurrence in rectal cancer [40]. It is therefore important to identify those patients with a potentially positive circumferential resection margin, which is defined as tumour within 1 mm of the mesorectal fascia [41]. The distance from the closest tumour margin to the mesorectal fascia should be measured and recorded (Fig. 18.12). Lymph nodes considered to be metastatic, tumour deposits or extramural vascular invasion (EMVI) lying within 1 mm of the CRM also threaten the margin and should be recorded separately.

Low rectal tumours require special consideration, as the anatomy in this area is different to the rest of the rectum, and outcomes for patients treated with abdominoperineal excision (APE) are worse in terms of margin involvement and local recurrence than those treated by anterior resection (AR) [42]. The mesorectum at this level tapers in a V shape down to top of the sphincter complex, just deep (or superior) to the levator muscles. The internal anal sphincter is formed from the circular muscle layer of the muscularis propria. At the top of the sphincter, muscle fibres from the puborectalis sling join with the fibres of the outer longitudinal muscle layer of the

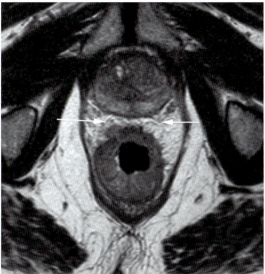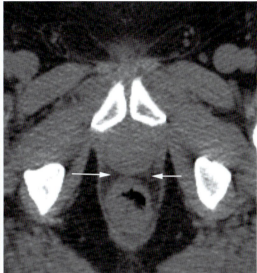

Fig. 18.12 CT and MRI showing tumour distance to mesorectal fascia. Transaxial views through a tumour at the same level on MRI (*left*) and CT (*right*). The anterior margin (*white arrows*) appears involved on CT, but a clear margin can be seen on MRI

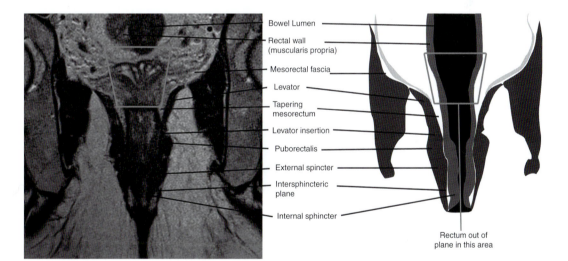

Bowel Lumen

Rectal wall
(muscularis propria)

Mesorectal fascia

Levator

Tapering
mesorectum

Levator insertion

Puborectalis

External spincter

Intersphincteric
plane

Internal sphincter

Rectum out of
plane in this area

Fig. 18.13 MRI showing anatomy of the sphincter complex. Coronal image and accompanying diagram demonstrating the anatomy of the sphincter complex as seen on MRI. Note that the rectum goes out of plane and therefore is not seen in the middle portion of the image (*grey box*)

muscularis propria to form a thin muscular layer between the internal and external sphincters. The external sphincter consists of voluntary muscle fibres which are continuous superiorly with the levator ani muscles (Fig. 18.13).

Tumours 1 mm or more from the mesorectal fascia may be safely treated by low anterior resection. The continuation of this plane is the intersphincteric plane, and tumours 1 mm or more from the outer border of the internal sphincter may be safely excised by a conventional intersphincteric APE [43]. However, if the tumour extends into the levator muscles or the intersphincteric plane, then the patient would require

Table 18.2 Staging and operative management of low rectal cancers

Level	Tumour height	Tumour depth	Operative plane
1	Between levator origin and puborectalis sling	Confined to muscularis propria	LAR/intersphincteric APE
		Beyond muscularis propria, >1 mm from mesorectal fascia/levator muscle	LAR/intersphincteric APE
		Within 1 mm of mesorectal fascia/levator muscle	Extra-levator APE
		Extending into levator muscle	Extra-levator APE
2	Tumour at or below puborectalis sling	Submucosa/partial thickness of muscularis propria	Intersphincteric APE
		Into the intersphincteric plane	Extra-levator APE
		Into the external sphincter	Extra-levator APE
		Beyond the external sphincter into ischiorectal tissue	Pelvic exenteration

Adapted from Shihab et al. [43], with permission
LAR low anterior resection, *APE* abdominoperineal excision

downstaging long-course chemoradiotherapy or an extra-levator APE as described by Holm et al. [44]. Tumours with extensive local invasion into adjacent structures may require pelvic exenteration. Table 18.2 shows a scheme described by Brown et al. for staging low rectal tumours, with appropriate surgical management.

The sharp tapering of the mesorectum at the level of the levator muscles, coupled with their oblique angle, can make image interpretation and accurate staging at this level difficult using only axial views. The addition of high-resolution – sagittal and coronal images can be helpful to avoid overstaging.

Nodal Staging

An assessment should be made of the mesorectal lymph nodes to determine whether or not they are likely to contain metastases. Unfortunately size alone, which has been the most common criteria used to decide whether lymph nodes contained metastases on MRI, is unreliable, and there has been no consensus about what size cutoff to use (criteria ranging from all identified lymph nodes to lymph nodes >10 mm in the long axis have been used) [25, 45]. A cutoff of 10 mm has a high specificity but low sensitivity, whereas a cutoff of 3 mm has a high sensitivity but low specificity. If lymph nodes are considered metastatic when they have either a heterogeneous

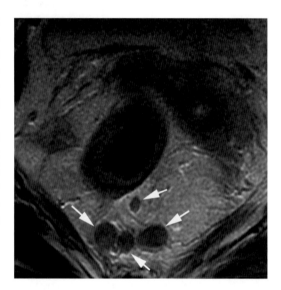

Fig. 18.14 MRI showing metastatic lymph nodes with signal heterogeneity. Transaxial image through the rectum demonstrating lymph node metastases with heterogeneous signal intensity (*white arrows*)

signal intensity or an irregular border, then a sensitivity of 85 % and a specificity of 96 % were achieved in a study of 42 patients where 281 lymph nodes identified on MRI were correlated with histological findings [27]. Similar results were obtained in a separate study of 75 patients [46]. We would therefore recommend denoting lymph nodes with signal heterogeneity (Fig. 18.14) or an irregular border (Fig. 18.15) as containing metastases.

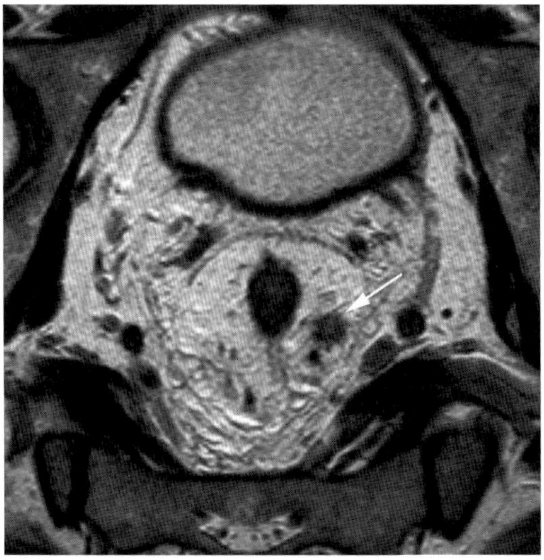

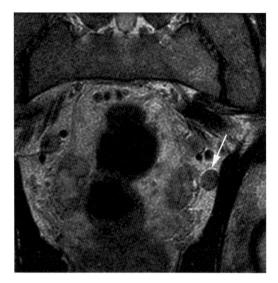

Fig. 18.15 MRI showing metastatic lymph node with irregular border. Transaxial image through the rectum demonstrating a lymph node metastasis with an irregular border (*white arrow*)

Fig. 18.16 MRI demonstrating pelvic sidewall lymph node metastasis. Coronal image demonstrating a pelvic sidewall lymph node metastasis with heterogeneous signal intensity (*white arrow*) lying outside the mesorectal fascia

Patients with no lymph nodes fitting the criteria for metastases are recorded as N0, patients with 1–3 involved lymph nodes within the mesorectal fascia are described as N1, and patients with four or more involved nodes are described as N2. Lymph nodes likely to contain metastases lying within 1 mm of the mesorectal fascia potentially threaten the CRM and a separate note of this should be made. Pelvic sidewall lymph node metastases (Fig. 18.16) lie outside the TME plane of excision and for this reason should also be recorded separately; some authorities regard these as distant rather than nodal metastases.

Extramural Vascular Invasion

Extramural vascular invasion (EMVI) has been demonstrated to be an important independent prognostic factor [47]. It can be reliably identifiable on rectal MRI [48] and should be reported to aid decision making with regard to neoadjuvant therapy.

Vessels can be identified on MRI as tubular structures with a signal void (due to blood flow), and these can frequently be followed between slices on high-resolution rectal MRI. Tumour

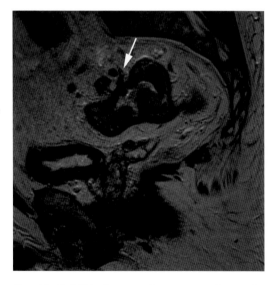

Fig. 18.17 MRI demonstrating extramural vascular invasion. Sagittal image showing tongue of extramural vascular invasion (EMVI) (*white arrow*) extending from the main tumour mass

extension into these vessels can be recognised when intermediate signal intensity tumour extends into these structures (Fig. 18.17). EMVI should first be recorded as present or absent and if present should be subdivided into large (extension

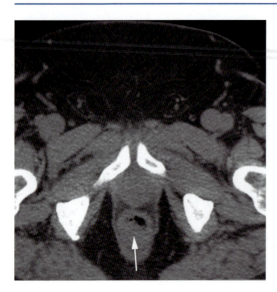

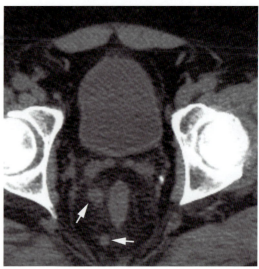

Fig. 18.18 CT demonstrating rectal tumour and meso-rectal fascia. Transaxial CT image demonstrating a rectal tumour (*white arrow*). The wall is greater than 6 mm thick and significantly thicker posteriorly than anteriorly. The mesorectal fascia cannot be defined

Fig. 18.19 CT demonstrating two large mesorectal lymph node metastases (*white arrows*)

into recognisable named vessels) or small (extension into small vessels which cannot be identified). Note should also be made if EMVI is within 1 mm of the mesorectal fascia, in which case the CRM is threatened.

Image Interpretation for CT Staging of Rectal Cancer

The tumour is usually identified within the rectum by focal thickening of the rectal wall, with a thickness of 6 mm or more considered abnormal [49], particularly if this thickening is asymmetrical (Fig. 18.18).

T Stage

The layers of the bowel wall are not clearly demonstrated on CT, which lacks the contrast resolution of MRI in soft tissues. However, the morphological appearances give some suggestion of tumour T stage. Intraluminal projection of a lesion without any apparent distortion of the rectal wall is likely to represent a T1 lesion.

Asymmetrical thickening of the bowel wall without disturbance of the contour of the outer edge of the muscularis propria is likely to represent T2 disease. Disruption of the outer contour of the bowel wall with smooth or nodular extension of the mass into the perirectal fat represents a T3 tumour. Localised loss of the fat plane between the advancing edge of the tumour mass and adjacent organs is likely to represent T4a invasion of adjacent organs. The involvement of the peritoneal surface with tumour represents T4b disease.

Nodal Staging

CT has relied primarily on size criteria for the identification of lymph node metastases (Fig. 18.19). However, with the wide overlap in size between malignant and benign nodes described previously, this technique has inherent limitations. The size criteria used have varied considerably, with some studies considering all nodes over 5 mm to be metastatic [13] and others considering lymph nodes over 10 mm or a cluster of three or more nodes to be metastatic [50]. Reported accuracy in predicting metastases using size criteria ranges from 62 % to 80 %. Other criteria suggested have included contrast enhancement of >100HU in the venous phase [51] and short-axis/long-axis ratio of greater than 0.8 [52]. These criteria have achieved lymph node staging accuracy of up to 80 % in fairly small series.

Extramural Vascular Invasion

Burton et al. have described the identification of EMVI on CT in colonic cancer with an accuracy of 55 % to 61 % [53]. This can be identified as thickened and irregular vessels with nodular enhancement. Although this accuracy is lower than that achieved by high-resolution rectal MRI, the same criteria (thickened and irregular vessels with nodular enhancement) can be used to recognise this important prognostic factor in rectal cancer on CT.

Circumferential Resection Margin

Wolberink et al. recently reported on the ability of MDCT to recognise the mesorectal fascia and to measure the distance of the tumour to the mesorectal fascia [14]. The mesorectal fascia can usually be identified as a thin line surrounding the perirectal fat, with signal intensity similar to that of the normal bowel wall (Fig. 18.18). The closest distance of the nodular or smooth tumour border to this line should be measured, and the mesorectal fascia should be considered involved if this distance is less than 1 mm. Wolberink et al. found that assessment of the mesorectal fascia was less accurate in cases of limited mesorectal fat. This measurement is also less accurate for low rectal tumours, a finding corroborate by Maizlin et al. [54].

Future Developments

The pace of technological development in diagnostic imaging is relentless, and this will doubtless continue to improve our ability to preoperatively stage rectal cancer.

Incremental improvements in existing imaging technology are likely to improve the speed and spatial resolution of both MRI and CT scanning. These include higher field strengths and increasing number of receiver coils for MRI and increasing number of detectors and dual-source scanners for CT.

Beyond simple improvements in the spatial and contrast resolution of anatomical imaging, there is great promise in functional imaging for staging colorectal cancer. This includes diffusion-weighted imaging (DWI) in MRI and FDG-PET/CT fusion. Although the spatial resolution of these technologies currently makes them more useful in staging metastatic disease, it is possible that in the future they may be helpful in lymph node staging. They also show promise in predicting and measuring response to neoadjuvant therapies.

Novel contrast agents may also be of future benefit. Ultrasmall super-paramagnetic iron oxide (USPIO) may increase the accuracy of lymph node staging in MRI, although it has not found widespread adoption in clinical practice. Ligand-targeted contrast agents may be of future benefit in the USS assessment of lymph nodes. The development of targeted nuclear imaging agents for PET and SPECT imaging may also help future preoperative assessment of lymph node metastases.

Summary

The accurate preoperative staging of rectal cancer is becoming ever more important, as the selective use of neoadjuvant therapy and choice of surgical approach (local excision, conventional AR or APE, extra-levator APE or exenteration) require accurate preoperative staging. The assessment of very early tumours when considering local excision is frequently performed with endoscopic ultrasound, although the increasing ability of high-resolution MRI to delineate the muscularis propria has recently expanded its role in this area. In all other cases, MRI is the modality of choice for local staging.

All rectal cancer patients should therefore undergo local staging with high-resolution rectal MRI to inform the MDT discussion unless there is an absolute contraindication. Prognostic features such as EMVI and depth of extramural tumour invasion should be reported in addition to TNM staging and CRM involvement.

In patients unable to undergo MRI, contrast-enhanced MDCT with multiplanar reconstruction is the second-line investigation for local staging of rectal tumours, and the same features should be reported.

References

1. Petrovic J, Stanojevic G, Barisic G, Dimitrijevic I, Micev M, Stojanovic S, et al. Influence of long-term radiotherapy on symptoms and signs of locally advanced primary rectal cancer of distant localisation. Acta Chir Iugosl. 2008;55(3):61–6.
2. MacFarlane JK, Ryall RD, Heald RJ. Mesorectal excision for rectal cancer. Lancet. 1993;341(8843): 457–60.
3. Wibe A, Rendedal PR, Svensson E, Norstein J, Eide TJ, Myrvold HE, et al. Prognostic significance of the circumferential resection margin following total mesorectal excision for rectal cancer. Br J Surg. 2002; 89(3):327–34.
4. Heald RJ, Moran BJ, Ryall RD, Sexton R, MacFarlane JK. Rectal cancer: the Basingstoke experience of total mesorectal excision, 1978–1997. Arch Surg. 1998;133(8):894–9.
5. Pahlman L, Glimelius B. Pre- or postoperative radiotherapy in rectal and rectosigmoid carcinoma. Report from a randomized multicenter trial. Ann Surg. 1990;211(2):187–95.
6. Sauer R, Becker H, Hohenberger W, Rodel C, Wittekind C, Fietkau R, et al. Preoperative versus postoperative chemoradiotherapy for rectal cancer. N Engl J Med. 2004;351(17):1731–40.
7. Sebag-Montefiore D, Stephens RJ, Steele R, Monson J, Grieve R, Khanna S, et al. Preoperative radiotherapy versus selective postoperative chemoradiotherapy in patients with rectal cancer (MRC CR07 and NCIC-CTG C016): a multicentre, randomised trial. Lancet. 2009;373(9666):811–20.
8. Blackstock W, Russo SM, Suh WW, Cosman BC, Herman J, Mohiuddin M, et al. ACR Appropriateness Criteria: local excision in early-stage rectal cancer. Curr Probl Cancer. 2010;34(3):193–200.
9. Chang AJ, Nahas CS, Araujo SE, Nahas SC, Marques CF, Kiss DR, et al. Early rectal cancer: local excision or radical surgery? J Surg Educ. 2008;65(1):67–72.
10. Thoeni RF, Moss AA, Schnyder P, Margulis AR. Detection and staging of primary rectal and rectosigmoid cancer by computed tomography. Radiology. 1981;141(1):135–8.
11. Holdsworth PJ, Johnston D, Chalmers AG, Chennells P, Dixon MF, Finan PJ, et al. Endoluminal ultrasound and computed tomography in the staging of rectal cancer. Br J Surg. 1988;75(10):1019–22.
12. Chapuis P, Kos S, Bokey L, Dent O, Newland R, Hinder J. How useful is pre-operative computerized tomography scanning in staging rectal cancer? Aust N Z J Surg. 1989;59(1):31–4.
13. Sinha R, Verma R, Rajesh A, Richards CJ. Diagnostic value of multidetector row CT in rectal cancer staging: comparison of multiplanar and axial images with histopathology. Clin Radiol. 2006;61(11):924–31.
14. Wolberink SV, Beets-Tan RG, de Haas-Kock DF, van de Jagt EJ, Span MM, Wiggers T. Multislice CT as a primary screening tool for the prediction of an involved mesorectal fascia and distant metastases in primary rectal cancer: a multicenter study. Dis Colon Rectum. 2009;52(5):928–34.
15. Chan TW, Kressel HY, Milestone B, Tomachefski J, Schnall M, Rosato E, et al. Rectal carcinoma: staging at MR imaging with endorectal surface coil. Work in progress. Radiology. 1991;181(2):461–7.
16. Torricelli P, Lo Russo S, Pecchi A, Luppi G, Cesinaro AM, Romagnoli R. Endorectal coil MRI in local staging of rectal cancer. Radiol Med. 2002;103(1–2): 74–83.
17. Drew PJ, Farouk R, Turnbull LW, Ward SC, Hartley JE, Monson JR. Preoperative magnetic resonance staging of rectal cancer with an endorectal coil and dynamic gadolinium enhancement. Br J Surg. 1999; 86(2):250–4.
18. Meyenberger C, Huch Boni RA, Bertschinger P, Zala GF, Klotz HP, Krestin GP. Endoscopic ultrasound and endorectal magnetic resonance imaging: a prospective, comparative study for preoperative staging and follow-up of rectal cancer. Endoscopy. 1995;27(7):469–79.
19. Brown G, Radcliffe AG, Newcombe RG, Dallimore NS, Bourne MW, Williams GT. Preoperative assessment of prognostic factors in rectal cancer using high-resolution magnetic resonance imaging. Br J Surg. 2003;90(3):355–64.
20. Beets-Tan RG, Beets GL, Vliegen RF, Kessels AG, Van Boven H, De Bruine A, et al. Accuracy of magnetic resonance imaging in prediction of tumour-free resection margin in rectal cancer surgery. Lancet. 2001;357(9255):497–504.
21. MERCURY Study Group. Extramural depth of tumor invasion at thin-section MR in patients with rectal cancer: results of the MERCURY study. Radiology. 2007;243(1):132–9.
22. Jao SY, Yang BY, Weng HH, Yeh CH, Lee LW. Evaluation of gadolinium-enhanced T1-weighted MRI in the preoperative assessment of local staging in rectal cancer. Colorectal Dis. 2009;12(11):1139–48.
23. Vliegen RF, Beets GL, von Meyenfeldt MF, Kessels AG, Lemaire EE, van Engelshoven JM, et al. Rectal cancer: MR imaging in local staging–is gadolinium-based contrast material helpful? Radiology. 2005;234(1):179–88.
24. Futterer JJ, Yakar D, Strijk SP, Barentsz JO. Preoperative 3T MR imaging of rectal cancer: local staging accuracy using a two-dimensional and three-dimensional T2-weighted turbo spin echo sequence. Eur J Radiol. 2008;65(1):66–71.

25. Okizuka H, Sugimura K, Yoshizako T, Kaji Y, Wada A. Rectal carcinoma: prospective comparison of conventional and gadopentetate dimeglumine enhanced fat-suppressed MR imaging. J Magn Reson Imaging. 1996;6(3):465–71.

26. Bipat S, Glas AS, Slors FJ, Zwinderman AH, Bossuyt PM, Stoker J. Rectal cancer: local staging and assessment of lymph node involvement with endoluminal US, CT, and MR imaging–a meta-analysis. Radiology. 2004;232(3):773–83.

27. Brown G, Richards CJ, Bourne MW, Newcombe RG, Radcliffe AG, Dallimore NS, et al. Morphologic predictors of lymph node status in rectal cancer with use of high-spatial-resolution MR imaging with histopathologic comparison. Radiology. 2003;227(2):371–7.

28. Akasu T, Iinuma G, Takawa M, Yamamoto S, Muramatsu Y, Moriyama N. Accuracy of high-resolution magnetic resonance imaging in preoperative staging of rectal cancer. Ann Surg Oncol. 2009;16(10):2787–94.

29. Iannaccone R, Laghi A, Passariello R. Colorectal carcinoma: detection and staging with multislice CT (MSCT) colonography. Abdom Imaging. 2005;30(1):13–9.

30. Dewey M, Schink T, Dewey CF. Frequency of referral of patients with safety-related contraindications to magnetic resonance imaging. Eur J Radiol. 2007; 63(1):124–7.

31. Brown G, Daniels IR, Richardson C, Revell P, Peppercorn D, Bourne M. Techniques and troubleshooting in high spatial resolution thin slice MRI for rectal cancer. Br J Radiol. 2005;78(927):245–51.

32. Johnson W, Taylor MB, Carrington BM, Bonington SC, Swindell R. The value of hyoscine butylbromide in pelvic MRI. Clin Radiol. 2007;62(11):1087–93.

33. Kim SH, Lee JM, Lee MW, Kim GH, Han JK, Choi BI. Diagnostic accuracy of 3.0-Tesla rectal magnetic resonance imaging in preoperative local staging of primary rectal cancer. Invest Radiol. 2008;43(8):587–93.

34. Aigner F, Zbar AP, Ludwikowski B, Kreczy A, Kovacs P, Fritsch H. The rectogenital septum: morphology, function, and clinical relevance. Dis Colon Rectum. 2004;47(2):131–40.

35. Heald RJ. Total mesorectal excision. The new European gold standard. G Chir. 1998;19(6–7):253–5.

36. Bjerkeset T, Morild I, Mork S, Soreide O. Tumor characteristics in colorectal cancer and their relationship to treatment and prognosis. Dis Colon Rectum. 1987;30(12):934–8.

37. Grinnell RS. The grading and prognosis of carcinoma of the colon and rectum. Ann Surg. 1939;109(4): 500–33.

38. Sasaki O, Atkin WS, Jass JR. Mucinous carcinoma of the rectum. Histopathology. 1987;11(3):259–72.

39. Taylor FG, Swift RI, Blomqvist L, Brown G. A systematic approach to the interpretation of preoperative staging MRI for rectal cancer. AJR Am J Roentgenol. 2008;191(6):1827–35.

40. Quirke P, Durdey P, Dixon MF, Williams NS. Local recurrence of rectal adenocarcinoma due to inadequate surgical resection. Histopathological study of lateral tumour spread and surgical excision. Lancet. 1986; 2(8514):996–9.

41. MERCURY. Diagnostic accuracy of preoperative magnetic resonance imaging in predicting curative resection of rectal cancer: prospective observational study. BMJ. 2006;333(7572):779.

42. Marr R, Birbeck K, Garvican J, Macklin CP, Tiffin NJ, Parsons WJ, et al. The modern abdominoperineal excision: the next challenge after total mesorectal excision. Ann Surg. 2005;242(1):74–82.

43. Shihab OC, Moran BJ, Heald RJ, Quirke P, Brown G. MRI staging of low rectal cancer. Eur Radiol. 2009;19(3):643–50.

44. Holm T, Ljung A, Haggmark T, Jurell G, Lagergren J. Extended abdominoperineal resection with gluteus maximus flap reconstruction of the pelvic floor for rectal cancer. Br J Surg. 2007;94(2):232–8.

45. Zerhouni EA, Rutter C, Hamilton SR, Balfe DM, Megibow AJ, Francis IR, et al. CT and MR imaging in the staging of colorectal carcinoma: report of the Radiology Diagnostic Oncology Group II. Radiology. 1996;200(2):443–51.

46. Kim JH, Beets GL, Kim MJ, Kessels AG, Beets-Tan RG. High-resolution MR imaging for nodal staging in rectal cancer: are there any criteria in addition to the size? Eur J Radiol. 2004;52(1):78–83.

47. Courtney ED, West NJ, Kaur C, Ho J, Kalber B, Hagger R, et al. Extra-mural vascular invasion is an adverse prognostic indicator of survival in patients with colorectal cancer. Colorectal Dis. 2008;11(2):150–6.

48. Smith NJ, Shihab O, Arnaout A, Swift RI, Brown G. MRI for detection of extramural vascular invasion in rectal cancer. AJR Am J Roentgenol. 2008;191(5): 1517–22.

49. Thoeni RF. Colorectal cancer. Radiologic staging. Radiol Clin North Am. 1997;35(2):457–85.

50. Ashraf K, Ashraf O, Haider Z, Rafique Z. Colorectal carcinoma, preoperative evaluation by spiral computed tomography. J Pak Med Assoc. 2006;56(4): 149–53.

51. Hundt W, Braunschweig R, Reiser M. Evaluation of spiral CT in staging of colon and rectum carcinoma. Eur Radiol. 1999;9(1):78–84.

52. Kanamoto T, Matsuki M, Okuda J, Inada Y, Tatsugami F, Tanikake M, et al. Preoperative evaluation of local invasion and metastatic lymph nodes of colorectal cancer and mesenteric vascular variations using multidetector-row computed tomography before laparoscopic surgery. J Comput Assist Tomogr. 2007;31(6):831–9.

53. Burton S, Brown G, Bees N, Norman A, Biedrzycki O, Arnaout A, et al. Accuracy of CT prediction of poor prognostic features in colonic cancer. Br J Radiol. 2008;81(961):10–9.

54. Maizlin ZV, Brown JA, So G, Brown C, Phang TP, Walker ML, et al. Can CT replace MRI in preoperative assessment of the circumferential resection margin in rectal cancer? Dis Colon Rectum. 2010;53(3): 308–14.

Endorectal Ultrasonography of Rectal Tumours

19

J. Nonner, J.E.R. Waage, P.E.A. Hermsen,
Gunnar Baatrup, P.G. Doornebosch,
and E.J.R. de Graaf

Abstract

The use of endorectal ultrasonography is becoming increasingly popular for evaluating rectal tumours. It is valuable in differentiating rectal adenomas from carcinomas, in preoperative staging of rectal cancer and in the follow-up after resection of rectal tumours. Use of endorectal ultrasonography plays an essential role in tailor-made treatment of rectal tumours, and new ultrasound-based methods might further increase the value of endorectal ultrasound evaluation.

Introduction

In the rectum, adenomas can be excised locally, whereas cancer is treated with radical resection. For early rectal cancer (T1), transanal endoscopic

J. Nonner • P.E.A. Hermsen • P.G. Doornebosch
E.J.R. de Graaf (✉)
Department of Surgery, IJsselland Hospital,
Capelle a/d IJssel, The Netherlands
e-mail: jnonner@ysl.nl; pleunhermsen@gmail.co;
pdoornebosch@ysl.nl; edgraaf@ysl.nl

J.E.R. Waage
Department of Surgery,
Haukeland University Hospital, Bergen, Norway
e-mail: dr.waage@gmail.com

G. Baatrup, DMSC
Department of Surgery, OUH Svendborg Hospital,
Svendborg, Denmark

Institute of Regional Health Science,
University of Southern Denmark, Odense, Denmark
e-mail: baatrupgunnar@baatrup.com

microsurgery (TEM) might provide good long-term results as well [1–4]. Preoperatively, it can be difficult to differentiate between adenomas and carcinomas. In 21–34 % of patients with benign preoperative biopsies from large rectal tumours, definitive histopathology after resection reveals a malignancy [5–7 include Baatrup et al. Int. J. Colorect. Dis.]. Local excision based on false-negative biopsies might burden subsequent radical resection [8].

Depth of invasion into the rectal wall and lymph node involvement are important prognostic factors for rectal cancer [9, 10]. Accurate preoperative assessment of these prognostic factors is important for assigning patients to the most suitable therapy [11, 12]. However, routine diagnostics such as computed tomography (CT) and magnetic resonance imaging (MRI) are known to have limited accuracy, especially in T-staging of early rectal cancer and lymph node involvement.

Endoluminal ultrasonography allows close acoustic contact between the transducer and the structures to be visualized. Over the past two decades, endoluminal ultrasonography of the rectum has gained popularity and is now considered to be an integral part of the preoperative staging of rectal tumours [13].

This review gives a description of the use of endorectal ultrasonography (ERUS) techniques in rectal tumours and its value in preoperative decision-making.

Anatomy of the Rectum

Rectal Wall

The ultrasonographic anatomy of the rectal wall was originally described by Hildebrandt and Feifel [14] and by Beynon [15]. Hildebrandt and Feifel proposed a model with three anatomical layers and two interfaces between these two layers. Beynon presented a model in which all five layers represent anatomical structures, as a result of differences in acoustic impedance. The basic ultrasonographic anatomy of the normal rectal wall can be seen in Fig. 19.1. The inner hyperechoic, mostly white line, represents the interface between the balloon covering the probe and the mucosa. The inner hypoechoic, grey line, represents the mucosa and muscularis mucosa. The middle white line represents the submucosa. The outer grey line represents the muscularis propria, and the outer white line represents the perirectal fat. In Fig. 19.2, the different layers are shown schematically. It appears that there might not be an accurate correlation between ultrasonography layers and true anatomical layers. This is due to the enhanced signals created by interfaces between different anatomical layers.

At the anterior side, the urinary bladder, prostate and seminal vesicles can be identified in men. In women, the urinary bladder, uterus and vagina can be identified but less well appreciated.

Lymph Nodes

Endosonographically, lymph nodes appear as round or oval structures that are hypoechoic

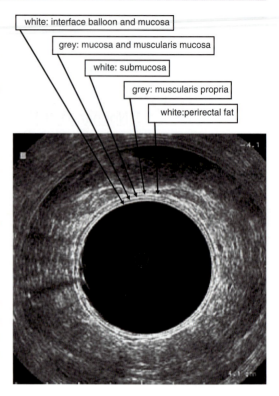

white: interface balloon and mucosa

grey: mucosa and muscularis mucosa

white: submucosa

grey: muscularis propria

white:perirectal fat

Fig. 19.1 Ultrasonographic anatomy of the normal rectal wall

compared with the surrounding perirectal fat [16]. It is difficult to differentiate between benign and metastatic lymph nodes by ERUS. Consequently, a number of criteria are used for identifying metastatic lymph nodes as proximity to tumour, hypoechogenicity, round shape and size larger than 3 mm or 5 mm [13, 17].

Equipment

In literature, mostly Brüel and Kjaer (Brüel & Kjaer Medical Systems Inc., Naerum, Denmark) equipment is used. In our hospital, we used up to 2007 the B&K Medical Scanner® type 2001 with a type 1850 endoscopic probe with a 10-MHz crystal. Recently, we changed to the B&K Medical Scanner® type 2052 Pro Focus with a type 2052 rotating endosonic probe with a 10–16-MHz transducer (Fig. 19.3). Inside the transducer is a double-crystal assembly where 2 crystals located back to back. The assembly can rotate inside the transducer to give a 360° field of view and can be moved forwards and

Fig. 19.2 Schematic overview of anatomy of the normal rectal wall

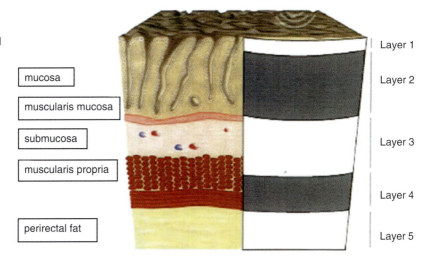

mucosa

muscularis mucosa

submucosa

muscularis propria

perirectal fat

Layer 1

Layer 2

Layer 3

Layer 4

Layer 5

Fig. 19.3 BK Medical 2052 Pro Focus scanner with type 2050 endosonic probe

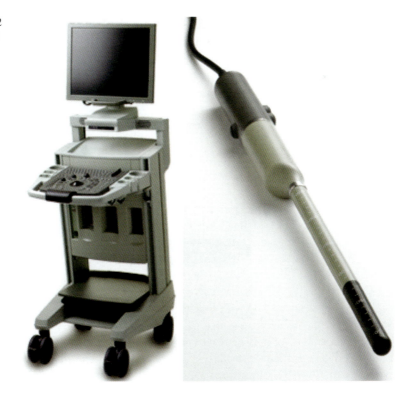

backwards by control buttons over a length of 6 cm within the distal, black-coloured part of the shaft of the probe. An additional feature is the possibility to compose 3D reconstructions. A balloon is placed over the transducer and is filled with approximately 50 ml of water for optimal acoustic coupling. Alternatively, one can simply fill water into the rectum and use the hard anal probe without balloon. It is important to use degassed water to avoid artefacts on the ultrasound image.

Technique

Patients can be investigated in an outpatient setting, preferably in a specially designed colorectal unit. One to two hours before endorectal ultrasonography (ERUS), a cleansing enema is given to prevent reduced visibility by stool and avoid artefacts on the images. Patients are placed in lithotomy position, or left lateral decubitus position. First, digital rectal examination is performed to determine sphincter tone and, if within reach of index finger, tumour size, position, mobility and distance from anal verge. Next, a rigid rectoscope (RectoLution® System, Richard Wolf Medical Devices, Knittlingen, Germany), with an outer diameter of 23 mm, is introduced for inspection of the tumour (Fig. 19.4). The rectoscope is then positioned proximal to the upper margin of the tumour, followed by the removal of the inner tube with hand piece. The endosonic probe, with a diameter of 20 mm, is introduced via the rectoscope with the tip of the probe just outside the rectoscope. The rectoscope is then pulled back over the remaining 6 cm of the endosonic probe. Consequently, the distal 6 cm of the probe,

coloured black and containing the 10–16-MHz transducer, is outside the rectoscope at the level of the tumour (Fig. 19.5). The balloon is now filled with degassed water for acoustic coupling. Ultrasonographic examination of the entire tumour is now performed and documented in a data file.

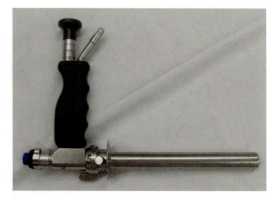

Fig. 19.4 RectoLution system 3 rectoscope

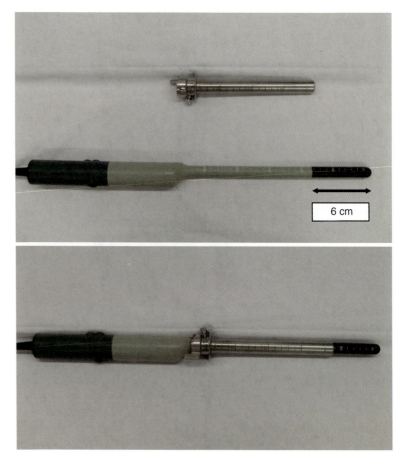

6 cm

Fig. 19.5 Rectoscope with endosonic probe

Staging of Rectal Tumours

ERUS for Differentiating Between Rectal Adenoma and Carcinoma

Local excision of rectal tubulovillous and villous adenomas (TVA) is a validated treatment modality. Concern has been made regarding local recurrences, but with the introduction of transanal endoscopic microsurgery (TEM), the risk has become minimal, and even larger and more proximal located TVA can be excised [18, 19]. In these larger, presumed benign, rectal lesions, based on preoperative biopsy, definite histopathology reveals carcinoma in 21–34 % of tumours [5–7]. When an invasive carcinoma is misdiagnosed as a benign TVA, a suboptimal procedure may be performed for a potentially curable malignant tumour [20]. Although evidence is lacking, previous local excision may burden immediate radical surgery with possible higher morbidity, including increased risk of a (permanent) stoma. Moreover, patient's satisfaction is impeded by this unexpected histopathologic finding and the need for additional surgery. Finally, oncologic outcome in this subgroup of patients is questionable [21, 22].

Extensive efforts have been made to improve preoperative diagnosis of rectal tumours, with computerized tomography (CT), magnetic resonance imaging (MRI) and ERUS. Two large meta-analysis studies found ERUS to be the most accurate modality when compared with CT and MRI in the assessment of wall penetration of rectal cancer [11, 23]. Results in differentiating adenoma from carcinoma were not mentioned. In a retrospective analysis by Zorcolo et al., 81 patients treated with TEM for rectal tumours were investigated [24]. Of these, 21 cases with preoperative biopsy showing adenoma presented foci of carcinoma at final pathology. In 13 of these (62 %), infiltration of the submucosal layer was correctly demonstrated by ERUS. In a prospective study by Doornebosch et al., 264 patients with preoperative diagnosis of TVA (by tissue biopsy) were included [7]. In 231 tumours, endorectal ultrasonography was technically feasible. Of these 231 assessable tumours, ERUS was considered conclusive in 210 tumours (91 %). All patients were operated and

Table 19.1 Agreement of preoperative endorectal ultrasonography with definitive histopathologic stage (Doornebosch et al.) [7]

	Histopathologic T-staging				
	pTVA	pT1	pT2	pT3	Total
ERUS T-staging					
uTVA	147	4	1	1	153
uT1	14	22	4	0	40
uT2	4	2	7	0	13
uT3	1	2	1	0	4
Total	166	30	13	1	210

ERUS endorectal ultrasonography, *TVA* tubulovillous adenoma; overall accuracy 84 % (176/210); sensitivity in diagnosing: TVA, 89 % (147/166); T1 carcinomas, 73 % (22/30); T2 carcinoma 54 % (7/13)

definite histopathologic staging revealed TVA in 166 tumours (79 %), while 44 tumours were diagnosed as invasive carcinoma (21 %). Overall accuracy of ERUS was 84 %. ERUS correctly staged 147 tumours as TVA, with a corresponding sensitivity of 89 %. ERUS correctly staged 38 tumours as invasive with a corresponding sensitivity of 86 % (Table 19.1). With ERUS, the rate of missed carcinomas could be reduced from 21 to 3 % ($p < 0.01$).

Concluding, ERUS is of value in determining treatment strategy for rectal tumours.

ERUS for Staging of Rectal Carcinoma

In the majority of rectal cancer treatment, total mesorectal excision (TME) is the gold standard. This optimized and standardized surgical technique, combined with preoperative radiotherapy, has improved outcome [25, 26]. The prognosis of rectal cancer is closely related to the stage at diagnosis and the choice of treatment. Colorectal staging is currently based on clinical parameters, including degree of invasion of the intestinal wall, degree of lymph node involvement and the existence or not of metastases (TNM classification) [9, 10]. For rectal cancer, the circumferential resection margin is also an important prognostic factor [27]. For T1 rectal carcinomas, TEM is safer than TME, and survival is comparable, although local recurrence rate after TEM can be substantial (4–24 %) [1–4].

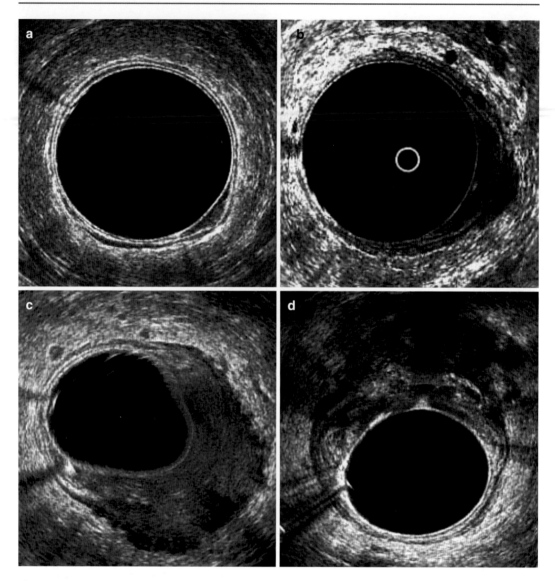

Fig. 19.6 Endoscopic ultrasonographic images of rectal cancer. (**a**) shows uT1 lesion, (**b**) uT2 lesion, (**c**) uT3 lesion and (**d**) uT4 lesion (with ingrowth in the vagina)

ERUS is a reliable method to stage rectal cancers preoperatively for degree of invasion of the rectal wall. Rectal cancer usually appears as a hypoechoic lesion that disrupts the normal five layer rectal wall structures (see Fig. 19.6a–d). Drawbacks are the inability to diagnose distant lymph node and liver metastases and to determine the circumferential resection margin. Hildebrandt and Feifel proposed a modification of the TNM system to stage rectal cancer by ERUS (Table 19.2) [14]. The prefix u is used to indicate the use of ultrasound.

In a meta-analysis by Kwok et al. [23], in determining rectal wall penetration, the sensitivity of ERUS was 93 % and specificity 78 %. In a meta-analysis by Bipat et al. [11], for muscularis propria invasion (uT2), ERUS had a sensitivity of 94 % and a specificity of 86 %. For perirectal fat infiltration (uT3), sensitivity and specificity were 90 and 75 %, and for adjacent organ invasion (uT4) 70 and 97 %, respectively.

Regarding lymph node involvement, ERUS is less accurate. In determining nodal involvement by tumour, the sensitivity of ERUS was 71 % and

Table 19.2 Staging of rectal cancer by endorectal ultrasonography

uT0	Confined to the mucosa
uT1	To but not through the submucosa
uT2	Into but not through the muscularis propria
uT3	Through the bowel wall into the perirectal fat
uT4	Involving adjacent structures
uNo	No definable lymph nodes
uN1	Ultrasonographically apparent lymph nodes

specificity 76 % in the study by Kwok et al. Bipat et al. showed sensitivity and specificity of 67 and 78 % respectively concerning lymph node involvement. A study by Landmann et al. found an overall accuracy of 70 % for nodal staging, with a 16 % false-positive and 14 % false-negative rate [17]. They observed that size of nodal metastases is related to pT stage and that the ability of ERUS to correctly identify nodal disease was related to the size of the affected lymph nodes and metastatic deposits. Early rectal cancers (T1 and T2) are more likely to have small lymph node metastases (diameter smaller than 3 mm) that are not easily identified by ERUS.

ERUS for Restaging Rectal Carcinoma After Neoadjuvant Therapy

Patients with locally advanced rectal carcinoma are commonly treated with neoadjuvant chemoradiotherapy followed by resection. This approach is aimed to downsize and/or downstage rectal cancers with intention to enhance resectability, allow sphincter-preserving surgery, reduce local recurrence and improve long-term survival. ERUS can be used to restage rectal carcinoma after neoadjuvant therapy, although accuracy is questionable. Neoadjuvant therapy can lead to tumour regression and necrosis and fibrotic and inflammatory changes in the rectal wall [28], which can lead to misinterpretation of ERUS images. In a study by Mezzi et al., after neoadjuvant chemoradiation, ERUS correctly classified 46 % (18/39) of patients in line with their histological T-stage [29]. Radovanovic et al. found a good accuracy rate for staging rectal cancer after neoadjuvant chemoradiation (75 %) [30]. However, ERUS could not identify complete pathological response.

Overall, there is little literature concerning restaging after neoadjuvant treatment, and it appears very difficult.

ERUS for Follow-Up After Resection of Rectal Tumours

In patients treated for rectal cancer with local resection, local recurrence occurs in 4–24 % [1–4], usually within the first 2 years after resection. Because local recurrences also arise extraluminally, ERUS may be useful in detection of recurrences when no mucosal lesions are seen during rectoscopy. In a study to recurrences after TEM for T1 rectal cancer by Doornebosch et al., 18 local recurrences occurred [31]. Of these, 6 were found extraluminally and were only visible with ERUS. In a prospective study in 275 patients with invasive rectal cancer treated with local excision or TME, 48 patients (17 %) developed local recurrence [32]. Of these patients, 30 (63 %) were asymptomatic. ERUS detected one-third of these asymptomatic local recurrences that were missed by digital examination or proctoscopic examination. Muller et al. also found ERUS to be highly sensitive (>90 %) in detecting local tumour recurrence [33].

In our hospital, ERUS is used for the follow-up of patients with T1N0 rectal carcinoma, treated with TEM with curative intent. In the first 2 years, digital examination, rectoscopy and ERUS are performed every 3 months, hereafter every 6 months for 3 years and then annually for another 5 years. The regimen of ultrasonography of the liver and pelvic MRI is the same as patients with more advanced cancer, treated with TME.

Limitations

The accuracy of tumour and nodal staging depends on the experience and expertise of the operator [34, 35]. One study showed that at least 50 examinations are required before the operator reaches optimal accuracy [36].

Another problem with ERUS is difficulty in interpreting differences between different stages in rectal wall penetration. ERUS tends to over-stage cancer due to inflammatory infiltrate adjacent to the tumour, that is, endosonographically indistinguishable from the tumour itself [37]. Understaging may be caused by failure to detect microscopic cancer invasion. Preoperative radiotherapy and previous biopsies also diminish the accuracy of T-staging.

If ERUS is considered essential in preoperative staging, accuracy however is not the only relevant issue. Feasibility in all rectal tumours is equally important. If the tumour cannot be reached or passed completely during rectoscopy, or if technical problems occur, such as inability of cleansing the rectum or equipment failure, the tumour is considered not assessable. In series of our hospital, ERUS, with the help of a rigid rectoscope, was technically feasible in 86 % of all rectal tumours. If not feasible, distance from the dentate line (higher percentage in more proximal tumours) proved to be a significant contributing factor [7]. Proper interpretation of ERUS imaging was possible in 78 % of all tumours. The only significant factor negatively influencing interpretation in ERUS imaging was residual or recurrent disease, especially after recent (endoscopic) manipulation.

Novel Ultrasound Methods

In order to improve the decision process for patients with early rectal cancer, there is an obviate need for new methods providing better tissue characterization. The technology of ultrasonography diagnostics is rapidly increasing both concerning the quality of the B-mode image and novel ultrasonography-based methods. As ultrasound waves travel through tissue, harmonic waves from a nonlinear distortion of the signal are generated. These signals are called higher harmonic echo signals and are the background for tissue harmonic imaging and improve both axial and lateral resolution. Tissue harmonic imaging is also shown to improve signal-to-noise ratio and reduce artefacts [38]. Second-order ultrasound field (SURF) imaging

takes further advantage of higher harmonic echo signals by adding a low-frequency manipulation pulse to the high-frequency imaging pulse [39]. SURF technology is able to increase the performance of another novel imaging modality, contrast-enhanced ultrasonography (CEUS) [40, 41]. Ultrasound contrast agents are gas microbubbles dissolved in fluid designed for intravenous injection. The microbubbles are typically smaller than the blood cells, but large enough to stay within the vascular system. In response to emitted ultrasound waves, the size of the microbubbles decrease/increase, and this resonance creates a signal detectable by the ultrasound probe. Consequently, they act as an intravascular contrast agent. Several studies have assessed the methods' ability to evaluate focal liver lesions, and the method has demonstrated higher diagnostic accuracy for focal liver lesions than that of contrast-enhanced CT and MRI [42–44]. The method has also shown promising results for the evaluation lymph node metastasis in breast cancer [45] and the evaluation of prostate cancer [46], but the method is yet to be implemented in routine evaluation for these indications.

Real-time elastography (RTE) is another ultrasonography-based method for tissue evaluation that is now commercially available. RTE displays a colour-coded strain map called elastogram, which is superimposed on the B-mode image. Elastographic evaluation of tissues has been introduced for the assessment of pathological transformation in several organs over the past few years [47–55]. Most clinical RTE studies have applied categorical scales based on colour distribution within the lesion or compared to adjacent tissue. Several different clinical scoring regimes have been reported [49, 52, 53, 56]. More recently, strain ratio (SR) measurements have been introduced as a method for making elastogram interpretation less subjective, providing semiquantitative data on relative tissue strain [57, 58].

To our knowledge, the only RTE method available in association with a 360° endorectal probe

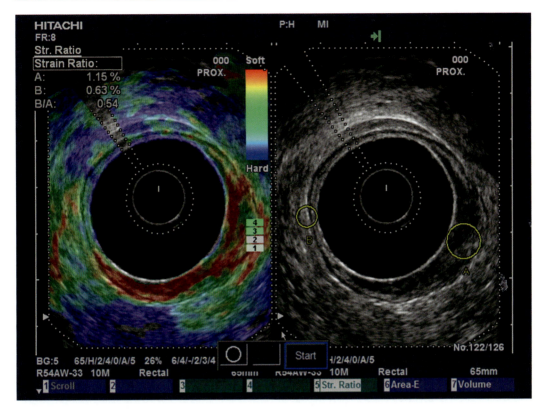

Fig. 19.7 Split-screen image of elastography and B-mode ERUS on right and left hand side, respectively. Tumour from 2 to 7 o'clock suspicious of uT1 on ERUS, but soft (red) on elastography with a strain ratio of 0.54 (upper left corner), indicative of adenoma. Histopathology following surgical resection (TEM) showed pT0 tumour

is the extended combined autocorrelation method (ECAM) [59, 60]. External compression in a compression-decompression cycle is necessary in order to update the elastogram. A water-filled balloon covering the ultrasound probe is used to create strain by inflating and deflating water via a connected syringe during the elastographic examination.

In a study performed at our institution, we evaluated the feasibility of routine evaluation of rectal tumours by endorectal RTE and established a cut-off value for separating adenomas and adenocarcinomas using strain ratio measurements. Sixty-nine patients referred to our outpatient clinic for diagnostic evaluation of rectal tumours were included prospectively. The patients were examined with endorectal elastography, and a strain ratio between tumour tissue strain and adjacent reference tissue strain was calculated. No examination was aborted due to patient discomfort, and a single examiner could perform the examination without assistance. From the recorded strain ratio data, the best separation between malignant and benign lesions was obtained using a strain ratio cut-off value of 1.25, yielding a sensitivity, specificity and accuracy of 0.93, 0.96 and 0.94, respectively. Although the potential for improving preoperative T- and N-staging remains to be investigated in more detail, endorectal elastography is a promising modality that may improve the preoperative evaluation of rectal tumours (Figs. 19.7 and 19.8).

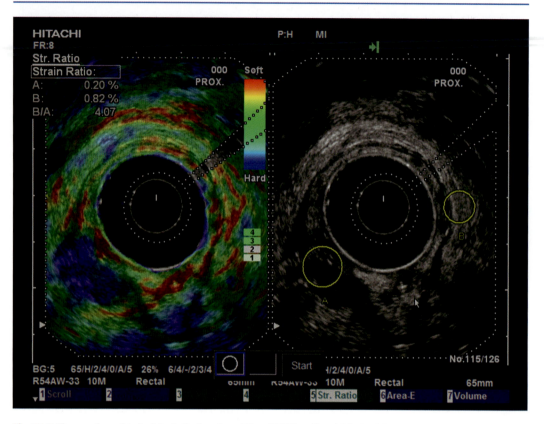

Fig. 19.8 Tumour from 6 to 9 o'clock displayed as uT3 on ERUS and hard (blue) with a strain ratio of 4.07 on elastography. Histopathology confirmed a pT3 adenocarcinoma

Conclusion

ERUS is feasible in most rectal tumours and is of added value in preoperative decision-making for rectal tumours. On the other hand, it has a relatively long learning curve and is operator dependent.

With the introduction of new scanners, with the ability to generate 360° and three-dimensional images, and tissue harmonic imaging, the accuracy of ERUS is likely to become even higher. Novel methods as contrast-enhanced ultrasonography and real-time elastography might also contribute to increased diagnostic accuracy. New research is needed to objectify this.

References

1. Winde G, et al. Surgical cure for early rectal carcinomas (T1). Transanal endoscopic microsurgery vs. anterior resection. Dis Colon Rectum. 1996;39(9):969–76.

2. Baatrup G, et al. Transanal endoscopic microsurgery in 143 consecutive patients with rectal adenocarcinoma: results from a Danish multicenter study. Colorectal Dis. 2009;11(3):270–5.

3. De Graaf EJ, et al. Transanal endoscopic microsurgery versus total mesorectal excision of T1 rectal adenocarcinomas with curative intention. Eur J Surg Oncol. 2009;35(12):1280–5.

4. Bentrem DJ, et al. T1 adenocarcinoma of the rectum: transanal excision or radical surgery? Ann Surg. 2005;242(4):472–7; discussion 477–9.

5. Galandiuk S, et al. Villous and tubulovillous adenomas of the colon and rectum. A retrospective review, 1964–1985. Am J Surg. 1987;153(1):41–7.

6. Taylor EW, et al. Limitations of biopsy in preoperative assessment of villous papilloma. Dis Colon Rectum. 1981;24(4):259–62.

7. Doornebosch PG, et al. The role of endorectal ultrasound in therapeutic decision-making for local vs. transabdominal resection of rectal tumors. Dis Colon Rectum. 2008;51(1):38–42.

8. Borschitz T, Heintz A, Junginger T. The influence of histopathologic criteria on the long-term prognosis of locally excised pT1 rectal carcinomas: results of local excision (transanal endoscopic microsurgery) and immediate reoperation. Dis Colon Rectum. 2006;49(10):1492–506; discussion 1500–5.

9. Sobin LH. TNM: principles, history, and relation to other prognostic factors. Cancer. 2001;91(8 Suppl): 1589–92.

10. Greene FL, Sobin LH. A worldwide approach to the TNM staging system: collaborative efforts of the AJCC and UICC. J Surg Oncol. 2009;99(5): 269–72.

11. Bipat S, et al. Rectal cancer: local staging and assessment of lymph node involvement with endoluminal US, CT, and MR imaging–a meta-analysis. Radiology. 2004;232(3):773–83.

12. Beets-Tan RG, Beets GL. Rectal cancer: review with emphasis on MR imaging. Radiology. 2004;232(2): 335–46.

13. Schaffzin DM, Wong WD. Surgeon-performed ultrasound: endorectal ultrasound. Surg Clin North Am. 2004;84(4):1127–49, vii.

14. Hildebrandt U, Feifel G. Preoperative staging of rectal cancer by intrarectal ultrasound. Dis Colon Rectum. 1985;28(1):42–6.

15. Beynon J, et al. The endosonic appearances of normal colon and rectum. Dis Colon Rectum. 1986;29(12): 810–3.

16. Giovannini M, Ardizzone S. Anorectal ultrasound for neoplastic and inflammatory lesions. Best Pract Res Clin Gastroenterol. 2006;20(1):113–35.

17. Landmann RG, et al. Limitations of early rectal cancer nodal staging may explain failure after local excision. Dis Colon Rectum. 2007;50(10):1520–5.

18. Langer C, et al. Surgical cure for early rectal carcinoma and large adenoma: transanal endoscopic microsurgery (using ultrasound or electrosurgery) compared to conventional local and radical resection. Int J Colorectal Dis. 2003;18(3):222–9.

19. de Graaf EJ, et al. Transanal endoscopic microsurgery is feasible for adenomas throughout the entire rectum: a prospective study. Dis Colon Rectum. 2009;52(6): 1107–13.

20. Worrell S, et al. Endorectal ultrasound detection of focal carcinoma within rectal adenomas. Am J Surg. 2004;187(5):625–9; discussion 629.

21. Baron PL, et al. Immediate vs. salvage resection after local treatment for early rectal cancer. Dis Colon Rectum. 1995;38(2):177–81.

22. Hahnloser D, et al. Immediate radical resection after local excision of rectal cancer: an oncologic compromise? Dis Colon Rectum. 2005;48(3):429–37.

23. Kwok H, Bissett IP, Hill GL. Preoperative staging of rectal cancer. Int J Colorectal Dis. 2000;15(1): 9–20.

24. Zorcolo L, et al. Preoperative staging of patients with rectal tumors suitable for transanal endoscopic microsurgery (TEM): comparison of endorectal ultrasound and histopathologic findings. Surg Endosc. 2009;23(6): 1384–9.

25. Kapiteijn E, Putter H, van de Velde CJ. Impact of the introduction and training of total mesorectal excision on recurrence and survival in rectal cancer in The Netherlands. Br J Surg. 2002;89(9):1142–9.

26. Peeters KC, et al. The TME trial after a median follow-up of 6 years: increased local control but no survival benefit in irradiated patients with resectable rectal carcinoma. Ann Surg. 2007;246(5): 693–701.

27. Gosens MJ, et al. Circumferential margin involvement is the crucial prognostic factor after multimodality treatment in patients with locally advanced rectal carcinoma. Clin Cancer Res. 2007;13(22 Pt 1): 6617–23.

28. Napoleon B, et al. Accuracy of endosonography in the staging of rectal cancer treated by radiotherapy. Br J Surg. 1991;78(7):785–8.

29. Mezzi G, et al. Endoscopic ultrasound and magnetic resonance imaging for re-staging rectal cancer after radiotherapy. World J Gastroenterol. 2009;15(44): 5563–7.

30. Radovanovic Z, et al. Accuracy of endorectal ultrasonography in staging locally advanced rectal cancer after preoperative chemoradiation. Surg Endosc. 2008;22(11):2412–5.

31. Doornebosch PG, et al. Treatment of recurrences after Transanal Endoscopic Microsurgery (TEM) for T1 recal cancer. Dis Colon Rectum. 2010;53(9): 1234–9.

32. de Anda EH, et al. Endorectal ultrasound in the follow-up of rectal cancer patients treated by local excision or radical surgery. Dis Colon Rectum. 2004;47(6): 818–24.

33. Muller C, Kahler G, Scheele J. Endosonographic examination of gastrointestinal anastomoses with suspected locoregional tumor recurrence. Surg Endosc. 2000;14(1):45–50.

34. Herzog U, et al. How accurate is endorectal ultrasound in the preoperative staging of rectal cancer? Dis Colon Rectum. 1993;36(2):127–34.

35. Carmody BJ, Otchy DP. Learning curve of transrectal ultrasound. Dis Colon Rectum. 2000;43(2):193–7.

36. Mackay SG, et al. Assessment of the accuracy of transrectal ultrasonography in anorectal neoplasia. Br J Surg. 2003;90(3):346–50.

37. Katsura Y, et al. Endorectal ultrasonography for the assessment of wall invasion and lymph node metastasis in rectal cancer. Dis Colon Rectum. 1992;35(4): 362–8.

38. Choudhry S, et al. Comparison of tissue harmonic imaging with conventional US in abdominal disease. Radiographics. 2000;20(4):1127–35.

39. Nasholm SP, et al. Transmit beams adapted to reverberation noise suppression using dual-frequency SURF imaging. IEEE Trans Ultrason Ferroelectr Freq Control. 2009;56(10):2124–33.

40. Masoy SE, et al. SURF imaging: in vivo demonstration of an ultrasound contrast agent detection technique. IEEE Trans Ultrason Ferroelectr Freq Control. 2008;55(5):1112–21.

41. Hansen R, Angelsen BA. SURF imaging for contrast agent detection. IEEE Trans Ultrason Ferroelectr Freq Control. 2009;56(2):280–90.

42. Leen E, et al. Multi-centre clinical study evaluating the efficacy of SonoVue (BR1), a new ultrasound contrast agent in Doppler investigation of focal hepatic lesions. Eur J Radiol. 2002;41(3):200–6.

43. Leen E. The role of contrast-enhanced ultrasound in the characterisation of focal liver lesions. Eur Radiol. 2001;11 Suppl 3:E27–34.

44. Dietrich CF, et al. Assessment of metastatic liver disease in patients with primary extrahepatic tumors by contrast-enhanced sonography versus CT and MRI. World J Gastroenterol. 2006;12(11):1699–705.

45. Ouyang Q, et al. Detecting metastasis of lymph nodes and predicting aggressiveness in patients with breast carcinomas. J Ultrasound Med. 2010;29(3):343–52.

46. Wink M, et al. Contrast-enhanced ultrasound and prostate cancer; a multicentre European research coordination project. Eur Urol. 2008;54(5):982–92.

47. Itoh A, et al. Breast disease: clinical application of US elastography for diagnosis. Radiology. 2006;239(2):341–50.

48. Zhu QL, et al. Real-time ultrasound elastography: its potential role in assessment of breast lesions. Ultrasound Med Biol. 2008;34(8):1232–8.

49. Ueno E. Breast ultrasound. Gan To Kagaku Ryoho. 1996;23 Suppl 1:14–23.

50. Saftoiu A, et al. Neural network analysis of dynamic sequences of EUS elastography used for the differential diagnosis of chronic pancreatitis and pancreatic cancer. Gastrointest Endosc. 2008;68(6):1086–94.

51. Pallwein L, et al. Real-time elastography for detecting prostate cancer: preliminary experience. BJU Int. 2007; 100(1):42–6.

52. Janssen J, Schlorer E, Greiner L. EUS elastography of the pancreas: feasibility and pattern description of the normal pancreas, chronic pancreatitis, and focal pancreatic lesions. Gastrointest Endosc. 2007;65(7): 971–8.

53. Giovannini M, et al. Endoscopic ultrasound elastography: the first step towards virtual biopsy? Preliminary results in 49 patients. Endoscopy. 2006; 38(4):344–8.

54. Garra BS, et al. Elastography of breast lesions: initial clinical results. Radiology. 1997;202(1):79–86.

55. Allgayer H, Ignee A, Dietrich CF. Endosonographic elastography of the anal sphincter in patients with fecal incontinence. Scand J Gastroenterol. 2010;45(1): 30–8.

56. Alam F, et al. Accuracy of sonographic elastography in the differential diagnosis of enlarged cervical lymph nodes: comparison with conventional B-mode sonography. AJR Am J Roentgenol. 2008;191(2): 604–10.

57. Thomas A, et al. Significant differentiation of focal breast lesions: calculation of strain ratio in breast sonoelastography. Acad Radiol. 2010;17(5): 558–63.

58. Waage JER, et al. Endorectal elastography in the evaluation of rectal tumours. Colorectal Dis. 2010;13(10): 1130–7.

59. Shiina T, Yamakawa M. Fast reconstruction of tissue elastic modulus image by ultrasound. Conf Proc IEEE Eng Med Biol Soc. 2005;1:976–80.

60. Shiina T, Doyley M, Bamber J. Strain imaging using combined RF and envelope autocorrelation processing. Ultrason Symp. 1996;2:1331–6.

Part V

Pathology

Introduction to the Pathology of Colorectal Cancer

Iris D. Nagtegaal

Abstract

Contribution from pathologist to the MDT meeting does not only include decision on malignancy, staging of tumor, and risk assessment based upon histological features. Also evaluation of tumor response to neoadjuvant or adjuvant treatment is important. Criteria for complete resection of cancers are also becoming more complex. The pathologist should deliver data for the prediction of clinical outcome. In screening programs, the key challenges are evaluation of risk factors in polyps and early cancers and identification of indicators of hereditary syndromes.

In the multidisciplinary treatment of colorectal cancer, various disciplines are involved in making treatment decisions. Pathology is one of them, being involved in both preoperative and postoperative patient evaluation. This evaluation is not only the assessment of tumor invasion, margins, and lymph node status, but effects of neoadjuvant therapy and surgical technique can be judged as well and have profound clinical value. Moreover, based on certain histological characteristics, further treatment decisions can be made.

In the era of potential extensive neoadjuvant therapy, the histological diagnosis of rectal adenocarcinoma on pretreatment biopsies has become even more important. Not only is a definite diagnosis on invasive adenocarcinoma required before treatment can start, but the destructive effects of the therapy on tumor cells make this biopsy essential for further (molecular) testing. Up to now, prediction can be made based on the biopsy about the response to therapy, although a number of attempts have been made to do so.

While in the twentieth century, the evaluation of treatment was limited to the assessment of the resection margins of the operation specimen, in the current century, innovations in the multimodality treatment of colorectal cancer patients are reflected in the increasingly complex evaluation of the specimen (Chap. 22), both on the macroscopic and microscopic levels. Studies in recently completed large multicenter trials have confirmed the importance of evaluation of the resection specimen and the assessment of the circumferential margin. These trials increasingly include

I.D. Nagtegaal, MD, PhD
Department of Pathology, Radboud University
Nijmegen Medical Center,
Nijmegen, The Netherlands
e-mail: iris.nagtegaal@radboudumc.nl

neoadjuvant therapy challenging the pathologist to improve the information obtained from the resection specimen. The main challenges lie in the evaluation of treatment response and the prediction of clinical outcomes based on these data (Chap. 23).

With the widespread introduction of population screening in Europe, the detection of early colorectal cancer as well as the evaluation of colorectal polyps has become increasingly important. The detection of patients at risk, be it due to one high-risk lesion that is not completely removed or due to the detection of multiple lesions that are suggestive of hereditary syndromes, is one of the key challenges for the next couple of years (Chap. 21).

The role of pathology in the multidisciplinary treatment of colorectal cancer has expanded during the last 20 years. The modern pathologist is a key member of the multidisciplinary team, and the information provided from traditional histology is integrated with macroscopic and molecular analyses in order to optimize treatment choices for each individual patient.

Early Colorectal Cancer

21

Cord Langner and Michael Vieth

Abstract

This chapter explains the terminology and classification of colorectal neoplastic precursor lesions, with focus on serrated lesions: hyperplastic polyp, sessile serrated adenoma/polyp (or lesion), mixed polyp and traditional serrated adenoma. We refer to practical issues, such as the measurement of polyp size and the grading of intraepithelial neoplasia/dysplasia (low grade vs. high grade). The definition of invasion is driven by the World Health Organization and defined as invasion into the submucosal layer. Risk assessment of pT1 colorectal cancers is the prerequisite of clinical decision making ranging from follow-up only to additional endoscopic and surgical procedures. The evaluation is based upon the following parameters: depth of invasion (for sessile lesions reported according to Kikuchi levels sm1–sm3; for polypoid/pedunculated lesions reported according to Haggitt levels I–IV), tumour grade, vascular invasion, margin involvement, budding (tumour cell dissociation at the invasion front) and (possibly) perineural invasion.

Introduction

In the routine setting, pathologists are often confronted with biopsies or polypectomy specimens of the colorectum that show architectural and/or cytological features of a neoplastic precursor lesion. Traditionally, these lesions have been termed "dysplastic". In the year 2000, however, the World Health Organization (WHO) replaced the term "dysplasia" by "intraepithelial neoplasia" [1]. It is a matter of fact that this term was not accepted worldwide for various reasons leading to a parallel use of dysplasia and intraepithelial neoplasia in the gastrointestinal tract, while in the anus and pancreas, the term intraepithelial neoplasia was rather uniformly applied. In the 2010 edition of the WHO classification [2], the term intraepithelial neoplasia is used as an umbrella term for all kinds of neoplastic lesions

C. Langner (✉)
Institute of Pathology, Medical University of Graz,
Auenbruggerplatz 25, 8036 Graz, Austria
e-mail: cord.langner@medunigraz.at

M. Vieth
Klinikum Bayreuth, Institute of Pathology,
Preuschwitzerstraße 101, 95445 Bayreuth, Germany
e-mail: vieth.lkpathol@uni-bayreuth.de

G. Baatrup (ed.), *Multidisciplinary Treatment of Colorectal Cancer*,
DOI 10.1007/978-3-319-06142-9_21, © Springer International Publishing Switzerland 2015

that present with the classical histological and/or cytological features of dysplasia but also without. The key elements of the definition of intraepithelial neoplasia are that lesions are morphologically identifiable, have the potential to become malignant and are noninvasive. The term dysplasia was "reintroduced" in 2010 and is now mainly used for preinvasive neoplastic lesions that arise in chronic inflammatory conditions of the oesophagus, stomach and colon. To avoid ultimate confusion, we have to ensure that pathology diagnoses are clear to clinicians and that, based upon the pathology report, appropriate clinical decision making is possible, even if this might lead to national solutions that differ from worldwide classification systems.

Classification of Neoplastic Precursor Lesions

An adenoma is defined as a circumscribed benign epithelial lesion characterised by the presence of neoplastic (dysplastic) epithelium, but without evidence of invasion [3]. Classification of adenomas should include grading of neoplasia. A two-tiered system of low-grade and high-grade (intraepithelial) neoplasia is recommended [3, 4].

This system aims to minimise intra- and interobserver variation and facilitates management of endoscopically detected lesions. Classically, adenomas are divided into tubular, tubulovillous or villous types, and separation between the three is based on the relative proportions of tubular and villous components, according to the "25 % rule" described in the WHO classification: at least 25 % of the luminal surface of an adenoma should be villous, i.e. leaflike projections lined by dysplastic glandular epithelium, to classify the lesion as tubulovillous and more than 75 % to classify the lesion as villous, respectively; all other lesions are classified as tubular [3]. Upon endoscopy, adenomas may appear polypoid, non-polypoid or depressed. The term "flat" should be avoided. The definition of a non-polypoid adenoma refers to a lesion that is not thicker than 3 mm and does not exceed twice the height of the neighbouring normal mucosa. The

size of an adenoma, i.e. the maximum diameter, is important for risk estimation of inherent adenocarcinoma. The term "advanced" adenoma which was developed in screening programmes is sometimes used to categorise adenomas for clinical management. In this context, an advanced adenoma is defined by either size larger than 10 mm, presence of high-grade intraepithelial neoplasia/dysplasia or a villous component.

Classical histological criteria of neoplasticlesions in the colorectal mucosa include alterations of nuclear size and shape (nuclear enlargement, elongation, increased nuclear/cytoplasmic (N/C) ratio, hyperchromasia, clumped chromatin pattern, (multiple) enlargednucleoli, irregular nuclear membranes), nuclear pseudostratification and loss of nuclear polarity, increased number of (atypical) mitoses and dense or hyperbasophilic cytoplasm. Common architectural abnormalities include crypt distortion, branchingand dilatation, back-to-back gland formation, gland-in-gland pattern and villous growth.

The term "carcinoma in situ" refers to a cytologically malignant lesion that does not show invasion into the lamina propria or submucosa and is thus limited to the epithelium. Carcinoma in situ lesions are well recognised in stratified epithelia, and, within the gastrointestinal tract, the term is widely used in the classification of preinvasive neoplastic oesophageal lesions. In gastrointestinal columnar epithelia, although from a biological point of view the concept of carcinoma in situ appears valid ("adenocarcinoma in situ"), the use of this term is discouraged since criteria on how to diagnose carcinoma in situ and how to differentiate it from high-grade intraepithelial neoplasia/dysplasia are simply lacking. Therefore, to avoid overtreatment of affected patients, these lesions are currently summarised under the term high-grade intraepithelial neoplasia/dysplasia, in accordance with the current WHO practice guidelines [3]. Since both lesions lack features of invasion into the lamina propria or the submucosal layer, clinical implications including treatment are virtually the same.

The definition of "intramucosal carcinoma" varies worldwide. In the USA and in most European countries, the term is applied to lesions that show histological evidence of invasion into the lamina propria and/or muscularis mucosa, but not into the submucosa. Classical signs of invasion, such as infiltration of the stroma by single cells or small clusters of cells, complex glandular arrangements that are beyond those present in adenomas, presence of a stromal response such as desmoplasia and evidence of lymphovascular invasion are rarely seen in well-differentiated early carcinomas. According to the current WHO classification, the term intramucosal carcinoma is deemed appropriate in the upper gastrointestinal tract including the small bowel, but not in the colorectum [3]. In Japan, intramucosal (adeno)carcinomas are diagnosed both in the upper and in the lower gastrointestinal tract including the colorectum. According to the AJCC/UICC tumour node metastasis (TNM) classification system [5, 6], submucosal invasion represents a prerequisite for the diagnosis of invasion in colorectal neoplasia, but lesions confined to the mucosa may be classified as either high-grade neoplasia/dysplasia *or* carcinoma in situ (pTis). All these approaches have their pros and cons. But it appears that the worldwide use of the term intramucosal carcinoma for colorectal lesions is only a matter of time. Thus, in the Kyoto conference held in 2008, an international consensus was reached that colorectal carcinoma can be confined to the mucosal layer, and the members of the conference agreed upon the diagnostic term intramucosal carcinoma [4].

In the European guidelines for colorectal cancer screening, the main pathology chapter was written in parallel with the current WHO classification, stating that invasion is defined as invasion into the submucosal layer. In an annex to this chapter, this concept was supported, but it was also mentioned that from a biological point of view, the diagnosis of intramucosal carcinomas is reasonable [7, 8].

Recent advances in molecular pathology, particularly with genotype-phenotype correlation, caused pathologists to recognise a broader spectrum of precursor lesions of colorectal cancer which include lesions that do not necessarily show the classical histological and/or cytological features of intraepithelial neoplasia/dysplasia.

These lesions are summarised in the serrated pathway, ranging from hyperplastic polyps to serrated adenomas and, ultimately, to serrated adenocarcinomas [9]. These lesions may be difficult to diagnose, and knowledge of their natural history is still limited, albeit rapidly growing, since the "serrated route to cancer" currently represents a major research topic in the field of gastrointestinal pathology. Data, however, are controversial, the clinical implications are still ill defined, and the interobserver agreement of pathologists diagnosing these lesions is believed to be low. Further work is required in this field, and until we understand these lesions better, it is recommended that all serrated lesions, with the exception of small left-sided hyperplastic polyps, are fully removed.

Measurement of Adenoma Size

Size, in particular the largest diameter of an adenoma, represents an important objective tool in risk assessment. This method is auditable, accurate, simple to perform and able to assess the adenomatous component within a mixed lesion.

Although the level of evidence is low, literature data suggest that different ways to assess the size of a lesion (endoscopic measurement vs. the pathologist's measurement – before and after fixation and/or slide preparation) may affect diagnostic reproducibility and the detection rate of advanced adenomas. Over- or underestimation of polyp size is more likely to be important when the misjudgement crosses the 10-mm threshold. Overall, assessing adenoma size by the pathologist appears to be the most accurate tool [10] and is analogously recommended in the EU guidelines for breast cancer screening [11].

If the lesion is too large for the maximum dimension to be measured on a single slide, the measurement taken at the time of specimen dissection should be used. If a biopsy is received or if piecemeal resection is performed, it should be stated that the size of the lesion cannot be accurately assessed by the pathologist. In these cases, the endoscopist's measurement of the size of the lesion should be used with respect to surveillance and/or follow-up strategy. Of note, measurements should exclude the stalk if it is lined by normal, i.e. non-adenomatous, mucosa. The distance to the excision margin should be noted. In the routine setting, the largest diameter of the polyp's head is measured, and details regarding the stalk are given in length and diameter.

Tubular, Tubulovillous and Villous Adenomas: The Grading of "Villousness"

The 25 % rule only applies to wholly excised polyps and to intact sections of lesions large enough to enable reliable assessment. For small fragmented lesions or biopsy material, the presence of at least one clearly identifiable villus merits an adenoma to be classified as "at least tubulovillous" [7].

Serrated Lesions

Terminology
Depending on the criteria used for definition and/ or the inclusion of hyperplastic polyps in this group, literature data regarding the incidence (also prevalence) of serrated lesions are highly variable. Consequently, levels of evidence are still limited, and recommendations are not well established. Overall, these lesions have in common a serrated morphology, but their potential to progress to cancer varies considerably. Hence, the serrated lesions take part in the so-called serrated pathway ("serrated route") to adenocarcinoma and comprise *hyperplastic polyps, sessile serrated adenomas* (also referred to as *sessile serrated lesions/sessile serrated polyps*), *mixed polyps* and, as the ultimate lesion, *serrated adenocarcinoma. Traditional serrated adenomas* represent another distinct lesion in this group.

Hyperplastic Polyp
Hyperplastic polyps are often small (<5 mm in diameter), frequently found in the left (distal) colon and/or rectum and generally considered harmless and not an indicator for colorectal neo-

plasia. They are characterised by simple elongated crypts with normal proliferation in the basal (non-serrated) half of the crypts and serrated morphology in the upper half of the crypts, which has been attributed to decreased apoptosis. Hyperplastic polyps with perineurial-like stromal proliferation (perineurioma) are referred to as fibroblastic polyps. Cytological atypia is lacking, thus nuclei are small, regular and basally orientated.

Sessile Serrated Adenoma
Sessile serrated adenomas are morphologically similar to hyperplastic polyps and have for a long time been diagnosed as such. In fact, they are larger non-polypoid lesions that are predominantly, but not exclusively, encountered in the right colon. Histologically, they show marked structural alterations such as hyperserration, columnar dilatation and serration in the lower third of the crypts with and without crypt branching, formation of L- and T-shaped crypts above the muscularis mucosae and inverted crypts (pseudoinvasion) below the muscularis mucosae. Classical (cytological) features of intraepithelial neoplasia/dysplasia are not observed (Fig. 21.1a).

Notably, both the Kyoto classification [4, 12] and the European guidelines of colorectal carcinoma screening [7, 8] recommend the use of the term sessile serrated lesion for these lesions based upon the lack of classical (cytological) features of intraepithelial neoplasia/dysplasia. However, in the 2010 edition of the WHO classification, the term sessile serrated adenoma/ polyp (SSA/P) is recommended [9], even though these lesions are flat, belonging to the group of non-polypoid colorectal lesions.

Diagnosis of "serrated (historically hyperplastic) polyposis" should be considered in cases with (1) at least five histologically proven serrated polyps proximal to the sigmoid colon with two or more of these exceeding 10 mm in size; (2) any number of serrated polyps proximal to the sigmoid colon in an individual who has a first-degree relative with serrated polyposis; or (3) if more than 20 serrated polyps of any size are found distributed throughout the colon [9].

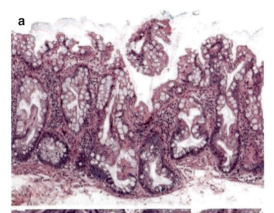

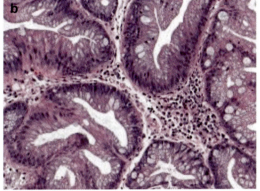

Fig. 21.1 Sessile serrated adenoma (**a**) showing marked structural alterations such as hyperserration, columnar dilatation and serration in the lower third of the crypts with crypt branching and formation of L- and T-shaped crypts above the muscularis mucosae. Traditional serrated adenoma (**b**) showing a serrated morphology but also classical (cytological) features of intraepithelial neoplasia/dysplasia

Mixed Polyp

According to current WHO guidelines, these are combinations of serrated lesions (mainly sessile serrated adenomas, rarely hyperplastic polyps) with conventional (tubular, tubulovillous, villous) as well as traditional serrated adenomas [9]. They were interpreted as collision tumours in the past. Nowadays, these lesions are considered serratedlesions, in particular SSA/Ps complicated by intraepithelial neoplasia/dysplasia, thereby indicating neoplasticprogression on the serrated route to cancer. Of note, both the European guidelines for colorectal cancer screening [7, 8] and the proposal of diagnostic criteria for serrated lesions presented by members of the

Working Group of Gastrointestinal Pathology of the German Society of Pathology [13] recommend to first describe the components of the "mixed polyp" and then include the term mixed polyp in parentheses, e.g. sessile serrated adenoma and tubular adenoma (mixed polyp) with low-grade intraepithelial neoplasia/dysplasia. As classical adenomas, these lesions should be removed completely.

Traditional Serrated Adenoma

Polyps that show a serrated morphology, but also classical (cytological) features of intraepithelial neoplasia/dysplasia, are termed traditional serrated adenomas (Fig. 21.1b). These lesions were recognised as a distinct entity by Longacre and Fenoglio-Preiser already in 1990 [14] and were given the name serrated adenoma at that time. They are rare and usually encountered in the left colon. In order to avoid confusion with sessile serrated adenomas, they were later given the name "traditional" serrated adenoma. Treatment and surveillance are considered to be the same as for classical (tubular, tubulovillous, villous) adenomas.

Grading of Intraepithelial Neoplasia/Dysplasia

Grading of a neoplastic lesion aims at translating biology, i.e. the multistep progress described in the adenoma-carcinoma sequence, into different levels of risk for progression and/or aggressiveness. It has to be noted that there is considerable interobserver variation in the final diagnoses worldwide, mainly due to poorly defined criteria and/or varying interpretation of criteria, causing different assessment of a lesion among different pathologists.

The Vienna classification aimed to group diagnoses with the same clinical consequences together in order to minimise interobserver variation. The system also improved the accuracy of biopsy diagnoses by minimising discrepancies between diagnoses obtained from biopsy material and subsequent resections, respectively [15]. One disadvantage is the use of several subcategories. The Kyoto classification [4, 12] and also the

European guidelines of colorectal carcinoma screening [7, 8] recommend a revised scheme of the Vienna classification meant to further simplify the system. These recommendations led to a 4-tiered system: no neoplasia, low-grade mucosal neoplasia (low-grade adenoma), high-grade mucosal neoplasia (high-grade adenoma, mucosal carcinoma) and carcinoma infiltrating the submucosal layer or beyond. This revision caused increased attention for intramucosal carcinoma and was felt to be a compromise, bringing Western and Asian standpoints closer together. The future will show whether these pragmatic approaches will become more accepted worldwide than previous systems.

Low-Grade Intraepithelial Neoplasia/ Dysplasia

Low-grade intraepithelial neoplasia is an unequivocal neoplastic condition confined to the glandular epithelium, not to be mistaken for inflammatory or regenerative changes. The earliest morphological precursor of intraepithelial neoplasia is the aberrant crypt focus (ACF), i.e. a "single-crypt adenoma" [16]. Microscopic examination of mucosal sheets dissected from the bowel wall in patients with familial adenomatous polyposis or mucosal examination with a magnifying endoscope reveals ACFs to have crypts of enlarged calibre and thickened epithelium with reduced mucin content [16]. Progression from ACF through adenoma to adenocarcinoma characterises carcinogenesis in the large intestine. The situation is more complex in individuals with chronic inflammatory bowel disease in which the diagnosis of a sporadic adenoma has clinical implications different from those of colitis-associated neoplasia.

Histologically, lesions characterised by low-grade intraepithelial neoplasia show reduced mucin content (reduced number of goblet cells) with increased cytoplasmic basophilia and a variety of nuclear changes, such as hyperchromasia, enlargement (spindle-like elongation) and pseudostratification (palisading). Although the number of mitotic figures is increased, atypical mitoses are generally not observed, and nuclear polarity is retained (Fig. 21.2a, b).

High-Grade Intraepithelial Neoplasia/Dysplasia

Morphological changes suggestive of high-grade intraepithelial neoplasia should involve more than just one or two crypts. In addition to the histological characteristics of low-grade intraepithelial neoplasia described above, high-grade intraepithelial neoplasia shows distinctive structural features: complex glandular crowding and irregularity (note that the word "complex" is important and excludes simple crowding of regular tubules that might result from crushing), prominent glandular budding, cribriform gland formation, back-to-back pattern as well as prominent intraluminal papillary tufting. Some of these criteria may be found in low-grade intraepithelial neoplasia/ dysplasia as well. This makes it necessary to use further cytological features: loss of cell and/or nuclear polarity and distinct nuclear changes such as vesicular and/or markedly enlarged irregular nuclei, often with a dispersed chromatin pattern and prominent nucleoli. Atypical mitotic figures are common, and prominent apoptosis, giving rise to intraluminal debris, may be found in some cases (Fig. 21.2c, d). Often several of the above-mentioned features are detected within the same lesion. Caution should be exercised if only a single criterion is observed in order to avoid over-interpretation. Since ordinary adenomas do not erode, erosions should always prompt thorough evaluation of an adenomatous lesion not to miss presence of high-grade intraepithelial neoplasia. However, overinterpretation of isolated surface changes that may be caused by trauma or prolapse needs to be excluded.

Misplacement (entrapment) of adenomatous epithelium into the submucosa of a polyp (pseudoinvasion) represents a well-known histopathological pitfall which needs to be distinguished from invasive carcinoma [17]. If in doubt, the relevant findings should be stated in the pathology report, and a second opinion and/or additional biopsies from the polypectomy site should be considered. Sigmoid polyps are particularly prone to inflammation, a feature which tends to exaggerate the histological features of neoplasia. When associated with epithelial misplacement, the potential for misdiagnosing these lesions as early

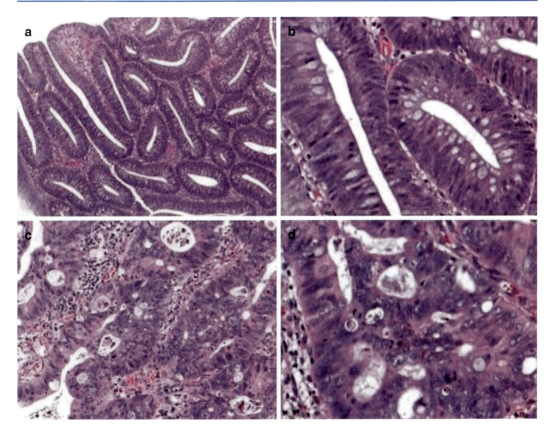

Fig. 21.2 Grading of intraepithelial neoplasia/dysplasia. Lesions characterised by low-grade intraepithelial neoplasia (**a, b**) show reduced mucin content (reduced number of goblet cells) and a variety of nuclear changes, such as hyperchromasia, spindle-like elongation and pseudostratification. Nuclear polarity, however, is retained. In high-grade intraepithelial neoplasia (**c, d**), complex glandular crowding and irregularity with cribriform gland formation and back-to-back pattern is seen (Note loss of nuclear polarity and distinct nuclear changes such as presence of vesicular markedly enlarged irregular nuclei, often with a dispersed chromatin pattern and prominent nucleoli)

carcinoma is evident. Histological changes suggestive of epithelial misplacement are acellular submucosal mucin lakes (not to be misinterpreted for mucinous adenocarcinoma) and hemosiderin-laden macrophages within the stroma.

Histological Evaluation of pT1 Colorectal Cancer

According to the AJCC/UICC TNM system [5, 6], pT1 cancers are those showing invasion through the muscularis mucosae into the submucosa but not beyond. Once again, it has to be stressed that in Japan the term mucosal carcinoma is used as a diagnostic term to describe a distinct tumour category. The discussion, however, seems to be somewhat academic, since all mucosal high-grade lesions, regardless of the terminology used, are adequately treated by endoscopic removal and are believed not to metastasize.

Definition of Invasion

The danger of surgical overtreatment due to misinterpretation of a lesion as invasive cancer must always be considered in biopsy diagnoses. Postoperative mortality (within 30 days) varies between 5 and 10 % in colonic cancers, depending on the population, age of the patient and quality of services available [18–20].

Achieving the optimum balance between removing all disease by resection and minimising harm is crucial. Since criteria of intramucosal criteria are currently not well defined in columnar epithelium, we strongly recommend to adhere to the definition given by the WHO classification of tumours of the digestive system [3], which regards invasion of neoplastic cells through the muscularis mucosae into the submucosa as prerequisite for diagnosing invasive adenocarcinoma at this site (Fig. 21.3a). It needs, however, to be recognised that diagnoses made on the basis of this definition will hamper comparison with series from Japan for which the diagnosis of intramucosal adenocarcinoma is possible. Of note, the AJCC/UICC TNM classification scheme [5, 6] allows to use the term carcinoma in situ (pTis) in columnar epithelium, but as pointed out above, this category is rather vague and ill defined, and, therefore, its use is discouraged by the European guidelines on colorectal cancer screening [7, 8].

Histological criteria of invasion, such as single tumour cells, are more likely to be seen in advanced carcinomas, but not in early carcinomas. Likewise, a desmoplastic stromal response is only rarely observed, particularly when carcinoma cells have just started to invade the submucosal layer (Fig. 21.3b). In addition, basal membranes are frequently discernible around invading glands in well-differentiated early carcinomas [21–23], and definitions using the term "invasion through the basement membrane" are for this reason misleading. Nevertheless, a subclassification of early carcinomas into low-risk and high-risk categories, based on the estimated risk of regional lymph node involvement, should always be performed.

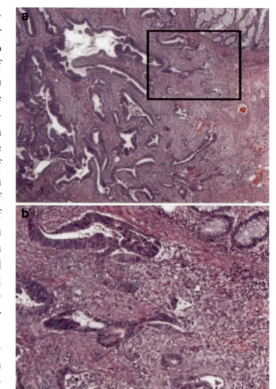

Fig. 21.3 Early colorectal cancer showing invasion of neoplastic cells through the muscularis mucosae into the submucosa (**a**). Note desmoplastic stromal response around invading glands in high-power view (**b**)

cells are usually large and tall, and the gland lumina may contain varying amounts of debris. The designation of mucinous adenocarcinoma is used when more than 50 % of the lesion is composed by pools of extracellular mucin. Signet ring cell carcinoma and adenosquamous carcinoma represent rare variants that are almost never observed as early cancer.

Typing of Early Colorectal Cancer

Histological typing of colorectal cancers is generally performed according to WHO guidelines and does not differ between early and advanced tumours [3]. Thus, most adenocarcinomas are gland forming, with variability in size and configuration of glandular structures. In well- and moderately differentiated cases, which make up the vast majority of early cancers, the epithelial

Risk Assessment in pT1 Colorectal Cancer

In early colorectal adenocarcinoma, discussions regarding optimal treatment of affected individuals (endoscopic vs. surgical) appear to be an integral part of multidisciplinary team meetings. To facilitate clinical decision making, the pathologist should always report on histological features that may indicate increased risk of local lymph node spread, thus enabling stratification of tumours into low- and high-risk categories [7, 24–28].

In colorectal adenocarcinoma, in general, several parameters have been correlated with adverse outcome, such as depth of invasion reflected by the AJCC/UICC TNM system, tumour size, tumour differentiation, lymph and blood vessel invasion, perineural invasion, tumour border configuration, incomplete tumour resection and tumour cell dissociation at the invasion front referred to as tumour budding [29–31]. Some of these parameters, e.g. lymph and blood vessel invasion as well as tumour budding, are potential predictors of increased risk of local lymph node spread (compare below).

For early colorectal cancer, the most appropriate method for risk estimation of lymph node involvement appears to be the assessment of depth of invasion which should be assessed depending on the overall morphology of the lesion, e.g. sessile (Kikuchi levels; [32]) or polypoid (Haggitt levels; [33]). Other parameters, such as vascular invasion and tumour budding, may serve as additional markers. In the following, we will refer to the main prognostic parameters in detail. Of note, the value of these markers has very recently been proven in two systematic meta-analyses [34, 35].

Subclassification of pT1 Adenocarcinomas According to Depth of Invasion

For submucosal carcinomas, substaging of pT1 is essential. The most widely used approach implies the pragmatic subdivision of the submucosal layer into three parts: a superficial, a middle and a deep third, also referred to as Kikuchi levels sm1, sm2 and sm3 [32]. The risk of lymph node involvement has been calculated to account for 1.4–5 % for sm1, 8 % for sm2 and 23 % for sm3 tumours, respectively [36, 37]. In polypoid lesions, the stalk always represents the upper third of the submucosal layer. Haggitt et al. [33] identified the level of invasion into the stalk of a pedunculated polyp as being important in predicting outcome.

The authors classified polypoid tumours as follows: "level 1" lesions show invasion of the submucosa limited to the head of the polyp, "level 2" lesions extend into the neck of the polyp, "level 3" lesions show invasion of any part of the stalk and "level 4" lesions invade beyond the stalk but still confined to the submucosal layer. An example illustrating the use of the Kikuchi and the Haggitt system is given in Fig. 21.4.

It has to be noted that both the Kikuchi (for sessile tumours) and the Haggitt (for polypoid or pedunculated tumours) classification systems may be difficult to apply, especially if there is fragmentation or suboptimal orientation of the tissue. Separation of Haggitt level 2 from levels 1 and 3 may be difficult even if the lesion is well preserved. Moreover, although level 4 invasion is generally accepted as a major risk factor for adverse outcome, regional lymph node metastasis may be observed also in level 2 or 3 lesions.

Thus, recent classification systems stressed the advantage of exact measurement of tumour invasion beyond the muscularis mucosae. Ueno et al. [38] suggested to assess both the depth (cut-off value 2,000 μm) and the width (cut-off value 4,000 μm) of invasion. The authors demonstrated that by doing so, a more objective and accurate assessment of the risk of lymph node metastasis is possible: 3.9 % vs. 17.1 %, when depth of submucosal invasion is lower or higher than 2,000 μm, as well as 2.5 % vs. 18.2 %, when width of submucosal invasion is lower or higher than 4,000 μm. According to other studies, tumours with submucosal invasion not deeper than 1,000 μm generally lack lymph node metastasis, thus rending the 1,000-μm cut-off value as major criterion for stratification of patients for endoscopic or surgical therapy [39, 40].

Each classification system has its advantages and disadvantages: (1) the Kikuchi system cannot reliably be used if the muscularis propria is not present (i.e. in most endoscopic resections), (2) the Haggitt levels are not applicable in non-polypoid (sessile) lesions and (3) exact measurement depends on the feasibility to identify the muscularis mucosae which may be difficult, if not impossible, when cancer tissue has destroyed this histological landmark. Lacking a worldwide

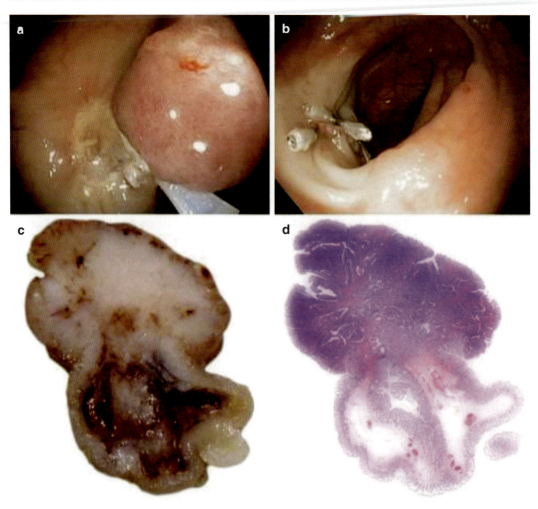

Fig. 21.4 Pedunculated early colorectal cancer. The lesion is completely removed by endoscopy (**a**, **b**; Images courtesy of Dr. Franz Siebert, Hospital of Barmherzige Brüder, St. Veit/Glan, Austria); all margins are free of cancer (R0 resection). The cut surface (**c–d**) shows invasion (marked by an *arrow*) extending into the upper third of the submucosal layer (sm1), as represented by the neck of the polyp (Haggitt level 2)

consensus, a definitive recommendation for one method or another can currently not be given. The European guidelines of colorectal cancer screening, however, recommend the Kikuchi system for non-polypoid (sessile) and the Haggitt system for polypoid (pedunculated) lesions [5, 6].

Tumour Grade in pT1 Adenocarcinomas

Grading of colorectal cancer is generally performed according to the WHO guidelines assessing the extent of glandular appearance and should be divided into well-, moderately and poorly differentiated or into low-grade (encompassing well- and moderately differentiated cancers) and high-grade (including poorly differentiated and undifferentiated cancers) tumours, respectively [3]. Poorly differentiated adenocarcinomas should at least show some gland formation or mucus production. When a carcinoma is heterogeneous, grading should be based on the least differentiated component, not including the leading front of invasion. The percentage of the tumour showing gland formation can be used to define the grade. According to the current WHO classification [3], well-differentiated tumours (grade 1) exhibit glandular structures in >95 % of the tumour area, moderately differentiated tumours (grade 2) in 50–95 % and poorly differentiated tumours (grade 3) in >0–49 %, respectively. By convention, morphological grading of tumours applies only to adenocarcinoma "NOS" (not otherwise specified). Other morphological variants (e.g. mucinous adenocarcinoma, signet ring cell carcinoma) carry their own prognostic significance and grading does not apply [3].

In general, no substantial differences exist between the grading of early and advanced cancers. In the absence of good evidence, the European guidelines for colorectal cancer screening recommend that a grade of poor differentiation should be applied in a polyp cancer when *any* area of the lesion is considered to show poor tumour differentiation [7]. As for advanced tumours, tumour cell dissociation at the leading edge of invasion ("budding") should not influence the grading of early cancers.

Recently, Ueno et al. [41] proposed "objective criteria for grade 3" in early colorectal cancer. In their experience, the incidence of nodal involvement differed most greatly between G3 (27 %) and non-G3 (4 %) tumours, when G3 was applied to lesions containing either or both of the following criteria: (1) ten or more solid cancer nests in the microscopic field of a 4× objective lens and (2) a mucin-producing component fully occupying the microscopic field of a 40× objective lens. This study, however, still warrants external validation.

Vascular Invasion in pT1 Adenocarcinomas

Invasion of endothelium-lined vascular spaces, i.e. lymphatic and/or venous invasion, is generally regarded as a significant risk factor for regional lymph node and/or distant metastasis in colorectal cancer, including early lesions. Thus, lymphatic invasion has repeatedly proven to be an independent predictor of local metastatic lymph node spread in early colorectal cancer [41–45].

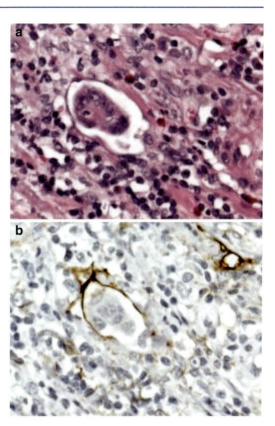

Fig. 21.5 Lymphatic invasion in early colorectal cancer, as assed by routine haematoxylin and eosin (**a**) and additional D2-40 (**b**) immunostaining which specifically labels endothelial cells of lymph vessels (serial sections)

Sometimes retraction artefact around invading tumour glands may mimic vascular spaces. In these cases additional histochemical and/or immunohistochemical staining may be helpful to prove true angioinvasion and rule out false-positive results. In addition, immunostaining with the monoclonal antibody D2-40 which is specific for lymphatic endothelial cells significantly increases the detection rate of lymphatic invasion compared to conventional haematoxylin and eosin staining (Fig. 21.5a, b) [46, 47], while Elastica van Gieson stain and CD31 and/or CD34 immunostaining for blood vessel endothelia facilitate detection of venous invasion [48–50]. Finally, interobserver agreement of vascular invasion is only moderate but cannot be improved by the use of immunohistochemistry, highlighting the need for strict criteria in the evaluation [51].

Of note, presence of blood vessel invasion has also been correlated with presence of regional lymph node metastasis [50, 52, 53]. The reason for this at first glance unexpected finding is unclear. Most probably, tumours with venous invasion do also harbour lymphatic invasion which may have been missed or may only be detected performing additional sections.

Margin Involvement in pT1 Adenocarcinomas

It is important to record whether the deep (basal) resection margin is involved by invasive tumour (which may be a reason for additional surgery) and whether the lateral mucosal resection margin is involved by carcinoma or by the neoplastic precursor lesion (for which extended local excision may be attempted) [7].

There has been considerable discussion and controversy in the literature regarding the degree of clearance (resection status) that might be acceptable after local excision of early carcinoma extending close to the deep submucosal margin [25]. All pathologists would possibly agree on 0 mm, most would regard a clearance of <1 mm as an indication for additional therapy, while others would use <2 mm. According to the European guidelines for colorectal cancer screening, clearance of 1 mm or less should be regarded as margin involvement [7, 8].

Anyhow, reporting on the degree of clearance (resection status) represents a major item in the pathology report, particularly after local excision, and the distance to the resection margin should be measured (reported in mm), regarding both deep submucosal and lateral margins.

Tumour Cell Dissociation ("Budding") in pT1 Adenocarcinomas

Tumour cell budding has been defined as the presence of isolated single cells or small clusters of cells (composed of fewer than five cells) scattered in the stroma at the invasive tumour margin and has been significantly associated with outcome in

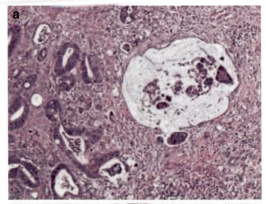

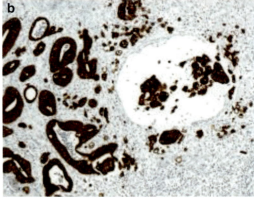

Fig. 21.6 High-grade tumour budding at the invasion front of early colorectal cancer, as assed by routine haematoxylin and eosin (**a**) and additional keratin (**b**) immunostaining which specifically labels single cancer cells and small clusters of invading cancer cells (serial sections)

colorectal cancer [38, 54–57]. Although criteria how to assess the extent of tumour budding have not been standardised, several studies reported upon its usefulness in predicting regional lymph node metastasis in early colorectal cancer [44, 58, 59]. Immunostaining using an antibody directed against keratin, the intermediate filament of epithelial cells and their tumours may facilitate its detection (Fig. 21.6a, b) [44, 60].

Perineural Invasion in pT1 Adenocarcinomas

Perineural invasion is a pathological process characterised by tumour invasion of nervous structures and spread along nerve sheaths which has recently been identified as a new promising marker in colorectal cancer. Presence of perineural invasion appears to be significantly associated with high tumour stage and grade and may serve as a predictor of local tumour relapse (higher risk of incomplete tumour resection) and regional lymph node metastasis [61, 62]. In addition, perineural invasion was found to be an independent predictor of disease-free and cancer-specific survival [61–63]. It is therefore strongly recommended to record presence of perineural invasion in routine pathological assessment of colorectal cancer. Future studies, however, are needed to define the role of perineural invasion in early cancers, since data are currently lacking in this regard.

References

1. Diagnostic terms and definitions. In: Hamilton SR, Aaltonen LA, editors. World Health Organization classification of tumours. Pathology & genetics. Tumours of the digestive system. Lyon: IARC; 2000. p. 8.
2. Odze RD, Riddell RH, Bosman FT, Carneiro F, Flejou JF, Geboes K, Genta RM, Hattori T, Hruban RH, van Krieken JH, Lauwers GY, Offerhaus GJA, Rugge M, Shimizu M, Shimoda T, Theise ND, Vieth M. Premalignant lesions of the digestive system. In: Bosman FT, Carneiro F, Hruban RH, Theise ND, editors. WHO classification of tumours of the digestive system. Lyon: IARC; 2010. p. 10–2.
3. Hamilton SR, Bosman FT, Boffetta P, Ilyas M, Morreau H, Nakamura SI, Quirke P, Riboli E, Sobin LH. Carcinoma of the colon and rectum. In: Bosman FT, Carneiro F, Hruban RH, Theise ND, editors. WHO classification of tumours of the digestive system. Lyon: IARC; 2010. p. 134–46.
4. Kudo S, Lambert R, Allen JI, Fujii H, Fujii T, Kashida H, Matsuda T, Mori M, Saito H, Shimoda T, Tanaka S, Watanabe H, Sung JJ, Feld AD, Inadomi JM, O'Brien MJ, Lieberman DA, Ransohoff DF, Soetikno RM, Triadafilopoulos G, Zauber A, Teixeira CR, Rey JF, Jaramillo E, Rubio CA, Van Gossum A, Jung M, Vieth M, Jass JR, Hurlstone PD. Nonpolypoid neoplastic lesions of the colorectal mucosa. Gastrointest Endosc. 2008;68(4 Suppl):S3–47.
5. Edge SB, Byrd DR, Compton CC, Fritz AG, Greene FL, Trotti A. AJCC cancer staging manual. 7th ed. New York: Springer; 2010.
6. Sobin LH, Gospodarowicz MK, Wittekind C. TNM classification of malignant tumours. 7th ed. New York: Wiley-Blackwell; 2009.
7. Quirke P, Risio M, Lambert R, von Karsa L, Vieth M, International Agency for Research on Cancer. Quality assurance in pathology in colorectal cancer screening and diagnosis. European recommendations. Virchows Arch. 2011;458:1–19.
8. Vieth M, Quirke P, Lambert R, von Karsa L, Risio M. Quality assurance in pathology in colorectal cancer screening and diagnosis: annotations of colorectal lesions. Virchows Arch. 2011;458:21–30.
9. Snover DC, Ahnen DJ, Burt RW, Odze RD. Serrated polyps of the colon and rectum and serrated polyposis. In: Bosman FT, Carneiro F, Hruban RH, Theise ND, editors. WHO classification of tumours of the digestive system. Lyon: IARC; 2010. p. 160–5.
10. Schoen RE, Gerber LD, Margulies C. The pathologic measurement of polyp size is preferable to the endoscopic estimate. Gastrointest Endosc. 1997;46:492–6.
11. EC Working Group on Breast Screening Pathology. Quality assurance guidelines for pathology. In: Perry N, Broeders M, de Wolf C, Törnberg S, Holland R, von Karsa L, editors. European guidelines for qualityassurance in cancer screening and diagnosis.4th ed.Vol 6. European Union; 2006. p. 219–312.
12. Lambert R, Kudo SE, Vieth M, Allen JI, Fujii H, Fujii T, Kashida H, Matsuda T, Mori M, Saito H, Shimoda T, Tanaka S, Watanabe H, Sung JJ, Feld AD, Inadomi JM, O'Brien MJ, Lieberman DA, Ransohoff DF, Soetikno RM, Zauber A, Teixeira CR, Rey JF, Jaramillo E, Rubio CA, Van Gossum A, Jung M, Jass JR, Triadafilopoulos G. Pragmatic classification of superficial neoplastic colorectal lesions. Gastrointest Endosc. 2009;70:1182–99.
13. Aust DE, Baretton GB, Members of the Working Group GI-Pathology of the German Society of Pathology. Serrated polyps of the colon and rectum (hyperplastic polyps, sessile serrated adenomas, traditional serrated adenomas, and mixed polyps)-proposal for diagnostic criteria. Virchows Arch. 2010;457:291–7.
14. Longacre TA, Fenoglio-Preiser CM. Mixed hyperplastic adenomatous polyps/serrated adenomas. A distinct form of colorectal neoplasia. Am J Surg Pathol. 1990;14:524–37.
15. Schlemper RJ, Riddell RH, Kato Y, Borchard F, Cooper HS, Dawsey SM, Dixon MF, Fenoglio-Preiser CM, Fléjou JF, Geboes K, Hattori T, Hirota T, Itabashi M, Iwafuchi M, Iwashita A, Kim YI, Kirchner T, Klimpfinger M, Koike M, Lauwers GY, Lewin KJ, Oberhuber G, Offner F, Price AB, Rubio CA, Shimizu M, Shimoda T, Sipponen P, Solcia E, Stolte M, Watanabe H, Yamabe H. The Vienna classification of gastrointestinal epithelial neoplasia. Gut. 2000;47:251–5.
16. Giardiello FM, Burt RW, Järvinen HJ, Offerhaus GJA. Familial adenomatous polyposis. In: Bosman FT, Carneiro F, Hruban RH, Theise ND, editors. WHO classification of tumours of the digestive system. Lyon: IARC; 2010. p. 147–51.

17. Muto T, Bussey HJ, Morson BC. The evolution of cancer of the colon and rectum. Cancer. 1975;36: 2251–70.

18. Ptok H, Marusch F, Schmidt U, Gastinger I, Wenisch HJ, Lippert H. Risk adjustment as basis for rational benchmarking: the example of colon carcinoma. World J Surg. 2011;35:196–205.

19. Marusch F, Koch A, Schmidt U, Wenisch H, Ernst M, Manger T, Wolff S, Pross M, Tautenhahn J, Gastinger I, Lippert H. Early postoperative results of surgery for rectal carcinoma as a function of the distance of the tumor from the anal verge: results of a multicenter prospective evaluation. Langenbecks Arch Surg. 2002;387:94–100.

20. Kessler H, Hermanek Jr P, Wiebelt H. Operative mortality in carcinoma of the rectum: results of the German Multicentre Study. Int J Colorectal Dis. 1993;8:158–66.

21. Borchard F, Heilmann KL, Hermanek P, Gebbers JO, Heitz PU, Stolte M, Pfeifer U, Schaefer HE, Wiebecke B, Schlake W. Definition and clinical significance of dysplasia in the digestive tract: results of a meeting of the Society of Gastroenterologic Pathology of the German Society of Pathology 1989 in Kronberg. Pathologe. 1991;12:50–6.

22. Borchard F. Forms and nomenclature of gastrointestinal epithelial expansion: what is invasion? Verh Dtsch Ges Pathol. 2000;84:50–61.

23. Vieth M, Stolte M. Distinction of high-grade intraepithelial neoplasia and tubular gastric adenocarcinoma. In: Kaminishi M, Takubo K, Mafune K, editors. The diversity of gastric carcinoma: pathogenesis, diagnosis and therapy. Tokyo: Springer; 2005. p. 109–16.

24. Coverlizza S, Risio M, Ferrari A, Fenoglio-Preiser CM, Rossini FP. Colorectal adenomas containing invasive carcinoma. Pathologic assessment of lymph node metastatic potential. Cancer. 1989;64:1937–47.

25. Cooper HS, Deppisch LM, Gourley WK, Kahn EI, Lev R, Manley PN, Pascal RR, Qizilbash AH, Rickert RR, Silverman JF. Endoscopically removed malignant colorectal polyps: clinicopathologic correlations. Gastroenterology. 1995;108:1657–65.

26. Volk EE, Goldblum JR, Petras RE, Carey WD, Fazio VW. Management and outcome of patients with invasive carcinoma arising in colorectal polyps. Gastroenterology. 1995;109:1801–7.

27. Hassan C, Zullo A, Risio M, Rossini FP, Morini S. Histologic risk factors and clinical outcome in colorectal malignant polyp: a pooled-data analysis. Dis Colon Rectum. 2005;48:1588–96.

28. Williams JG, Pullan RD, Hill J, Horgan PG, Salmo E, Buchanan GN, Rasheed S, McGee SG, Haboubi N. Management of the malignant colorectal polyp: ACPGBI position statement. Colorectal Dis. 2013;15 Suppl 2:1–38.

29. West NP, Morris EJ, Rotimi O, Cairns A, Finan PJ, Quirke P. Pathology grading of colon cancer surgical resection and its association with survival: a retrospective observational study. Lancet Oncol. 2008;9:857–65.

30. Zlobec I, Lugli A. Invasive front of colorectal cancer: dynamic interface of pro-/anti-tumor factors. World J Gastroenterol. 2009;15:5898–906.

31. Tilney HS, Rasheed S, Northover JM, Tekkis PP. The influence of circumferential resection margins on long-term outcomes following rectal cancer surgery. Dis Colon Rectum. 2009;52:1723–9.

32. Kikuchi R, Takano M, Takagi K, Fujimoto N, Nozaki R, Fujiyoshi T, Uchida Y. Management of early invasive colorectal cancer. Risk of recurrence and clinical guidelines. Dis Colon Rectum. 1995;38:1286–95.

33. Haggitt RC, Glotzbach RE, Soffer EE, Wruble LD. Prognostic factors in colorectal carcinomas arising in adenomas: implications for lesions removed by endoscopic polypectomy. Gastroenterology. 1985;89: 328–36.

34. Beaton C, Twine CP, Williams GL, Radcliffe AG. Systematic review and meta-analysis of histopathological factors influencing the risk of lymph node metastasis in early colorectal cancer. Colorectal Dis. 2013;15:788–97.

35. Bosch SL, Teerenstra S, de Wilt JH, Cunningham C, Nagtegaal ID. Predicting lymph node metastasis in pT1 colorectal cancer: a systematic review of risk factors providing rationale for therapy decisions. Endoscopy. 2013;45:827–34.

36. Nascimbeni R, Burgart LJ, Nivatvongs S, Larson DR. Risk of lymph node metastasis in T1 carcinoma of the colon and rectum. Dis Colon Rectum. 2002;45: 200–6.

37. Deinlein P, Reulbach U, Stolte M, Vieth M. Risk of lymph node metastasis from pT1 colon adenocarcinoma. Pathologe. 2003;24:387–93.

38. Ueno H, Mochizuki H, Hashiguchi Y, Shimazaki H, Aida S, Hase K, Matsukuma S, Kanai T, Kurihara H, Ozawa K, Yoshimura K, Bekku S. Risk factors for an adverse outcome in early invasive colorectal carcinoma. Gastroenterology. 2004;127:385–94.

39. Yasuda K, Inomata M, Shiromizu A, Shiraishi N, Higashi H, Kitano S. Risk factors for occult lymph node metastasis of colorectal cancer invading the submucosa and indications for endoscopic mucosal resection. Dis Colon Rectum. 2007;50:1370–6.

40. Fujimori T, Fujii S, Saito N, Sugihara K. Pathological diagnosis of early colorectal carcinoma and its clinical implications. Digestion. 2009;79 Suppl 1:40–51.

41. Ueno H, Hashiguchi Y, Kajiwara Y, Shinto E, Shimazaki H, Kurihara H, Mochizuki H, Hase K. Proposed objective criteria for "grade 3" in early invasive colorectal cancer. Am J Clin Pathol. 2010;134:312–22.

42. Egashira Y, Yoshida T, Hirata I, Hamamoto N, Akutagawa H, Takeshita A, Noda N, Kurisu Y, Shibayama Y. Analysis of pathological risk factors for lymph node metastasis of submucosal invasive colon cancer. Mod Pathol. 2004;17:503–11.

43. Okabe S, Shia J, Nash G, Wong WD, Guillem JG, Weiser MR, Temple L, Sugihara K, Paty PB. Lymph node metastasis in T1 adenocarcinoma of the colon and rectum. J Gastrointest Surg. 2004;8:1032–9.

44. Ishikawa Y, Akishima-Fukasawa Y, Ito K, Akasaka Y, Yokoo T, Ishii T, Toho Study Group for Cancer Biological Behavior. Histopathologic determinants of regional lymph node metastasis in early colorectal cancer. Cancer. 2008;112:924–33.

45. Rasheed S, Bowley DM, Aziz O, Tekkis PP, Sadat AE, Guenther T, Boello ML, McDonald PJ, Talbot IC, Northover JM. Can depth of tumour invasion predict lymph node positivity in patients undergoing resection for early rectal cancer? A comparative study between T1 and T2 cancers. Colorectal Dis. 2008;10:231–8.

46. Walgenbach-Bruenagel G, Tolba RH, Varnai AD, Bollmann M, Hirner A, Walgenbach KJ. Detection of lymphatic invasion in early stage primary colorectal cancer with the monoclonal antibody D2-40. Eur Surg Res. 2006;38:438–44.

47. Ishii M, Ota M, Saito S, Kinugasa Y, Akamoto S, Ito I. Lymphatic vessel invasion detected by monoclonal antibody D2-40 as a predictor of lymph node metastasis in T1 colorectal cancer. Int J Colorectal Dis. 2009;24:1069–74.

48. Kingston EF, Goulding H, Bateman AC. Vascular invasion is underrecognized in colorectal cancer using conventional hematoxylin and eosin staining. Dis Colon Rectum. 2007;50:1867–72.

49. Liang JT, Huang KC, Lai HS, Lee PH, Sun CT. Oncologic results of laparoscopic D3 lymphadenectomy for male sigmoid and upper rectal cancer with clinically positive lymph nodes. Ann Surg Oncol. 2007;14:1980–90.

50. Suzuki A, Togashi K, Nokubi M, Koinuma K, Miyakura Y, Horie H, Lefor AT, Yasuda Y. Evaluation of venous invasion by Elastica van Gieson stain and tumor budding predicts local and distant metastases in patients with T1 stage colorectal cancer. Am J Surg Pathol. 2009;33:1601–7.

51. Harris EI, Lewin DN, Wang HL, Lauwers GY, Srivastava A, Shyr Y, Shakhtour B, Revetta F, Washington MK. Lymphovascular invasion in colorectal cancer: an interobserver variability study. Am J Surg Pathol. 2008;32:1816–21.

52. Bayar S, Saxena R, Emir B, Salem RR. Venous invasion may predict lymph node metastasis in early rectal cancer. Eur J Surg Oncol. 2002;28:413–7.

53. Mitomi H, Mori A, Kanazawa H, Nishiyama Y, Ihara A, Otani Y, Sada M, Kobayashi K, Igarashi M. Venous invasion and down-regulation of p21(WAF1/CIP1) are associated with metastasis in colorectal carcinomas. Hepatogastroenterology. 2005;52:1421–6.

54. Hase K, Shatney C, Johnson D, Trollope M, Vierra M. Prognostic value of tumor "budding" in patients with colorectal cancer. Dis Colon Rectum. 1993;36:627–35.

55. Ueno H, Mochizuki H, Shinto E, Hashiguchi Y, Hase K, Talbot IC. Histologic indices in biopsy specimens for estimating the probability of extended local spread in patients with rectal carcinoma. Cancer. 2002;94:2882–91.

56. Prall F. Tumour budding in colorectal carcinoma. Histopathology. 2007;50:151–62.

57. Wang LM, Kevans D, Mulcahy H, O'Sullivan J, Fennelly D, Hyland J, O'Donoghue D, Sheahan K. Tumor budding is a strong and reproducible prognostic marker in T3N0 colorectal cancer. Am J Surg Pathol. 2009;33:134–41.

58. Ogawa T, Yoshida T, Tsuruta T, Tokuyama W, Adachi S, Kikuchi M, Mikami T, Saigenji K, Okayasu I. Tumor budding is predictive of lymphatic involvement and lymph node metastases in submucosal invasive colorectal adenocarcinomas and in non-polypoid compared with polypoid growths. Scand J Gastroenterol. 2009;44:605–14.

59. Homma Y, Hamano T, Otsuki Y, Shimizu S, Kobayashi H, Kobayashi Y. Severe tumor budding is a risk factor for lateral lymph node metastasis in early rectal cancers. J Surg Oncol. 2010;102:230–4.

60. Prall F, Nizze H, Barten M. Tumour budding as prognostic factor in stage I/II colorectal carcinoma. Histopathology. 2005;47:17–24.

61. Liebig C, Ayala G, Wilks J, Verstovsek G, Liu H, Agarwal N, Berger DH, Albo D. Perineural invasion is an independent predictor of outcome in colorectal cancer. J Clin Oncol. 2009;27:5131–7.

62. Poeschl EM, Pollheimer MJ, Kornprat P, Lindtner RA, Schlemmer A, Rehak P, Vieth M, Langner C. Perineural invasion: correlation with aggressive phenotype and independent prognostic variable in both colon and rectum cancer. J Clin Oncol. 2010;28:e358–60.

63. Marshall JL. Risk assessment in Stage II colorectal cancer. Oncology (Williston Park). 2010;24(1 Suppl 1):9–13.

Quality of Surgery

22

Nicholas P. West and Philip Quirke

Abstract

Pathologists closely interact with all members of the colorectal multidisciplinary team in order to improve patient outcomes. Consistent high-quality reporting is essential to communicate all relevant prognostic information so that the patient undergoes optimal management. Additional feedback on the interpretation of preoperative imaging, effectiveness of preoperative treatment and quality of surgery is now integral to the pathology report. For rectal cancer, the status of the circumferential resection margin and quality of the mesorectal dissection are already widely reported. However, evidence is accumulating for the benefit of pathological feedback on the quality of the sphincter dissection in abdominoperineal excision (APE) specimens and the mesocolic dissection for colon cancer. This chapter will address current best practice for the pathological approach to TME, APE and colon cancer specimens.

Introduction

Pathologists play a central role in the modern multidisciplinary management of colorectal cancer patients. In addition to the identification of important prognostic information, the pathologist must also feed back to other members of the multidisciplinary team regarding the quality of their services to facilitate audit as well as continued education and improvement.

Successful interaction between pathologists, gastroenterologists, radiologists, oncologists, nurses and surgeons is critical to improving patient outcomes. Feedback to gastroenterologists is important in bowel cancer screening programmes as well as in day-to-day practice. Pathologists can also help radiologists by confirming the accuracy of preoperative staging. Over recent years we have focussed on the use of magnetic resonance imaging (MRI) for rectal cancer, but preoperative staging of colon cancers is now increasingly being used and requires validation. Additionally, pathologists must feed

N.P. West (✉) • P. Quirke
Section of Pathology and Tumour Biology,
Leeds Institute of Cancer and Pathology, University of Leeds, Leeds, UK
e-mail: n.p.west@leeds.ac.uk; p.quirke@leeds.ac.uk

G. Baatrup (ed.), *Multidisciplinary Treatment of Colorectal Cancer*,
DOI 10.1007/978-3-319-06142-9_22, © Springer International Publishing Switzerland 2015

back to oncologists about the effectiveness of any neoadjuvant therapy if used and also whether there is a need for further adjuvant therapy based on findings in the resection specimen. Finally, and perhaps most importantly, the pathologist plays a crucial role in the quality control of colorectal cancer surgery as well as the primary staging of the tumour. The quality of surgery can be determined in part by a pathological assessment of the plane of dissection followed by the operating team. The importance of the circumferential resection margin (CRM) and the quality of the mesorectal dissection in total mesorectal excision (TME) for rectal cancer have already been proven to be important; however, recent evidence has suggested that quality control of the sphincters in abdominoperineal excision (APE) and the mesocolon in colon cancer may also be important.

Colorectal cancer pathologists must therefore produce a thorough and accurate report that contains all the important prognostic and quality control information required by other clinicians. We strongly recommend the use of a pro forma along the lines of the most recent United Kingdom Royal College of Pathologists dataset for colorectal cancer (http://www.rcpath.org/resources/worddocs/G049ColorectalDatasetAppendixC-Sep07.doc) [1]. This chapter will focus on the evidence for and the techniques used to pathologically assess the quality of colorectal cancer resection specimens.

Reporting Total Mesorectal Excision (TME)/Anterior Resection Specimens for Rectal Cancer

The muscularis propria of the rectum above the anal sphincter muscles is surrounded by a layer of fatty tissue known as the mesorectum. This structure is of crucial importance in rectal cancer surgery as it contains all the blood vessels, nerves, lymphatics and lymph nodes through which rectal cancers may disseminate. Above the peritoneal reflections, the anterior and part of the lateral mesorectum is covered by a layer of visceral peritoneum (Fig. 22.1). At its poste-

rior aspect and beneath the peritoneal reflections both anteriorly and laterally, the mesorectum is fixed and largely surrounded by a layer of fascia (Fig. 22.2). The elastic fibres of the mesorectal fascia fuse with elastic fibres beneath the peritoneum as well as with Denonvilliers fascia. The mesorectum is generally of greatest volume posteriorly with significantly less fat located anteriorly [2], particularly behind the prostate gland in males where it can be especially particularly thin. For this reason, incomplete removal of rectal tumours and intraoperative perforations most commonly occur in an anterior position [3]. The mesorectum gradually reduces in size beneath the peritoneal reflection to a point of maximal wasting 35–42 mm above the anal verge corresponding to the level of the puborectalis muscle [4].

Anterior resection specimens for rectal cancer contain a variable amount of mesorectum depending on the position of the tumour and the quality of the surgical dissection. There is also marked variation in the overall volume of the mesorectum and the height of the peritoneal reflections between individuals. During the operation, the surgeon should attempt to sharply dissect immediately outside the mesorectal fascia in the so-called holy plane of TME surgery described by Heald [5]. This ensures that the mesorectum is removed as an intact package that contains the entire primary tumour along with all possible routes of metastasis. The outer non-peritonealised surface of the specimen forms what is termed the CRM, a surgically created margin that should be extensively covered with mesorectal fascia if the dissection has been performed in the correct tissue plane.

Tumour involvement of the CRM, defined as tumour at or within 1 mm of the margin, is a poor prognostic feature and is strongly linked to local disease recurrence [6–10]. The method of involvement may be by direct spread or tumour deposit or within a vessel or nerve bundle with all showing a similarly poor prognosis [11]. A tumour deposit contained wholly within a lymph node may have a lesser risk, but this has yet to be proven. Others have suggested that tumour within 2 mm of the CRM is associated with a worse

Fig.22.1 Abdominoperineal excision specimen for low rectal cancer demonstrating the peritoneal reflections (marked by the *blue lines*) at the anterior (**a**) and posterolateral (**b**) aspects. *CRM* circumferential resection margin

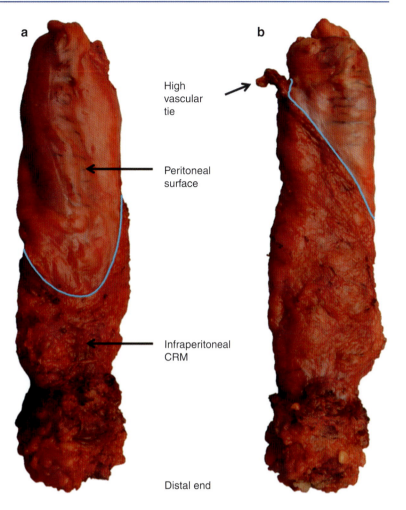

a   b

High vascular tie

Peritoneal surface

Infraperitoneal CRM

Distal end

outcome, but sufficient data does not currently exist to support this position [12]. Prior to the description of TME surgery, the rates of CRM involvement were as high as 36 % [6] and varied markedly between individual surgeons [11]. The introduction of TME over recent years has been shown to substantially reduce the rate of local disease recurrence and improve survival, initially in single-centre series [13, 14], followed by large-scale population series and clinical trials [15–17]. A recently published UK trial showed CRM involvement rates to be as low as 8 % in the latter patient cohort with an increase in the median distance between the tumour and the CRM from 5 to 8 mm over the duration of the study [18]. It is believed that a major factor in the success of TME surgery is the marked reduction in CRM involvement and tumour perforation associated with the technique [11]. However, the more advanced tumours may still extend to within 1 mm of the CRM or even breach the mesorectal fascia, and therefore, TME surgery on its own will not result in complete resection of the tumour. Surgeons may therefore attempt to perform a more extensive operation removing additional extra-fascial tissues or organs en bloc or more frequently use preoperative therapy to attempt to shrink the tumour into a surgically resectable state. Radiologists are now very good at predicting tumour involvement of the CRM using MRI [19, 20] and are therefore critical in selecting patients for neoadjuvant radiotherapy.

Fig. 22.2 Part of a haematoxylin and eosin-stained section from a whole mount rectal cancer block demonstrating the condensed fibrous tissue of the mesorectal fascia at the circumferential resection margin. Also demonstrated are blood vessels and a lymph node within the mesorectal fat, both of which are important routes of tumour dissemination

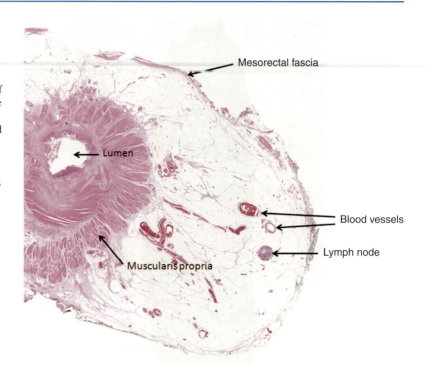

TME/anterior resection specimens for rectal cancer should be carefully examined and dissected by pathologists to ensure that all the important features are identified and described prior to irreversible slicing of the specimen. A meticulous and consistent approach is required to ensure that nothing is forgotten. We recommend the dissection protocol developed in Leeds [21] that has been adopted into the United Kingdom Royal College of Pathologists dataset for colorectal cancer [1]. It is important that the specimen is received intact and unopened, preferably in the fresh state, as any disruptions or incisions may impair the assessment of the CRM. On a fresh intact specimen, the CRM should be bound by mesorectal fascia, which appears as a shiny smooth layer that often becomes dulled and opaque after formalin fixation (Fig. 22.3). If the dissection extends as low as the prostate gland in males, an additional layer of fascia, the fascia of Denonvilliers, may also be noted [22].

An assessment by the pathologist of the integrity of the surface of the specimen forms an important component of the assessment of the quality of surgery that must be fed back to the surgical team. A three-point grading system was initially developed for the MRC CLASICC trial [23] and has subsequently been shown to predict CRM involvement, local recurrence and patient survival in both small series [24–26] and larger multicentre studies [18, 27]. The recommended mesorectal grading system is described in Table 22.1.

It is helpful if the specimen is photographed at this stage to form a permanent record of the plane of surgery (Fig. 22.4). Digital images should be taken of the front and back of the specimen alongside a metric scale, with additional close ups of any significant mesorectal defects or perforations. These images should be stored in a departmental archive and can be used to facilitate feedback to surgeons in multidisciplinary team meetings and utilised for subsequent research/audit. Feeding back the plane of surgery in such a way to the operating team has been shown to improve the planes of dissection over time leading to a

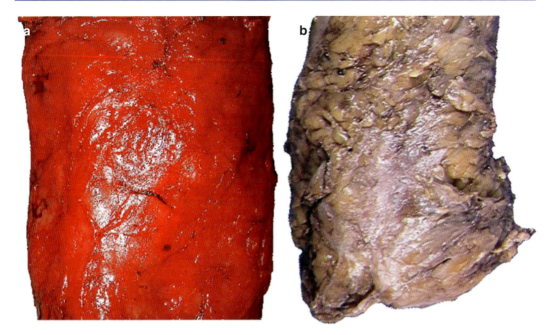

Fig. 22.3 The mesorectal fascia which appears as a shiny covering in the fresh specimen (**a**) and becomes a dull opaque colour after formalin fixation (**b**)

Table 22.1 Three-point grading system for the assessment of the plane of mesorectal dissection in TME/anterior resection specimens for rectal cancer

Grade	Short description	Long description
Mesorectal plane	Good surgery	Intact smooth mesorectal surface with only minor irregularities. Any defects must be no deeper than 5 mm. No coning of the specimen distally. Smooth CRM on slicing
Intramesorectal plane	Moderate surgery	Moderate bulk to mesorectum but irregularity of the mesorectal surface. Moderate distal coning. Muscularis propria not visible with the exception of levator insertion. Moderate irregularity of CRM
Muscularis propria plane	Poor surgery	Little bulk to mesorectum with defects down onto the muscularis propria and/or very irregular CRM. It includes infraperitoneal perforations

reduction in CRM involvement, which should ultimately improve patient outcomes [18].

Perforations, defined as a communication between the surface of the specimen and the lumen of the bowel, should similarly be documented in the report. Tumour perforations above the peritoneal reflections risk intraperitoneal recurrence and are associated with a poor prognosis [28, 29]. Under TNM staging rules, these tumours should be classified as pT4 [30].

However, infraperitoneal perforations are much more frequent and can occur at the time of surgery, often at the anterior aspect where the mesorectal thickness is at a minimum or in the area of the puborectalis. These surgical failures are not strictly pT4 tumours under TNM staging, but due to the high risk of local recurrence and reduced survival [31], we feel that they should be classified as pT4 on the basis of a poor anticipated prognosis.

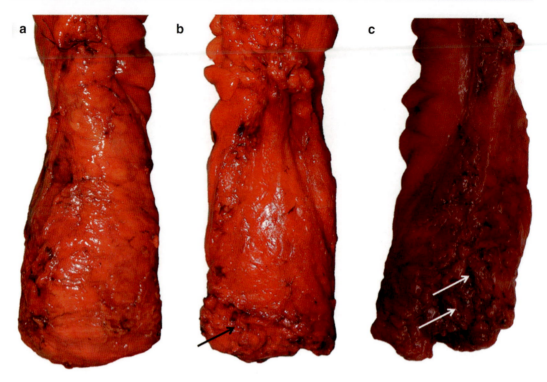

Fig. 22.4 Photographic documentation of the posterior surfaces of three anterior resection specimens showing good examples of the mesorectal plane (**a**), intramesorec- tal plane (**b**) and muscularis propria plane (**c**). Mesorectal defects are highlighted by *arrows*, which extend down to expose the muscularis propria in specimen C

Following a detailed macroscopic description, the specimen should be inked over the entire area of the CRM to allow for accurate histological measurement between the tumour and this margin. There should be no confusion between the CRM and the peritoneal surface as tumour involvement of both of these structures has different potential sequelae. Peritoneal disease, as described above, risks intraperitoneal recurrence in the abdominal cavity, whereas CRM involvement risks local pelvic recurrence. After inking, the tumour segment should undergo serial cross-sectional slicing at 3–5 mm intervals. The slices should be laid out in order and photographed to record the relationship between the tumour and the CRM and also to provide additional evidence for the plane of surgery. These images can be very useful for comparing to the radiological appearance of the tumour if any discrepancies arise. Ideally a minimum of five tumour blocks should be taken and at least one of these must demonstrate the tumour closest to the inked CRM. The pathological report must include a comment as to whether or not the CRM is involved by tumour so that the patient may be offered further adjuvant therapy, if appropriate, to reduce the chances of local disease recurrence. The distance between the tumour and the closest CRM to the nearest millimetre should be fed back to radiologists to allow them to audit the accuracy of their preoperative prediction of CRM status. If the MRI scan predicted a clear margin but the resection specimen shows evidence of tumour involvement, then it is helpful if the pathologist can indicate why this is so. Possible reasons include a tiny tumour deposit at the margin which would not be visible on MRI or alternatively that the area of CRM involvement relates

Fig. 22.5 Haematoxylin and eosin-stained tissue section through the anal sphincters demonstrating the internal and external sphincters separated by the intersphincteric space

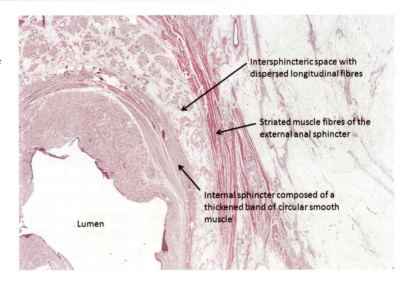

Intersphincteric space with dispersed longitudinal fibres

Striated muscle fibres of the external anal sphincter

Internal sphincter composed of a thickened band of circular smooth muscle

Lumen

to a region where the TME plane was not followed by the surgeon. In post-neoadjuvant therapy cases, it is also helpful for the pathologist to indicate whether any fibrosis extends beyond the tumour towards the CRM for correlation with the pre-radiotherapy MRI scan.

Reporting Abdominoperineal Excision (APE) Specimens for Low Rectal Cancer

APE of the rectum and anus is frequently utilised for the surgical treatment of advanced low rectal tumours (within 6 cm of the anal verge) where anatomical reconstruction is not possible or for reasons of poor predicted functionality. The specimen should include the rectum and mesorectum, as for a TME specimen, in continuity with the anal canal and a portion of perineal skin resulting in a permanent stoma for the patient. The anal sphincter muscles and levator ani muscles may be removed en bloc with the specimen depending on the radicality of the operation. The internal anal sphincter is a thickened continuation of the inner circular layer of smooth muscle from the rectal muscularis propria. Occasionally dispersed longitudinal fibres may also be seen. Immediately outside this layer the striated mus-

cle fibres of the external sphincter are seen (Fig. 22.5). Above the sphincter complex, some of these striated fibres fuse with the levator ani muscles of the pelvic floor.

Approximately 25 % of operations for primary rectal cancer will result in an APE [32], although there is wide variation in the frequency of this operation, which is considered by some to be unacceptable [33]. For this reason it has been proposed that APE rates themselves may be used as a surrogate marker of surgical quality. Obviously to provide a fair and meaningful comparison, these rates should be adjusted for factors such as tumour height [34] and specialist referral practice at the centre. In general, however, lower APE rates are considered to be a marker of good practice. This is because APE surgery for low rectal cancer is well recognised to be associated with poorer patient outcomes when compared to anterior resection for higher rectal tumours [2, 29, 35]. As stated in the section above, there is a natural reduction in mesorectal tissue volume when moving from the middle of the mesorectum down towards the commencement of the sphincters. For this reason, there is less protective tissue around lower rectal tumours when following the standard mesorectal fascial plane, which accounts for the higher CRM involvement rate with APE surgery [2]. Also, because much of the perineal dissection

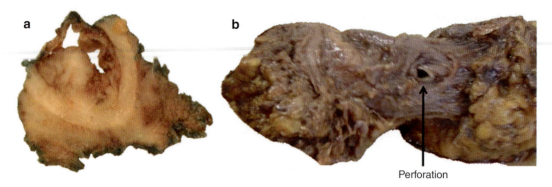

Fig. 22.6 Two examples of APE surgery performed in the wrong tissue planes. One specimen shows approximately one third of the circumferential resection margin being formed by submucosa resulting in a margin positive pT2 tumour (**a**) and the second shows a classic anterior intraoperative perforation at the level of the waist (**b**)

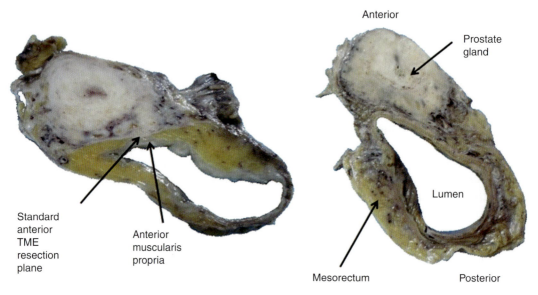

Fig. 22.7 Cross-sectional slices from two separate APE cases with en bloc prostatectomy showing the negligible amount of mesorectal tissue often seen between the anterior muscularis propria and the standard TME resection plane

during standard APE is performed under limited visualisation in the lithotomy position, surgeons often deviate into the wrong tissue plane which further increases the chances of an involved margin and may also result in an intraoperative perforation (Fig. 22.6). As has previously been stated, the most risky area for both CRM involvement and perforation is at the anterior aspect of the specimen where the mesorectum often reduces to a negligible amount [3, 36]. For this reason, en bloc prostatectomy or resection of the posterior vaginal wall may be performed in cases with advanced anterior tumours in order to protect the anterior CRM (Fig. 22.7).

Recent research has demonstrated improved clinical outcomes with more radical techniques termed extended APE and abdominosacral resection [37–40]. These procedures involve en bloc resection of the levator ani muscles along with the mesorectum and anal canal to create a more cylindrically shaped specimen as originally described by Miles [41]. Such 'extra-levator' surgery is

Table 22.2 Three-point grading system for assessment of the plane of anal canal/sphincter dissection in APE specimens for low rectal cancer

Grade	Short description	Long description
Extra-levator plane	Good surgery	The specimen has a cylindrical shape due to the presence of levator ani removed en bloc with the mesorectum and sphincters. Any defects must be no deeper than 5 mm. No waisting of the specimen. Smooth CRM on slicing
Sphincteric plane	Moderate surgery	The specimen is waisted and the CRM in this region is formed by the surface of the sphincter muscles which have been removed intact
Intrasphincteric	Poor surgery	The specimen is waisted and includes deviations into the sphincter muscles, submucosa and complete perforations

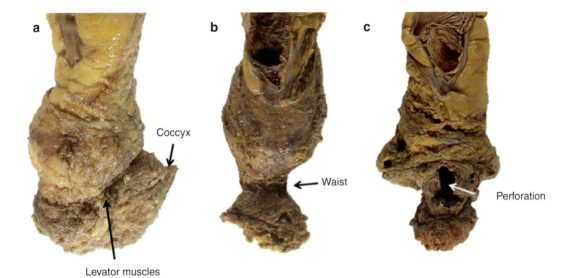

Fig. 22.8 Photographic documentation of the anterior surfaces of three formalin-fixed APE specimens showing good examples of the extra-levator plane (**a**), sphincteric plane (**b**) and Intrasphincteric plane (**c**). The extra-levator specimen shows no waisting due to the levators and coccyx being removed en bloc with the mesorectum. The sphincteric specimen shows a classical surgical waist in the area of the sphincters but a good quality mesorectal dissection. The intramucosal/submucosal specimen shows evidence of significant mesorectal defects with a large anterior perforation through the tumour in the classic danger area

usually carried out in the prone jackknife position to improve visualisation and has been shown to markedly reduce the rates of CRM involvement and intraoperative perforations compared to standard APE techniques [3, 36]. In turn this should improve outcomes towards those reported with anterior resection for higher rectal tumours.

Variables such as the mesorectal plane of dissection, presence of intraoperative perforations and CRM involvement should be reported for APE specimens in the same way as for TME/anterior resection specimens. However, in addition it has been proposed that the area of dissection around the sphincters should be separately graded [29]. This is of direct relevance to the rates of CRM involvement and patient outcomes because a beautiful mesorectal dissection will be offset by a perforation of the anal canal in the region of a low rectal tumour. The recommended anal canal/sphincter grading system is described in Table 22.2.

Photographs should be taken of the front and back of the whole specimen as for TME/anterior resection specimens and additional close ups of the anal canal/sphincter dissection are particularly useful for recording the plane of surgery in this area (Fig. 22.8).

Data obtained from the Dutch TME trial, which included 373 APE specimens, demonstrated that two thirds of specimens were in the sphincteric plane and one third in the intrasphincteric plane [29]. None of the cases were scored as being in the extra-levator plane. In a multicentre European study comparing a large series of extra-levator APE to standard APE specimens, extra-levator APE was shown to remove significantly more tissue around low rectal tumours with a reduction in CRM involvement from 50 to 20 % and intraoperative perforations from 28 to 8 % [36]. The need to modify an APE operation to the extra-levator plane can be accurately predicted by the radiologist using preoperative MRI [42], and pathological feedback to confirm this prediction from the resection specimen is again essential.

Reporting Colon Cancer Specimens

The colon and its mesentery, the mesocolon, are both invested by a layer of visceral peritoneum to a variable degree. The ascending colon has a broad attachment to the posterior abdominal wall that varies in both size and shape. A layer of fascia exists at the deep aspect of the ascending mesocolon, and dissection outside of this layer forms the retroperitoneal surgical margin in a right hemicolectomy specimen if the dissection is carried out in the correct tissue plane. The transverse colon is suspended by a true mesentery, the transverse mesocolon, which is a substantial structure often not resected in its entirety due to technical difficulties with the dissection. Similar to the ascending colon, the descending colon has a broad attachment at its posterior aspect that merges into the sigmoid colon, which again has a true suspensory mesentery. Over recent years it has become clear that the surgical principles of mesorectal surgery should be extended to include operations for colon cancer. Surgical removal of the colon and mesocolon in an intact package containing the lymphatics, lymph nodes and blood vessels is essential to guarantee the complete removal of primary colonic tumours along with the routes of potential dissemination.

An in-depth knowledge of colorectal vasculature is essential to appreciate the technical aspects of the chosen operation and to identify the relevant arteries which run with the draining lymphatics from the tumour [43]. Branches of the superior and inferior mesenteric arteries supply the colon; however, there is often marked variation between individuals which influences the type and extent of resection performed. The embryological midgut is supplied by branches of the superior mesenteric artery and the major vascular ties that may be visible in right and transverse colon resection specimens include the ileocolic artery, the right colic artery and the middle colic artery. The right colic artery shows considerable variation and often represents a branch of the middle colic rather than arising directly from the superior mesenteric artery [44]. The inferior mesenteric artery and its branches supply the majority of the hindgut.

The lymphatic drainage of the colon and consistent surgical approaches for adequate clearance of colon cancer were first described in 1909 [43]. The colonic lymph nodes are often classified as being present in three distinct layers [45]. The first line of drainage comes from a series of paracolic lymph nodes that lie close to the muscle wall in proximity to the marginal artery of Drummond. Colon cancers tend to demonstrate a small degree of lateral spread throughout these paracolic nodes before turning centrally into the second layer of intermediate nodes, which follow the supplying arteries towards their origin. Finally, the third layer of central lymph nodes are situated at the origin of the supplying vessels at either the branching of the inferior mesenteric artery from the aorta on the left or the major branches of the superior mesenteric artery on the right.

An optimal colon cancer resection specimen should therefore include the tumour with an adequate portion of non-diseased colon on either side, along with the associated mesocolon containing the blood vessels with high ligation of the supplying vessels and the paracolic, intermediate and central lymph nodes in an intact peritoneal and fascial bound package with no significant intraoperative defects. Surgeons practising this

Table 22.3 Three-point grading system for assessment of the plane of mesocolic dissection in specimens resected for colon cancer

Grade	Short description	Long description
Mesocolic plane	Good surgery	Intact smooth mesocolic surface with only minor irregularities. Any peritoneal or fascial defects must be no deeper than 5 mm. Smooth retroperitoneal and mesocolic margins on slicing
Intramesocolic plane	Moderate surgery	Moderate bulk to mesocolon but irregularity/tearing of the peritoneal or fascial surface. Muscularis propria not visible. Moderate irregularity of retroperitoneal and mesocolic margins on slicing
Muscularis propria plane	Poor surgery	Little bulk to mesocolon with extensive defects reaching down onto the muscularis propria

type of surgery, known as complete mesocolic excision with central vascular ligation (CME with CVL), report very impressive outcomes when compared to standard techniques [44, 46]. The majority of the survival benefit is believed to be derived from preventing mesocolic defects or tearing in the tumour drainage area, which could shed tumour cells into the peritoneal cavity and therefore risk intra-abdominal recurrence. Keeping the mesocolon intact has been shown to be associated with a 15 % overall survival benefit at 5 years compared to specimens with significant defects down on to the muscularis propria [47]. This difference rose to 27 % in stage III disease when all cases have tumour in the mesocolic lymph nodes and mesocolic disruptions are at their most dangerous.

Additional survival benefits when performing CME with CVL are likely to be derived from the optimum nodal clearance. The technique has been shown to be associated with the removal of an additional 10–12 lymph nodes in two independent colon cancer series [48, 49]. The majority of these extra nodes are likely to be pericolic and intermediate ones associated with the removal of a greater length of colon. The greatest benefit may be derived by removal of the central nodes in cases with downstaging of an otherwise Dukes C2 case into a Dukes C1. The majority of cancers display lateral nodal spread of up to 10 cm on either side of the lesion before the major drainage pathway heads centrally along the supplying arteries. However, occasionally the degree of lateral spread along the pericolic lymphatics can be

considerable, particularly in cases with extensive nodal disease and blockage of the central lymphatics [50]. Such advanced disease is likely to be already incurable and therefore CME with CVL is unlikely to significantly impact on overall outcomes in this group of patients.

As a pathologist, a variety of specimens may be received for cases of colon cancer depending on the site of the tumour, the number of lesions present and individual patient anatomy. Patients with multiple tumours may undergo panproctocolectomy including the entire large bowel and the mesocolon/mesorectum with high vascular ties for all major supplying vessels. Other frail patients with early tumours may undergo a much more limited segmental resection with very little mesentery to assess. Whatever type and size of resection is received, it is important as for rectal cancer that a meticulous macroscopic assessment of the specimen is performed prior to slicing through the tumour. It has recently been suggested that the plane of mesocolic dissection in colon cancer surgery can be assessed in a similar way to the mesorectum as described above [47]. The recommended mesocolic grading system is described in Table 22.3.

As for rectal cancer excisions, it is extremely helpful if photographs are taken of the macroscopic specimen at this time to provide a permanent record of the quality of surgery (Fig. 22.9). Other reproducible quality measures suggested in the literature include the distance between the tumour and the high vascular tie and the total number of lymph nodes resected. Surgeons

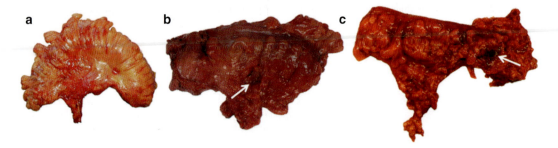

Fig. 22.9 Photographic documentation of three colon cancer specimens showing good examples of the mesocolic plane (**a**), intramesocolic plane (**b**) and muscularis propria plane (**c**). The mesocolic plane specimen shows a nice intact mesentery covered with peritoneum where appropriate and additionally shows a good central vascular tie. The intramesocolic plane specimen shows a significant mesocolic defect (*arrow*) which is well away from the primary tumour although almost certainly lies within its lymphatic drainage pathway. The muscularis propria plane specimen has a very irregular mesocolon with extensive defects (*arrow*) that expose large areas of muscularis propria in the region of the tumour

utilising the CME with CVL technique have been shown not only to operate more frequently in the mesocolic plane but also to remove more tissue between the tumour and the vascular resection margin and achieve a greater lymph node yield [48]. More importantly, evidence has recently emerged which suggests that the CME with CVL technique can be learned and adopted within a single surgical unit resulting in a instant improvement in the quality of the specimen produced [49]. In the Capital and Zealand regions of Denmark, we have been able to show that surgeons in one hospital who were trained in CME with CVL demonstrated a mesocolic plane resection rate of 75 % compared to only 48 % in the other hospitals that at that time utilised standard resection techniques. This was associated with a greater length of colon removed (315 vs. 247 mm), a greater distance between the tumour and the high vascular tie (105 vs. 84 mm) and a superior lymph node yield (28 vs. 18).

The concept of central vascular ligation and removal of the central lymph nodes is now over 100 years old [43], and while some studies have demonstrated an association with better outcomes [51–53], other studies have failed to demonstrate a clear benefit [54–57]. We strongly believe that a failure to standardise the plane of surgery is likely to offset any benefit derived from central ligation, which may well explain the conflicting evidence. Certainly we know that in a

small number of studies where careful mesocolic dissection was attempted in combination with central ligation, superior outcomes were reported [44, 58, 59].

Lymph node yields, while related to certain tumour and host factors, are largely dependent on both the surgeon and the pathologist [60]. Tumour and host factors cannot be easily influenced, but it is essential that high-quality surgery and pathology be delivered to ensure accurate staging so that patients who may benefit from adjuvant chemotherapy are identified. Poor nodal yields have been shown to markedly reduce the number of stage III cases thus denying many patients the adjuvant chemotherapy they need [60]. The number of lymph nodes required to accurately stage colorectal cancer has been debated over recent years. Present guidelines drawn up in the United Kingdom Royal College of Pathologists dataset for colorectal cancer suggest that all of the nodes within the specimen should be identified and examined [1]. With standardised high-quality pathology, we have been able to show in two independent series that CME with CVL removes significantly more lymph nodes compared to standard techniques [48, 49]. For centres where pathologists continually fail to achieve an adequate lymph node yield, particularly post-neoadjuvant therapy, accessory techniques including fat clearance and GEWF fixation may help [61–63]. While examining additional lymph nodes will not yield any positive nodes in bona fide stage II disease, studies have still demonstrated an association with improved outcomes [64, 65]. This has been suggested to be related to the overall quality of pathology in these centres and particularly an increased reporting of other high-risk features [66].

Conclusion

Over recent years outcomes for patients with rectal cancer have markedly improved following the description and dissemination of TME surgery [5, 13], the introduction of MRI for preoperative staging [67–69] and the use of neoadjuvant radiotherapy [70, 71]. Colorectal cancer pathologists have played a central role in improving outcomes through the identification of the importance of the CRM [6] and the description of surgical planes as a method of specimen-orientated quality control [18, 27]. Following surgical, radiological and pathological workshops concentrating on the need for consistent high-quality rectal cancer management, some countries actually improved outcomes to such a degree that the survival of rectal cancer patients actually overtook the traditionally better results for patients with colon cancer [72, 73]. Recent research has therefore tried to address this imbalance and carry the principles of optimal rectal cancer management into the colon and also additionally focus on the ongoing issue of poor outcomes for low rectal cancer patients treated by APE. Throughout this process, pathologists have remained critical in the identification of high-quality research data to support a widespread change in surgical, radiological, oncological and pathological practice.

Within this chapter, we have demonstrated that the quality of surgery in TME/anterior resection specimens can be assessed by a combination of the plane of mesorectal dissection, the presence of intraoperative perforations and the status of the CRM. In addition radiologists and oncologists benefit from feedback regarding the response of the tumour after neoadjuvant therapy with estimation as to the likely staging of the original

tumour if significant regression has occurred. Similarly the quality of surgery in APE specimens can be assessed by the plane of dissection around the sphincters, the presence of intraoperative perforations, the status of the CRM and the overall rate of APE procedures. Finally recent research has suggested that the quality of surgery in colon cancer resection specimens can be assessed by the plane of mesocolic dissection, the distance between the tumour and the high vascular tie and the total lymph node yield.

Pathologists continue to play an important part in the management of colorectal cancer patients through the production of a meticulous histopathology report containing all the necessary staging and prognostic data along with the above measures of specimen quality control. By consistently feeding back such data to the other members of the colorectal multidisciplinary team, outcomes can be expected to continue to improve in line with the current centres of excellence.

References

1. Williams GT, Quirke P, Shepherd N. Standards and datasets for reporting cancers: dataset for colorectal cancer. 2nd ed. London: The Royal College of Pathologists; 2007.
2. Marr R, Birbeck K, Garvican J, Macklin CP, Tiffin NJ, Parsons WJ, et al. The modern abdominoperineal excision: the next challenge after total mesorectal excision. Ann Surg. 2005;242:74–82.
3. West NP, Finan PJ, Anderin C, Lindholm J, Holm T, Quirke P. Evidence of the oncologic superiority of cylindrical abdominoperineal excision for low rectal cancer. J Clin Oncol. 2008;26:3517–22.
4. Salerno G, Chandler I, Wotherspoon A, Thomas K, Moran B, Brown G. Sites of surgical wasting in the abdominoperineal specimen. Br J Surg. 2008;95:1147–54.
5. Heald RJ, Husband EM, Ryall RD. The mesorectum in rectal cancer surgery–the clue to pelvic recurrence? Br J Surg. 1982;69:613–6.
6. Quirke P, Durdey P, Dixon MF, Williams NS. Local recurrence of rectal adenocarcinoma due to inadequate surgical resection: histopathological study of lateral tumour spread and surgical excision. Lancet. 1986;328:996–9.
7. Adam IJ, Mohamdee MO, Martin IG, Scott N, Finan PJ, Johnston D, et al. Role of circumferential margin

involvement in the local recurrence of rectal cancer. Lancet. 1994;344:707–11.

8. Wibe A, Rendedal PR, Svensson E, Norstein J, Eide TJ, Myrvold HE, et al. Prognostic significance of the circumferential resection margin following total mesorectal excision for rectal cancer. Br J Surg. 2002;89:327–34.

9. Martling A, Singnomklao T, Holm T, Rutqvist LE, Cedermark B. Prognostic significance of both surgical and pathological assessment of curative resection for rectal cancer. Br J Surg. 2004;91:1040–5.

10. Nagtegaal ID, Quirke P. What is the role for the circumferential margin in the modern treatment of rectal cancer? J Clin Oncol. 2008;26:303–12.

11. Birbeck K, Macklin CP, Tiffin NJ, Parsons W, Dixon MF, Mapstone NP, et al. Rates of circumferential resection margin involvement vary between surgeons and predict outcomes in rectal cancer surgery. Ann Surg. 2002;235:449–57.

12. Nagtegaal ID, Marijnen CA, Kranenbarg EK, van de Velde CJ, van Krieken JH. Circumferential margin involvement is still an important predictor of local recurrence in rectal carcinoma: not one millimeter but two millimeters is the limit. Am J Surg Pathol. 2002;26:350–7.

13. Heald RJ, Ryall RDH. Recurrence and survival after total mesorectal excision for rectal cancer. Lancet. 1986;327:1479–82.

14. Enker WE, Thaler HT, Cranor ML, Polyak T. Total mesorectal excision in the operative treatment of carcinoma of the rectum. J Am Coll Surg. 1995;181: 335–46.

15. Martling AL, Holm T, Rutqvist LE, Moran BJ, Heald RJ, Cedermark B. Effect of a surgical training programme on outcome of rectal cancer in the County of Stockholm. Stockholm Colorectal Cancer Study Group, Basingstoke Bowel Cancer Research Project. Lancet. 2000;356:93–6.

16. Kapiteijn E, Putter H, van de Velde CJH, Cooperative Investigators of the Dutch Colorectal Cancer Group. Impact of the introduction and training of total mesorectal excision on recurrence and survival in rectal cancer in the Netherlands. Br J Surg. 2002;89: 1142–9.

17. Wibe A, Møller B, Norstein J, Carlsen E, Wiig JN, Heald RJ, et al. A national strategic change in treatment policy for rectal cancer – implementation of total mesorectal excision as routine treatment in Norway. A national audit. Dis Colon Rectum. 2002; 45:857–66.

18. Quirke P, Steele R, Monson J, Grieve R, Khanna S, Couture J, et al. Effect of the plane of surgery achieved on local recurrence in patients with operable rectal cancer: a prospective study using data from the MRC CR07 and NCIC-CTG CO16 randomised clinical trial. Lancet. 2009;373:821–8.

19. MERCURY Study Group. Diagnostic accuracy of preoperative magnetic resonance imaging in predicting curative resection of rectal cancer: prospective observational study. BMJ. 2006;333:779–82.

20. Purkayastha S, Tekkis PP, Athanasiou T, Tilney HS, Darzi AW, Heriot AG. Diagnostic precision of magnetic resonance imaging for preoperative prediction of the circumferential margin involvement in patients with rectal cancer. Colorectal Dis. 2006;9:402–11.

21. Quirke P, Dixon MF. The prediction of local recurrence in rectal adenocarcinoma by histopathological examination. Int J Colorectal Dis. 1988;3:127–31.

22. Heald RJ, Moran BJ, Brown G, Daniels IR. Optimal total mesorectal excision for rectal cancer is by dissection in front of Denonvilliers' fascia. Br J Surg. 2004;91:121–3.

23. Quirke P, Thorpe H, Dewberry S, Brown J, Jayne D, Guillou P. Prospective assessment of the quality of surgery in the MRC CLASICC trial evidence for variation in the plane of surgery in colon cancer, local recurrence and survival. NCRI cancer conference abstract book. 2008. (http://www.ncri.org.uk/ncriconference/2008abstracts/abstracts/B115.htm).

24. Maslekar S, Sharma A, MacDonald A, Gunn J, Monson JRT, Hartley JE. Mesorectal grades predict recurrences after curative resection for rectal cancer. Dis Colon Rectum. 2006;50:168–75.

25. Garcia-Granero E, Faiz O, Munoz E, Flor B, Navarro S, Faus C, et al. Macroscopic assessment of mesorectal excision in rectal cancer: a useful tool for improving quality control in a multidisciplinary team. Cancer. 2009;115:3400–11.

26. Leite JS, Martins SC, Oliveira J, Cunha MF, Castro-Sousa F. Clinical significance of macroscopic completeness of mesorectal resection in rectal cancer. Colorectal Dis. 2009;13(4):381–6, published online.

27. Nagtegaal ID, van de Velde CJH, van der Worp E, Kapiteijn E, Quirke P, van Krieken JHJM, et al. Macroscopic evaluation of rectal cancer resection specimen: clinical significance of the pathologist in quality control. J Clin Oncol. 2002;20:1729–34.

28. Eriksen MT, Wibe A, Syse A, Haffner J, Wiig JN, Norwegian Rectal Cancer Group, Norwegian Gastrointestinal Cancer Group. Inadvertent perforation during rectal cancer resection in Norway. Br J Surg. 2004;91:210–6.

29. Nagtegaal ID, Van de Velde CJH, Marijnen CAM, van Krieken JHJM, Quirke P. Low rectal cancer: a call for a change of approach in abdominoperineal resection. J Clin Oncol. 2005;23:9257–64.

30. Sobin LH, Wittekind C, editors. UICC TNM classification on malignant tumours. 5th ed. New York: Wiley Liss; 1997.

31. Porter GA, O'Keefe GE, Yakimets WW. Inadvertent perforation of the rectum during abdominoperineal resection. Am J Surg. 1996;172:324–7.

32. Tilney HS, Heriot AG, Purkayastha S, Antoniou A, Aylin P, Darzi AW, et al. A national perspective on the decline of abdominoperineal resection for rectal cancer. Ann Surg. 2008;247:77–84.

33. Morris E, Quirke P, Thomas JD, Fairley L, Cottier B, Forman D. Unacceptable variation in abdominoperineal excision rates for rectal cancer – time to intervene? Gut. 2008;57:1690–7.

34. Morris E, Birch R, West N, Finan P, Forman D, Fairley L, et al. Low abdomino-perineal excision rates are associated with high workload surgeons and lower tumour height. Is further specialisation needed? Colorectal Dis. 2010;13(7):755–61, published online.

35. Wibe A, Syse A, Anderson E, Tretli S, Myrvold HE, Soreide O, et al. Oncological outcomes after total mesorectal excision for cure for cancer of the lower rectum: anterior vs. abdominoperineal resection. Dis Colon Rectum. 2004;47:48–58.

36. West NP, Anderin C, Smith KJ, Holm T, Quirke P, European Extralevator Abdominoperineal Excision Study Group. Multicentre experience with extraleva-tor abdominoperineal excision for low rectal cancer. Br J Surg. 2010;97:588–99.

37. Dehni N, McFadden N, McNamara DA, Guiguet M, Tiret E, Parc R. Oncologic results following abdomi-noperineal resection for adenocarcinoma of the low rectum. Dis Colon Rectum. 2003;46:867–74.

38. Bebenek M, Pudelko M, Cisarz K, Balcerzak A, Tupikowski W, Wojciechowski L, et al. Therapeutic results in low-rectal cancer patients treated with abdominosacral resection are similar to those obtained by means of anterior resection in mid- and upper-rectal cancer cases. Eur J Surg Oncol. 2007;33:320–3.

39. Holm T, Ljung A, Haggmark T, Jurell G, Lagergren J. Extended abdominoperineal resection with gluteus maximus flap reconstruction of the pelvic floor for rectal cancer. Br J Surg. 2007;94:232–8.

40. Davies M, Harris D, Hirst G, Beynon R, Morgan AR, Carr ND, et al. Local recurrence after abdomino-perineal resection. Colorectal Dis. 2009;11:39–43.

41. Miles WE. A method of performing abdomino-perineal excision for carcinoma of the rectum and of the terminal portion of the pelvic colon. Lancet. 1908;2:1812–3.

42. Shihab OC, Heald RJ, Rullier E, Brown G, Holm T, Quirke P, et al. Defining the surgical planes on MRI improves surgery for cancer of the low rectum. Lancet Oncol. 2009;10:1207–11.

43. Jamieson JK, Dobson JF. Lymphatics of the colon: with special reference to the operative treatment of cancer of the colon. Ann Surg. 1909;50:1077–90.

44. Hohenberger W, Weber K, Matzel K, Papadopoulos T, Merkel S. Standardized surgery for colonic cancer: complete mesocolic excision and central ligation–technical notes and outcome. Colorectal Dis. 2009; 11:354–64.

45. JSCCR. Japanese classification of colorectal carci-noma. 2nd ed. Tokyo: Kanehara & Co; 2009.

46. Higuchi T, Sugihara K. Complete mesocolic excision (CME) with central vascular ligation (CVL) as stan-dardised surgical technique for colonic cancer: a Japanese multicentre study (abstract). Dis Colon Rectum. 2010;53:646.

47. West NP, Morris EJ, Rotimi O, Cairns A, Finan PJ, Quirke P. Pathology grading of colon cancer surgical resection and its association with survival: a retro-spective observational study. Lancet Oncol. 2008;9: 857–65.

48. West NP, Hohenberger W, Weber K, Perrakis A, Finan PJ, Quirke P. Complete mesocolic excision with cen-tral vascular ligation produces an oncologically supe-rior specimen compared with standard surgery for carcinoma of the colon. J Clin Oncol. 2010;28:272–8.

49. West NP, Sutton KM, Ingeholm P, Hagemann-Madsen RH, Hohenberger W, Quirke P. Improving the quality of colon cancer surgery through a surgical education pro-gramme. Dis Colon Rectum. 2010;53(12):1594–603.

50. Grinnell RS. Lymphatic block with atypical and retro-grade lymphatic metastasis and spread in carcinoma of the colon and rectum. Ann Surg. 1966;163:272–80.

51. Rosi PA, Cahill WJ, Carey J. A ten-year study of hemicolectomy in the treatment of carcinoma of the left half of the colon. Surg Gynecol Obstet. 1962;114: 15–24.

52. Grinell RS. Results of ligation of inferior mesenteric artery at the aorta in resections of carcinoma of the descending and sigmoid colon and rectum. Surg Gynecol Obstet. 1965;120:1031–6.

53. Slanetz CA, Grimson R. Effect of high and intermedi-ate ligation on survival and recurrence rates following curative resection of colorectal cancer. Dis Colon Rectum. 1997;40:1205–19.

54. Pezim ME, Nicholls RJ. Survival after high or low ligation of the inferior mesenteric artery during cura-tive surgery for rectal cancer. Ann Surg. 1984;200: 729–33.

55. Surtees P, Ritchie JK, Phillips RKS. High versus low ligation of the inferior mesenteric artery in rectal can-cer. Br J Surg. 1990;77:618–21.

56. Rouffet F, Hay JM, Vacher B, Fingerhut A, Elhadad A, Flamant Y, et al. Curative resection for left colonic carcinoma: hemicolectomy vs. segmental colectomy. A prospective, controlled, multicenter trial. Dis Colon Rectum. 1994;37:651–9.

57. Tagliacozzo S, Tocchi A. Extended mesenteric exci-sion in right hemicolectomy for carcinoma of the colon. Int J Colorectal Dis. 1997;12:272–5.

58. Enker WE, Laffer UT, Block GE. Enhanced survival of patients with colon and rectal cancer is based upon wide anatomic resection. Ann Surg. 1979;190: 350–60.

59. Bokey EL, Chapuis PH, Dent OF, Mander BJ, Bissett IP, Newland RC. Surgical technique and survival in patients having a curative resection for colon cancer. Dis Colon Rectum. 2003;46:860–6.

60. Morris EJ, Maughan NJ, Forman D, Quirke P. Identifying stage III colorectal cancer patients: the influence of the patient, surgeon, and pathologist. J Clin Oncol. 2007;25:2573–9.

61. Wang H, Safar B, Wexner SD, Denoya P, Berho M. The clinical significance of fat clearance lymph node harvest for invasive rectal adenocarcinoma following neoadjuvant therapy. Dis Colon Rectum. 2009;52: 1767–73.

62. Hernanz F, Garcia-Somacarrera E, Fernandez F. The assessment of lymph nodes missed in mesenteric tis-sue after standard dissection of colorectal cancer specimens. Colorectal Dis. 2010;12:e57–60.

63. Iversen LH, Laurberg S, Hagemann-Madsen R, Dybdahl H. Increased lymph node harvest from colorectal cancer resections using GEWF solution: a randomised study. J Clin Pathol. 2008;61:1203–8.

64. Le Voyer TE, Sigurdson ER, Hanlon AL, Mayer RJ, Macdonald JS, Catalano PJ, et al. Colon cancer survival is associated with increasing number of lymph nodes analyzed: a secondary survey of intergroup trial INT-0089. J Clin Oncol. 2003;21:2912–9.

65. Chen SL, Bilchik AJ. More extensive nodal dissection improves survival for stages I to III of colon cancer: a population-based study. Ann Surg. 2006;244: 602–10.

66. Morris EJ, Maughan NJ, Forman D, Quirke P. Who to treat with adjuvant therapy in Dukes B/stage II colorectal cancer? The need for high quality pathology. Gut. 2007;56:1419–25.

67. Blomqvist L, Rubio C, Holm T, Machado M, Hindmarsh T. Rectal adenocarcinoma: assessment of tumour involvement of the lateral resection margin by MRI of resected specimen. Br J Radiol. 1999;72: 18–23.

68. Brown G, Richards CJ, Newcombe RG, Dallimore NS, Radcliffe AG, Carey DP, et al. Rectal carcinoma: thin-section MR imaging for staging in 28 patients. Radiology. 1999;211:215–22.

69. Beets-Tan RG, Beets GL, Vliegen RF, Kessels AG, Van Boven H, De Bruine A, et al. Accuracy of magnetic resonance imaging in prediction of tumour-free resection margin in rectal cancer surgery. Lancet. 2001;357:497–504.

70. Stockholm Rectal Cancer Study Group. Preoperative short-term radiation therapy in operable rectal carcinoma. A prospective randomized trial. Cancer. 1990;66:49–55.

71. Sauer R, Fietkau R, Wittekind C, Rödel C, Martus P, Hohenberger W, et al. Adjuvant vs. neoadjuvant radiochemotherapy for locally advanced rectal cancer: the German trial CAO/ARO/AIO-94. Colorectal Dis. 2003;5:406–15.

72. Birgisson H, Talba M, Gunnarsson U, Pahlman L, Glimelius B. Improved survival in cancer of the colon and rectum in Sweden. Eur J Surg Oncol. 2005;31: 845–53.

73. Iversen LH, Norgaard M, Jepsen P, Jacobsen J, Christensen MM, Gandrup P, et al. Trends in colorectal cancer survival in northern Denmark: 1985–2004. Colorectal Dis. 2007;9:210–7.

Staging of Colorectal Cancer (Including Staging After Neoadjuvant Therapy)

23

Iris D. Nagtegaal

Abstract

Pathological examination of colorectal cancer is the basis for further treatment. Staging of the tumor predicts prognosis and indicates the necessity of adjuvant therapy. Neoadjuvant treatment may hamper staging and is subject to ongoing research.

Introduction

The tumor node metastasis (TNM) staging system, derived from the Dukes classification, has been of major importance over the past 50 years. Although this system was initially developed to predict patients' prognosis, its function has expanded, and it is now used to select patients for adjuvant therapy and to determine inclusion in clinical trials.

Throughout the years, TNM has been challenged by the detection of new tumor markers as well as tumor profiles, but it still remains the hallmark of diagnosis and treatment. However, treatment of rectal cancer has changed dramatically over the past 20 years, and one should wonder whether this change in treatment, accompanied by a shift from adjuvant to neoadjuvant therapy, should lead to profound changes in TNM staging.

In the current chapter, pathological staging of colorectal carcinomas is discussed with special attention to the problematic features. Staging after neoadjuvant treatment is explained together with tumor regression grading.

Traditional Staging

Invasion Depth

TNM staging is based on the invasion depth of the primary *T*umor, the presence of lymph *N*ode metastases, and the presence of distant *M*etastases. The subclassification for the early (T1) tumors is described in Chap. 20.

I.D. Nagtegaal, MD, PhD
Department of Pathology,
Radboud University Nijmegen Medical Center,
Geert Grooteplein 2,
Nijmegen 6500 HB, The Netherlands
e-mail: iris.nagtegaal@radboudumc.nl

G. Baatrup (ed.), *Multidisciplinary Treatment of Colorectal Cancer*,
DOI 10.1007/978-3-319-06142-9_23, © Springer International Publishing Switzerland 2015

Lymph Nodes

The Trouble with Tumor Deposits

Although the 5th edition [1] of the TNM has been replaced by the 6th edition [2] in 2002 and the 7th edition [3] in 2010, a number of national guidelines for treatment and diagnosis of colorectal cancer prefers the 5th edition for reasons of reproducibility and uniformity. In the 6th edition of the TNM staging system, tumor deposits are considered positive lymph nodes if they have the form and smooth contour of lymph nodes [2], whereas in the 5th edition, they are considered as lymph nodes if they are 3 mm or more in size [1]. In any other case, the deposits should be considered as part of the primary tumor and thus be included in the T stage. In the 7th edition, it is left to the discretion of the pathologist to determine whether a deposit is actually a lymph node; no definitions are given. Moreover, all deposits may be placed in a new N subcategory, N1c, immediately upgrading all patients with deposit to stage III disease. This massive stage migration might have large effects on treatment and health-care costs without any evidence of benefit for patients and society.

Staging After Neoadjuvant Therapy

Neoadjuvant therapy has, at least in a large number of cases, profound effects on tumor stage and tumor histology, dependent on its *components* and *time frame* in which it has been applied. Not all treatment regimens are equally effective in causing downstaging. After short-term (5×5 Gy) radiotherapy, with surgery within 5 days after the radiotherapy, no downstaging is observed [4]. Despite the fact that in the radiotherapy, arm tumors were significantly smaller, no difference in T stage was observed. In addition, fewer lymph nodes were examined but the N stage was not different either. In contrast, a study from the Swedish rectal cancer trial using the same radiotherapy regimen did report downstaging in a subgroup of patients [5]. However, the overall treatment time in this subgroup was more than 10 days. A recent paper by Rado et al.

[6] demonstrates that even in T4 tumors, a pathological complete response can be achieved with 5×5 Gy with delayed surgery. Of the 24 patients treated with curative intent, 88 % had a R0 resection.

Increased downstaging and tumor regression can be seen in almost all longer radiotherapy and chemotherapy regimens with delayed surgery [7–10]. For the record, downstaging is not automatically correlated with better local control. In fact, in some studies downstaging does not lead to improved local control, whereas in other studies it does. These seemingly contradicting results can be explained by careful looking at the radiobiology underlying the mechanism of downstaging. For neoadjuvant treatment with a short interval, downstaging cannot be expected and is as such of no prognostic value. In addition, increased downstaging obtained by a longer interval between radiotherapy and surgery is of no importance for better local control. Obviously, cell death either occurs or does not occur, and a longer interval will make the cell death clinically and histopathologically more apparent but will have no additional benefit for local control. In contrast, increased downstaging obtained by a different mechanism (e.g., the addition of chemotherapy to radiotherapy) will indeed lead to an increase in local control.

Problems with the Current TNM System

Since the current TNM system is essentially unchanged since early modifications of the Dukes staging system, the accompanying effects of neoadjuvant therapy are not fully considered. The addition of the prefix "y" or "yp" to the TNM stage does indicate that neoadjuvant therapy has been applied, nothing more and nothing less. However, the often profound histological changes caused by the neoadjuvant treatment are confusing when standard rules are applied. Should mucinous lakes be considered in the T staging? When do we declare a complete response and how do we determine this? How do we define involved lymph nodes? Most of these issues have been signaled before, but there is as of yet no standard method available as how to solve these problems.

Mucinous Lakes

The appearance of acellular mucinous lakes, also called colloid response, is frequently observed after neoadjuvant therapy of a rectal tumor, both in the areas of the primary tumor and in the surrounding lymph nodes (see also the paragraph on ex-positive lymph nodes). In addition, an increased number of mucinous carcinomas, where mucinous lakes contain *vital* tumor cells, are frequently observed after neoadjuvant therapy. However, these tumors do not cause any diagnostic problems. The discussion should be focused on acellular mucinous lakes and whether to include these in T staging. In 20–55 % [11, 12] of neoadjuvantly treated cases, acellular mucinous lakes are observed. Results on its relation with prognosis are conflicting; Shia et al. [12] did not observe a relation with recurrence-free survival, while Rullier et al. [11] demonstrated that the prognosis of patients with a colloid response (5-year DFS 64 %) is in between those for patients with downstaging (5-year DFS 80 %) and without any response (5-year DFS 54 %). In a series of patients with a pCR, acellular mucin was present in 27 % of cases. Its presence did not influence prognosis [13]. However, no studies have evaluated the difference between prognostic value of T stage including and excluding mucinous lakes, so real evidence is lacking. For practical reasons, we advise to mention the presence of mucinous lakes in the report and as it can be seen as tumor response, not to include these in the T stage.

Complete Response

Clinical complete response (cCR) is often a clinical end point in trials but is only well defined in a limited number of studies. The correlation with a pathological complete response is variable; a recent review [14] demonstrated that in 8 studies this correlation was described and that a cCR results in a pCR in approximately 30 % of cases. There is confusion about what exactly constitutes a pCR: Is an ypT0 resection enough or is an ypT0N0 resection required? In up to 7.1 % of ypT0 cases, lymph node metastases are still present.

Moreover, the process of determining a pCR is not standardized, and the probability of finding vital tumor cells in resections after neoadjuvant therapy is dependent on the enthusiasm of the pathologist and how many tissue blocks and section levels are investigated. In order to standardize response determination, we advised the following procedure:

- Initially, five blocks of the tumor area are required.
- If no tumor is found in these first five blocks, the whole tumor area should be included for histological examination.
- If still no tumor is found, three levels of each block should be cut to exclude tumor involvement.

Further research is needed to evaluate the usefulness of this procedure.

Ex-Positive Lymph Nodes

The presence of positive lymph nodes is the most important prognostic factor in colorectal cancer and an indication for adjuvant therapy. Downstaging due to neoadjuvant therapy can cause positive lymph nodes to become negative. It is not clear whether, in these cases, the cN is more accurate in predicting prognosis than ypN. Theoretically, one could assume that any node that was positive is an indication of early metastasis, and thus also ex-positive lymph nodes have an increased risk on metastatic disease. On the other hand, the fact that the tumor in these lymph nodes reacts so well might be an indication for a good prognosis. A problem that so far has not been solved is the adequate pretreatment imaging of lymph nodes. Although the nodes can often be seen on MRI, predicting nodal involvement remains difficult.

Numbers of ex-positive lymph nodes are not frequently reported. Prall et al. [15] described in

10 out of 24 negative lymph nodes signs of tumor regression after chemoradiotherapy (fibrosis or acellular mucin lakes); Perez et al. [16] saw mucin lakes in 6 lymph nodes (1.2 % of all negative lymph nodes). Morgan et al. [17] describe necrotic tumor in lymph nodes in 2 of their 21 patients. In an MRI study [18], regressive changes were followed radiologically. Out of 29 positive lymph nodes, 3 became mucinous on MRI, while final pathological examination confirmed negative lymph nodes with acellular mucin lakes. These series are too small to draw any conclusion about the prognostic impact of ex-positive lymph nodes.

In a study with 165 patients, Valentini et al. [19] describe three different groups: 34 cN0ypN0, 72 cN+ypN0, and 56 ypN+patients, with a distant metastases-free 5-year survival of, respectively, 87.5, 82.9, and 47.9 %, suggesting that not initial N stage but rather final pathology makes the difference. However, with the limited possibilities of reliable clinical N staging, one can question which part of the cN0ypN0 group in reality should have belonged to the cN+ypN0 group. This might have affected the prognosis in this group and thus obscure the difference between the first two groups. Moreover, more studies are needed to confirm this finding. For now it seems reasonable to describe ex-positive lymph nodes as an additional item, but staging should be done on those lymph nodes with evident tumor present.

Number of Nodes

Neoadjuvant therapy influences the number of examined lymph nodes, either by decreasing their size below the observation limit [20] or by a complete disappearance of lymphocytes. Part of lymph nodes will be replaced by fibrosis [12]. In a randomized trial with short-term radiotherapy (5×5 Gy), fewer lymph nodes were examined in the radiotherapy arm (7.7 versus 9.7, $p < 0.001$) [4]. In a large population-based study with 5647 patients [21], after radiotherapy, 7.0 lymph nodes were examined, compared to ten nodes in the surgery-only group ($p < 0.0001$). Bujko et al.

demonstrated that the type of neoadjuvant treatment also makes a difference, with 11.4 nodes after 5×5 Gy compared to 7.6 nodes after radiochemotherapy ($p < 0.001$) [22]. Several studies demonstrated that the number of lymph nodes is not correlated with treatment response [23, 24].

Previously considered adequate lymph node numbers (12 in TNM, 10 by ASCO guidelines) are often not met after neoadjuvant therapy, with mean numbers of lymph nodes of 8.4 after 5×5 Gy ($n = 744$) [4, 22], 7.0 nodes after long-term radiotherapy ($n = 1034$) [21], and 10.8 nodes after radiochemotherapy ($n = 1,570$) [16, 22, 25–29]. In a considerable number of cases, no lymph nodes are investigated: 16 % after long-term radiotherapy (compared to 7.5 % in the surgery-only group) [21] and 6.1–22 % after radiochemotherapy [29–31]. These cases are sometimes wrongly coded as Nx. However, this classification is restricted for use in cases in which no lymph nodes are resected, i.e., local excisions. When no positive lymph nodes are found, the stage should still be coded as N0, irrespective of the number of examined lymph nodes.

Tumor Deposits

A confusing problem occurs after neoadjuvant therapy when considering tumor deposits [32]. In cases of regression, small tumor remnants, sometimes called microfoci, can be considered tumor deposits and, consequently, counted as positive lymph nodes. Since these are often the remains of advanced tumors, the presence of microfoci is indicative of a good prognosis. It is not advisable to use the tumor deposit rules after neoadjuvant therapy, but one should rather count the presence of microfoci in T staging, i.e., T3 accompanied by the comment *with signs of tumor regression present.*

Tumor Regression Grading

Tumor regression grading (TRG) in rectal carcinoma has been derived from a system developed for squamous cell carcinoma of the esophagus.

This system grades the amount of regressive changes along a 5-tiered scale, from 0 to 4 or 5 to 1, depending on the author. Several critical remarks considering the use of TRG should be made.

Firstly, differences between the various grades are subjective, as can be judged from definitions applied to TRG2 versus TRG3: tumor cells are easy to find versus tumor cells are difficult to find. Indeed, reproducibility of grading, as can be measured using kappa statistics, is between 0.29 and 0.47, which is considered only fair to moderate agreement between different pathologists. Moreover, in a study [33] where, in addition to the neoadjuvant arm, the surgery-only arm was graded for regression, one (3 %) patient showed TRG2 (considerable regression) and 12 (30 %) patients showed TRG4 (little regression), demonstrating the subjectivity of this system.

Moreover, sometimes definitions are used with percentage of regression [34], in analogy with clinical regression grading. However, for pathologists this is hard to achieve, since there is no before and after situation available for investigation, making it impossible to determine the percentage of regression.

Secondly, features that determine the presence of regression, like fibrosis or desmoplastic reaction, are in the surgery-only setting associated with a poor prognosis [35], whereas these features are correlated with regression and as such with good prognosis after neoadjuvant treatment.

Lastly, various studies have used TRG or one of its modifications to determine a correlation with prognosis. Unfortunately, different cutoff points are used between the different studies to prove the prognostic significance of the regression grade. In several multifactorial analyses, TRG is less important than CRM.

So, why do we want to use this system? Indeed, it is reasonable to expect some information about the grade of regression or response in a tumor after neoadjuvant therapy, not only because of the possible link with prognosis but also as an indication for the possible success of adjuvant therapy. Both prognosis and future therapy success will be most pronounced in those tumors with a complete or near-complete response. Taking into account the poor reproducibility between the middle grades (tumor cells easy to find and obvious signs of treatment, i.e., fibrosis and/or vasculopathy) and the fact that their prognosis does not really seem to differ much makes it acceptable to group these together. Tumors without any response should be considered as a separate group.

Conclusion

Cancer staging is one of the key requirements in the modern multidisciplinary treatment of colorectal cancer. Evidence-based medicine is built on the histological staging of tumors and the stage groups that are created. Information about prognosis has been derived from large groups of patients that are staged according to standardized definitions. Recent changes in TNM are confusing and decrease the reproducibility of the nodal staging. There is a need for more evidence before any changes in staging systems are made.

Although neoadjuvant therapy for rectal carcinoma has been applied for a number of years and is in many countries considered standard of care, essential problems in staging have not been properly investigated. Application of staging systems that have been developed in the era before neoadjuvant therapy has several disadvantages. There are large differences between types of treatment and the implications of the different stages. Moreover, a number of practical problems arise when investigating neoadjuvantly treated tumors. Recommendations in the current paper are not always based on evidence, simply because there is no evidence available. However, in order to be able to compare different studies and to collect evidence for future guidelines, it would be helpful to standardize procedures. These are the following:

1. *ypTNM* is useful to indicate that there has been neoadjuvant therapy and that downstaging might occur. However, in this view it seems reasonable not to classify cases with short-course radiotherapy and immediate surgery as such. These should be coded as pTNM instead.

2. *Invasion depth (T stage)* should be determined on vital tumor only; acellular mucinous lakes should not be included in T staging. Tumor microfoci should be included in T staging; when present, they are indicative of tumor response.
3. *Lymph node status* is very important for prognosis. Cases should be coded N0 if no positive nodes are detected, irrespective of the number of lymph nodes. Lymph nodes with signs of regression, but without vital tumor cells, should be separately noted. After neoadjuvant therapy, tumor deposits should be coded in the T stage.
4. The *CRM* should always be reported given its importance for diagnosis.
5. It is important to determine the presence and grade of *tumor response*. A 3-tiered system is proposed based for practical reasons, including reproducibility and possible prognostic and predictive impact: A, complete response or near-complete response; B, obvious signs of tumor response; and C, no response.

References

1. Sobin LH, Wittekind C. UICC TNM classification of malignant tumours. 5th ed. New York: Wiley; 1997.
2. Sobin LH, Greene FL. TNM classification. Cancer. 2001;92(2):452.
3. Sobin LH, Gospodarowicz M, Wittekind C. TNM classification of malignant tumours. 7th ed. New York: Wiley-Blackwell; 2009.
4. Marijnen CAM, Nagtegaal ID, Klein Kranenbarg E, Hermans J, van de Velde CJH, Leer JWH, et al. No downstaging after short-term preoperative radiotherapy in rectal cancer patients. J Clin Oncol. 2001;19(7):1976–84.
5. Graf W, Dahlberg M, Osman MM, Holmberg L, Pahlman L, Glimelius B. Short-term preoperative radiotherapy results in down-staging of rectal cancer: a study of 1316 patients. Radiother Oncol. 1997;43:133–7.
6. Radu C, Berglund K, Pahlman L, Glimelius B. Short-course preoperative radiotherapy with delayed surgery in rectal cancer – A retrospective study. Radiother Oncol. 2008;87(3):343–9.
7. Francois Y, Nemoz CJ, Baulieux J, Vignal J, Grandjean JP, Partensky C, et al. Influence of the interval between preoperative radiation therapy and surgery on downstaging and on the rate of sphincter-sparing surgery for rectal cancer: the Lyon R90-01 randomized trial. J Clin Oncol. 1999;17(8):2396–402.
8. Bujko K, Nowacki MP, Nasierowska-Guttmejer A, Michalski W, Bebenek M, Kryj M. Long-term results of a randomized trial comparing preoperative short-course radiotherapy with preoperative conventionally fractionated chemoradiation for rectal cancer. Br J Surg. 2006;93(10):1215–23.
9. Gerard JP, Conroy T, Bonnetain F, Bouche O, Chapet O, Closon-Dejardin MT, et al. Preoperative radiotherapy with or without concurrent fluorouracil and leucovorin in T3-4 rectal cancers: results of FFCD 9203. J Clin Oncol. 2006;24(28):4620–5.
10. Bosset JF, Collette L, Calais G, Mineur L, Maingon P, Radosevic-Jelic L, et al. Chemotherapy with preoperative radiotherapy in rectal cancer. N Engl J Med. 2006;355(11):1114–23.
11. Rullier A, Laurent C, Vendrely V, Le BB, Bioulac-Sage P, Rullier E. Impact of colloid response on survival after preoperative radiotherapy in locally advanced rectal carcinoma. Am J Surg Pathol. 2005; 29(5):602–6.
12. Shia J, Guillem JG, Moore HG, Tickoo SK, Qin J, Ruo L, et al. Patterns of morphologic alteration in residual rectal carcinoma following preoperative chemoradiation and their association with long-term outcome. Am J Surg Pathol. 2004;28(2):215–23.
13. Smith KD, Tan D, Das P, Chang GJ, Kattapogu K, Feig BW, et al. Clinical significance of acellular mucin in rectal adenocarcinoma patients with a pathologica complete response to preoperative chemoradiation. Ann Surg. 2010;251(2):261–4.
14. Glynne-Jones R, Wallace M, Livingstone JI, Meyrick-Thomas J. Complete clinical response after preoperative chemoradiation in rectal cancer: is a "wait and see" policy justified? Dis Colon Rectum. 2008;51(1):10–20.
15. Prall F, Wohlke M, Klautke G, Schiffmann L, Fietkau R, Barten M. Tumour regression and mesorectal lymph node changes after intensified neoadjuvant chemoradiation for carcinoma of the rectum. APMIS. 2006;114(3):201–10.
16. Perez RO, Habr-Gama A, Nishida Arazawa ST, Rawet V, Coelho Siqueira SA, Kiss DR, et al. Lymph node micrometastasis in stage II distal rectal cancer following neoadjuvant chemoradiation therapy. Int J Colorectal Dis. 2005;20(5):434–9.
17. Morgan MJ, Koorey DJ, Painter D, Findlay M, Tran K, Stevens G, et al. Histological tumour response to preoperative combined modality therapy in locally advanced rectal cancer. Colorectal Dis. 2002;4(3):177–83.
18. Koh DM, Chau I, Tait D, Wotherspoon A, Cunningham D, Brown G. Evaluating mesorectal lymph nodes in rectal cancer before and after neoadjuvant chemoradiation using thin-section T2-weighted magnetic resonance imaging. Int J Radiat Oncol Biol Phys. 2008;71(2):456–61.
19. Valentini V, Coco C, Picciocchi A, Morganti AG, Trodella L, Ciabattoni A, et al. Does downstaging predict improved outcome after preoperative chemoradiation for extraperitoneal locally advanced rectal cancer? A long-term analysis of 165 patients. Int J Radiat Oncol Biol Phys. 2002;53(3):664–74.

20. Wijesuriya RE, Deen KI, Hewavisenthi J, Balawardana J, Perera M. Neoadjuvant therapy for rectal cancer down-stages the tumor but reduces lymph node harvest significantly. Surg Today. 2005;35(6):442–5.

21. Baxter NN, Morris AM, Rothenberger DA, Tepper JE. Impact of preoperative radiation for rectal cancer on subsequent lymph node evaluation: a population-based analysis. Int J Radiat Oncol Biol Phys. 2005;61(2):426–31.

22. Bujko K, Nowacki MP, Nasierowska-Guttmejer A, Kepca L, Winkler-Spytkowska B, Suwinski R, et al. Prediction of mesorectal nodal metastases after chemoradiation for rectal cancer: results of a randomised trial: implication for subsequent local excision. Radiother Oncol. 2005;76(3):234–40.

23. Suarez J, Vera R, Balen E, Gomez M, Arias F, Lera JM et al. Pathologic response assessed by Mandard grade is a better prognostic factor than down staging for disease-free survival after preoperative radiochemotherapy for advanced rectal cancer. Colorectal Dis. 2008;10(6):563–8.

24. Biondo S, Navarro M, Marti-Rague J, Arriola E, Pares D, Del RC, et al. Response to neoadjuvant therapy for rectal cancer: influence on long-term results. Colorectal Dis. 2005;7(5):472–9.

25. Stipa F, Zernecke A, Moore HG, Minsky BD, Wong WD, Weiser M, et al. Residual mesorectal lymph node involvement following neoadjuvant combined-modality therapy: rationale for radical resection? Ann Surg Oncol. 2004;11(2):187–91.

26. Pucciarelli S, Capirci C, Emanuele U, Toppan P, Friso ML, Pennelli GM, et al. Relationship between pathologic T-stage and nodal metastasis after preoperative chemoradiotherapy for locally advanced rectal cancer. Ann Surg Oncol. 2005;12(2):111–6.

27. Kuo LJ, Liu MC, Jian JJ, Horng CF, Cheng TI, Chen CM, et al. Is final TNM staging a predictor for survival in locally advanced rectal cancer after preoperative chemoradiation therapy? Ann Surg Oncol. 2007; 14(10):2766–72.

28. Kim DW, Kim DY, Kim TH, Jung KH, Chang HJ, Sohn DK, et al. Is T classification still correlated with lymph node status after preoperative chemoradiotherapy for rectal cancer? Cancer. 2006;106(8): 1694–700.

29. Habr-Gama A, Perez RO, Proscurshim I, Rawet V, Pereira DD, Sousa AH, et al. Absence of lymph nodes in the resected specimen after radical surgery for distal rectal cancer and neoadjuvant chemoradiation therapy: what does it mean? Dis Colon Rectum. 2008;51(3):277–83.

30. Hughes R, Glynne-Jones R, Grainger J, Richman P, Makris A, Harrison M, et al. Can pathological complete response in the primary tumour following pre-operative pelvic chemoradiotherapy for T3-T4 rectal cancer predict for sterilisation of pelvic lymph nodes, a low risk of local recurrence and the appropriateness of local excision? Int J Colorectal Dis. 2006;21(1):11–7.

31. Shivnani AT, Small Jr W, Stryker SJ, Kiel KD, Lim S, Halverson AL, et al. Preoperative chemoradiation for rectal cancer: results of multimodality management and analysis of prognostic factors. Am J Surg. 2007; 193(3):389–93.

32. Nagtegaal ID, Quirke P. Colorectal tumour deposits in the mesorectum and pericolon; a critical review. Histopathology. 2007;51(2):141–9.

33. Vironen J, Juhola M, Kairaluoma M, Jantunen I, Kellokumpu I. Tumour regression grading in the evaluation of tumour response after different preoperative radiotherapy treatments for rectal carcinoma. Int J Colorectal Dis. 2005;20(5):440–5.

34. Rodel C, Martus P, Papadoupolos T, Fuzesi L, Klimpfinger M, Fietkau R, et al. Prognostic significance of tumor regression after preoperative chemoradiotherapy for rectal cancer. J Clin Oncol. 2005; 23(34):8688–96.

35. Halvorsen TB, Seim E. Association between invasiveness, inflammatory reaction, desmoplasia and survival in colorectal cancer. J Clin Pathol. 1989;42(2):162–6.

Part VI

The Palliative Team

Multidisciplinary Treatment of Colorectal Cancer: The Palliative Team Introduction

24

Dagny Faksvåg Haugen

Abstract

Approximately 40 % of colorectal cancer patients will eventually die of metastatic disease. Patients with advanced, incurable disease often present a high symptom burden and psychosocial challenges and will benefit from an evaluation by an interdisciplinary palliative care team. The palliative care team and the palliative medicine consultant may contribute valuable expertise in assessment of needs and symptoms, symptom management, communication and goal setting, prognostication and decision-making, and practical, emotional, and spiritual support for patients and their families. The palliative care team holds a natural place in the MDT of advanced colorectal cancer.

Despite advances in diagnostics and treatment, a relatively high proportion of patients with colorectal cancer are diagnosed with incurable disease [1]. This fact may be due to a locally advanced, inoperable tumour or metastatic disease at the time of diagnosis or to comorbidity or age-dependent changes prohibiting a curative approach. In Norway, 23 % of patients with colon cancer and roughly 18 % with rectal cancer have distant metastases at the time of diagnosis, and only approximately 14 % in this group will survive 5 years [1]. Also, roughly 10 % of patients diagnosed with a localised tumour, and 25 % diagnosed with regional lymph node metastases, will have recurrent disease and die within 5 years. These figures mean that even if the relative survival of colorectal cancer is steadily increasing, approximately 40 % of the patients still will eventually die of metastatic disease [1].

A patient may be diagnosed with stage IV disease and die within weeks or a few months [2], or he or she may die after receiving different life-prolonging treatments for years [3, 4]. In both cases, effective palliative care is needed to relieve symptoms and maintain the best possible quality of life [5].

D.F. Haugen, MD, PhD
Regional Centre of Excellence for Palliative Care, Western Norway, Haukeland University Hospital, Haukelandsbakken 2, N-5021 Bergen, Norway

European Palliative Care Research Centre, Department of Cancer Research and Molecular Medicine, Faculty of Medicine, Norwegian University of Science and Technology, Trondheim, Norway
e-mail: dagny.haugen@helse-bergen.no

G. Baatrup (ed.), *Multidisciplinary Treatment of Colorectal Cancer*, DOI 10.1007/978-3-319-06142-9_24, © Springer International Publishing Switzerland 2015

Characteristics of Patients with Advanced Colorectal Cancer

Patients with advanced cancer experience many distressing symptoms [6]. The symptoms are principally disease related but may also be related to morbidity and toxicity from past treatment – surgery, chemotherapy, and radiation [7]. The most common symptoms are lack of appetite, fatigue, sleepiness, pain, nausea, dry mouth, constipation, dyspnea, anxiety, and depression [6]. In addition, patients with colorectal malignancies often present typical challenges related to tumours in the bowels, liver, or peritoneum, such as cachexia with weight loss and muscle wasting, abdominal or pelvic pain, ascites, jaundice, or bowel obstruction [5]. The pain may be difficult to relieve due to neuropathic components caused by pelvic tumour infiltration into the lumbosacral nerve plexi. Further, distant metastases to the bones, lungs, and brain may give rise to bone pain, dyspnea, neurological deficits, or cognitive failure. The picture is often complex and becomes additionally complicated by social, occupational, and economic challenges and problems of a psychological, spiritual, and existential nature. Indeed, the last phase of the colorectal cancer trajectory may be the most challenging and demanding of all.

Palliative Care

Palliative care is the active, total care of patients with advanced, incurable disease and short life expectancy [8]. However, palliative care should not be withheld until all treatment alternatives for the underlying disease have been exhausted. The palliative care approach should be included in treatment and care from the time the patient is diagnosed with an incurable illness, regardless of prognosis. Palliative care is an approach that improves the quality of life of patients and their families facing the problem associated with life-threatening illness, through the prevention and relief of suffering by means of early identification and impeccable assessment and treatment of pain and other problems, physical, psychosocial, and spiritual [9]. This approach is also applicable early in the course of cancer in conjunction with other therapies that are intended to prolong life, such as surgery, chemotherapy, and radiation therapy. Palliative care may also include investigations that are required to better understand and manage distressing clinical complications [9].

Living with advanced cancer affects so many aspects of life; therefore, it is rarely, if ever, possible for any one professional to meet all of the needs of a patient or family. Consequently, teamwork is an inherent feature of palliative care [8].

The Palliative Care Team

The palliative care team is found in any setting providing specialist palliative care [10]. The core members may vary between countries and settings but usually include nurses, doctors, a physiotherapist, social worker, and chaplain. Other professions may be included in the team as needed. The typical palliative care team is the hospital consult team serving the hospital wards and possibly the nearby communities. The team may also staff an in-patient specialist palliative care unit, in which case the team assumes full responsibility for the patients admitted to the unit. The palliative care consult team seeks to influence and improve patient care by giving advice to the health professionals in charge of the care. The consult team members work alongside the hospital ward teams, giving advice on symptom control and psychosocial and spiritual issues, and supporting relatives and staff in difficult decisions. The team has an important role in assessing the needs and priorities of patients and families and helping to set goals and lay out plans for care [11]. The consult team must have an overview of all relevant services regardless of whether the hospital team also has outreach programmes or liaises with community teams. Important functions of the team are discharge planning and facilitating care transitions.

Consultations are also provided for cancer patients receiving disease-modifying treatment.

This role gives the palliative care team a unique opportunity to act as the interface between palliative medicine and other medical specialties [12]. Speaking in terms of teams, the consultant, advanced nurse practitioner, or other members of the palliative care team will be part of the extended medical team in the intensive care unit, department of oncology, or surgical ward.

The Role of the Palliative Care Team in MDT of Colorectal Cancer

Within the shared care of MDT for colorectal cancer, all team members bring their own expertise to the decision-making process. At the risk of oversimplifying the topic, one can say that the main focus of the radiologist and pathologist is diagnosis, and the main focus of the surgeon and oncologist is treatment. The main focus of the palliative care team is directed towards the needs and concerns of the patient and family [13, 14]. All of these different aspects are necessary when setting up an individual treatment plan; however, the closer to the end of life, the less important the disease and the more important the patient becomes.

The contributions of the palliative care team and the palliative medicine consultant are especially important in the following areas [5, 10–13]:

1. Assessment of needs and symptoms
   A thorough assessment is a prerequisite for optimal symptom control. The team will perform repeated assessments of the needs, symptoms, functioning, and quality of life. General symptom assessment tools, such as the Edmonton Symptom Assessment System (ESAS) [15], or more specific tools for colorectal cancer may be used [16, 17]. The ESAS should also be used routinely on the ward.
2. Symptom management
   The team has wide expertise in the control of physical symptoms, such as pain, nausea and vomiting, anorexia, dyspnea, and confusion. The palliative care team can work with the ward team to develop a pain and symptom management care plan, which also deals with nonmedical issues faced by the patient and family.
3. Communication and goal setting
   To reach the goal of best possible quality of life, the most important tool for the palliative care team is close, clear communication, valuing the patient and family's concerns, needs, and goals and taking into account all available prognostic information. Communication includes guidance with difficult and complex treatment choices, advance care planning, and maintaining realistic hope.
4. Prognostication and decision-making
   Predicting survival is important when making treatment decisions, as well as for giving guidance to patients and those close to them. Although prognostication continues to be a challenge, the palliative care physician may supplement the surgeon and oncologist, basing his or her judgement on a thorough assessment of the general condition of the patient and incorporating predictive parameters.

   Bowel obstruction is one example of a situation that requires careful clinical evaluation. This condition should always be discussed in a multidisciplinary team that includes a palliative care consultant. The palliative care physician spends a lot of time discussing end-of-life issues with patients and families, and is experienced in decision-making and handling ethical dilemmas.
5. Practical, emotional, and spiritual support for patients and families
   The multi-professional composition of the palliative care team allows for counselling and support for patients and their families in diverse areas, including detailed practical information and assistance, emotional backing and advice, and spiritual support.

In conclusion, the palliative care team holds a natural place in the MDT of advanced colorectal cancer. In cases with high symptom burden and complex psychosocial challenges, the patient should be transferred to a palliative care unit. However, all patients with incurable disease will benefit from an evaluation by the palliative care team.

References

1. Cancer Registry of Norway. Cancer in Norway 2011 – Cancer incidence, mortality, survival and prevalence in Norway. Oslo: Cancer Registry of Norway; 2013.
2. Sigurdsson HK, Körner H, Dahl O, Skarstein A, Søreide JA, Norwegian Rectal Cancer Group. Clinical characteristics and outcomes in patients with advanced rectal cancer: a national prospective cohort study. Dis Colon Rectum. 2007;50:285–91.
3. Fornaro L, Masi G, Loupakis F, Vasile E, Falcone A. Palliative treatment of unresectable metastatic colorectal cancer. Expert Opin Pharmacother. 2010;11:63–77.
4. Amersi F, Stamos MJ, Ko CY. Palliative care for colorectal cancer. Surg Oncol Clin N Am. 2004;13: 467–77.
5. Dunn GP. Palliating patients who have unresectable colorectal cancer: creating the right framework and salient symptom management. Surg Clin North Am. 2006;86:1065–92.
6. Teunissen SC, Wesker W, Kruitwagen C, de Haes HC, Voest EE, de Graeff A. Symptom prevalence in patients with incurable cancer: a systematic review. J Pain Symptom Manage. 2007;34:94–104.
7. Griffin-Sobel JP. Symptom management of advanced colorectal cancer. Surg Oncol Clin N Am. 2006;15: 213–22.
8. Doyle D, Woodruff R. The IAHPC manual of palliative care. 2nd ed. Houston: IAHPC Press; 2008.
9. National Cancer Control Programmes. Policies and Managerial Guidelines. 2nd ed. Geneva: WHO; 2002.
10. Haugen DF, Nauck F, Caraceni A. The core team and the extended team. In: Hanks G, Cherny NI, Christakis NA, Fallon M, Kaasa S, Portenoy RK, editors. Oxford textbook of palliative medicine. 4th ed. Oxford: Oxford University Press; 2009. p. 167–76.
11. Cintron A, Meier DE. The palliative care consult team. In: Bruera E, Higginson I, von Gunten D, Ripamonti C, editors. Textbook of palliative medicine. Oxford: Oxford University Press; 2006. p. 259–65.
12. Glare PA, Auret KA, Aggarwal G, Clark KJ, Pickstock SE, Lickiss JN. The interface between palliative medicine and specialists in acute-care hospitals: boundaries, bridges and challenges. Med J Aust. 2003;179:S29–31.
13. Aggarwal G, Glare P, Clarke S, Chapuis PH. Palliative and shared care concepts in patients with advanced colorectal cancer. ANZ J Surg. 2006;76:175–80.
14. Baile WF, Palmer JL, Bruera E, Parker PA. Assessment of palliative care cancer patients' most important concerns. Support Care Cancer. 2011;19:475–81.
15. Bruera E, Kuehn N, Miller MJ, Selmser P, Macmillan K. The Edmonton Symptom Assessment System (ESAS): a simple method for the assessment of palliative care patients. J Palliat Care. 1991;7(2):6–9.
16. Blazeby JM, Fayers P, Conroy T, Sezer O, Ramage J, Rees M. European Organization for Research and Treatment of Cancer (EORTC) Quality of Life Group. Validation of the European Organization for Research and Treatment of Cancer QLQ-LMC21 questionnaire for assessment of patient-reported outcomes during treatment of colorectal liver metastases. Br J Surg. 2009;96:291–8.
17. Hassan I, Cima RC, Sloan JA. Assessment of quality of life outcomes in the treatment of advanced colorectal malignancies. Gastroenterol Clin North Am. 2006;35:53–64.

Surgical Treatment in Palliative Care

Multidisciplinary Treatment of Colorectal Cancer

Hartwig Kørner and Jon Arne Søreide

Abstract

Palliative surgery aims to relieve symptoms in patients with incurable disease by interventions. Traditionally, palliative surgery has been understood as non-curative surgery, i.e. non-resectional or R2 procedures, without sufficient attention to the impact on patients' quality of life (QoL).

Palliative surgical procedures are indicated to relieve – or prevent – symptoms in patients with incurable disease in order to keep or improve the QoL. These interventions should fit into the patient's general situation within the disease trajectory. Effective and empathic communication is essential to achieve a common understanding of the clinical situation, the individual treatment goals and expectations with regard to the effects of an intervention. Severe complications or any futile procedure, which may jeopardise the patient's QoL, should be prevented. Palliative surgical procedures comprise any interventions, including conventional open surgery, minimally invasive procedures and endoscopic and percutaneous techniques. Indications and benefits have to be evaluated by patient-reported outcomes, e.g. by validated symptom scores.

H. Kørner, MD, PhD (✉)
Division of Colorectal Surgery, Department of Gastrointestinal Surgery, Stavanger University Hospital, 8100, N-4068 Stavanger, Norway

Department of Clinical Medicine, University of Bergen, Bergen, Norway

Regional Centre of Excellence for Palliative Care Western Norway, Haukeland University Hospital, N-5021 Bergen, Norway
e-mail: hartwig.korner@kir.uib.no

J.A. Søreide, MD, PhD, FACS
Department of Clinical Medicine, University of Bergen, Bergen, Norway

Division of HPB Surgery, Department of Gastrointestinal Surgery, Stavanger University Hospital, N-4068 Stavanger, Norway

G. Baatrup (ed.), *Multidisciplinary Treatment of Colorectal Cancer*,
DOI 10.1007/978-3-319-06142-9_25, © Springer International Publishing Switzerland 2015

Frequent palliative surgical scenarios include patients with surgically resectable but asymptomatic primary tumours with incurable metastatic disease or malignant bowel obstruction. Most patients will benefit from a multidisciplinary approach, which takes into account not only the physical but also the psychosocial and spiritual needs. The surgeon, as a part of the multidisciplinary palliative team, should add to the mutual efforts to improve the care for patients along a challenging last part of life.

Introduction

Palliative surgery aims to improve a patient's quality of life by using various interventions to relieve symptoms. Traditionally, surgery in its earliest attempts in human civilisation most likely focused on symptom relief, i.e. to modify illness, rather than the removal of tissues or organs [1]. Nevertheless, surgical efforts to treat malignant tumours, such as breast cancer, have been reported since the post-Hippocrates era.

In the sixteenth century, the French surgeon Ambroise Paré (1510–1590), who is considered to be one of the fathers of modern surgery, outlined the duties of surgery as "to remove what is superfluous, to restore what has been dislocated, to separate what has grown together, to reunite what has been divided, and to redress defects of nature". However, unfavourable outcomes made the people and society sceptical. Accordingly, the *primum non nocere* principle of Hippocrates (above all, do no harm!) governed surgical practice until the first part of the nineteenth century.

With a better understanding of anatomy, physiology, and pathology during the second part of the nineteenth century, a paradigm shift eventually took place in modern medicine. The introduction of modern antisepsis and anaesthesia was an important prerequisite for successful cancer surgery and was the basis for surgical treatment to cure malignant tumours. Surgeons like Billroth (1829–1894) in Vienna, Halsted (1852–1922) at Johns Hopkins Hospital, Kocher (1841–1917) in Berne, and Miles (1869–1947) at St. Mark's pioneered and introduced various operative techniques that are still in use, albeit partly modified, for the surgical curative treatment of cancer.

During this shift in treatment focus from a limited modification of illness to curative intent, less attention was paid to the treatment of patients with incurable cancer. The suffering of this group of patients, frequently with an impaired quality of life (QoL), was less than well recognised as a surgical responsibility.

However, since the 1960s, broad attention on the clinical importance of symptom relief in patients with incurable cancer enabled the introduction of palliative medicine as a separate discipline [2, 3]. The increasing incidence of cancer in our older populations and the introduction of new and more effective systemic cancer treatments increase the need for palliative care in general. In addition, a large proportion of these patients may benefit from various surgical interventions to improve QoL and relieve symptoms caused by their malignant disease.

As a consequence, the American College of Surgeons was the first surgical association to formalise palliative surgery, establishing the Palliative Surgical Care Task Force [4, 5]. In 2003, Principles Guiding Care at the End of Life were presented as the ethical base for palliative surgery (Table 25.1) [6]. Some of the most central principles are to respect the patient's dignity; to seek measures to alleviate physical, psychological, social, and spiritual symptoms; and to forego any futile treatment. Though surgeons may be regarded by most health-care providers as having limited knowledge regarding palliative care, they experience a lack of understanding and knowledge of palliative surgical care from their nonsurgical colleagues [7]. We think this dynamic emphasises the need for surgeons to be part of the palliative multidisciplinary team. Caring for patients with progressive, incurable, or terminal

Table 25.1 The ten principles of guiding care at the end of life, as defined by the Palliative Care Task Force of the American College of Surgeons [6]

1. Respect the dignity of both patient and caregivers
2. Be sensitive to and respectful of the patient's and family's wishes
3. Use the most appropriate measures that are consistent with the choices of the patient or the patient's legal surrogate
4. Ensure alleviation of pain and management of other physical symptoms
5. Recognize, assess, and address psychological, social, and spiritual problems
6. Ensure appropriate continuity of care by the patient's primary and/or specialist physician
7. Provide access to therapies that may realistically be expected to improve the patient's quality of life
8. Provide access to appropriate palliative care and hospice care
9. Respect the patient's right to refuse treatment
10. Recognize the physician's responsibility to forego treatments that are futile

Table 25.2 Examples of interventions, which might be considered for palliative treatment of symptoms in patients with incurable disease

Technique	Example of indication
Conventional open surgery	Bowel resection for obstruction or bleeding
Laparoscopic surgery	Bowel resection, creation of ostomy
Endoscopic surgery	
Transanal endoscopic surgery (TEM)	Local resection of rectal tumour
Self-expanding metal stent	Bowel obstruction, icterus
Argon plasma coagulation	Tumour reduction, bleeding
Interventional radiology	
Percutaneous drainage	Fluid collections
Stenting procedures	Common bile duct
Endovascular procedures	Embolization

illness is part of the practice of most surgeons, and surgeons will frequently see patients for whom "there is not much to do". However, surgeons should appreciate the clinical challenge and surgical opportunity in the context of the individual patient, even when a cure is not possible [8]. Surgeons can make important contributions to improve the QoL, and death, not only by palliative interventions but also by caring and staying with the patient when a cure is not possible [9].

Definition

Inconsistent definitions of palliative surgery have made comparing research results difficult, and clinical guidelines have suffered from blurred interpretations [10, 11]. *Palliative surgery is defined as any invasive procedure in which the main intention is to mitigate physical symptoms in patients with incurable disease without causing premature death* [12]. Accordingly, surgical palliative care comprises the complete spectrum from conventional open surgery to minimally invasive techniques such as endoscopic or percutaneous interventional radiological procedures

(Table 25.2). In this context, the traditional limits of surgery are blurred, which underlines the importance of a multidisciplinary approach to the palliative patient. Palliative surgical procedures may include treatment of the tumour, such as bowel resection due to cancer in the presence of incurable distant metastases, which may relieve symptoms and prolong life. However, the treatment of symptoms is the main focus of palliative surgery. The distinction with regard to incomplete tumour resection (e.g. R2 resection) in patients surgically treated with curative intent is important. An operation with primarily curative intent that results in incomplete removal of the tumour and without a main focus on symptom relief is better categorised as non-curative surgery [13].

The Scientific Evidence for Palliative Surgery

The scientific literature on this topic is complicated by numerous retrospective studies, often with small and heterogeneous study populations and ill-defined end points. In addition, validated QoL instruments have been employed only sporadically [14]. Because of various practical and ethical aspects related to clinical research on this group of patients, prospective randomised controlled trials (RCT) used to be the exception [12]. Accordingly, the lack of scientific evidence is a concern when many important clinical questions are addressed. The everyday clinical practice of palliative surgery has probably been guided more by the surgeons' personal experience and traditions in many institutions, rather than true scientific evidence. Nevertheless, results from some well-designed prospective (randomised) studies or systematic reviews have provided useful and reliable clinical information, such as celiac plexus block in patients with non-resectable pancreatic cancer [15], the treatment of asymptomatic colorectal cancer with non-resectable synchronous colorectal metastases [16], and palliative relief of gastric outlet syndrome [14, 17]. Yet, the appropriate and timely clinical implementation of this knowledge remains a challenge in many institutions.

Research and Outcome Measures

In modern medicine, treatment effects are evaluated by outcome measures, which are often defined by the treatment provider, i.e. the physician. Common outcome measures to describe the effectiveness of the chosen treatment mostly include postoperative mortality and morbidity, disease-free cancer-specific or overall survival, response rates, and cure rates. Notably, none of these variables are suitable for evaluating QoL. Optimally, the goal of palliative surgery is to meet the patient's individual needs and expectations [18]. Consequently, the effects of palliative treatment should be evaluated by *individual outcome measures*. Patients, relatives, and doctors tend to estimate QoL and treatment effects differently because doctors are biased by the wish to help and, necessarily, by judging the clinical situation and treatment effects from their own perspective [19, 20].

Various validated tools are available to measure QoL and assess symptoms. Spitzer et al. [21] published the *Quality of Life Index* in 1981, which is based on a physician-rated 5-item scale. Another used physician-rated score in

widespread use is the *ECOG Performance Status* [22], which is mainly based on the patient's ability to participate in daily life activities. Though these scores are helpful to describe the patient's functional state and fitness, they are unsuitable for measuring the QoL for an individual patient.

The most used symptom score for palliative patients is the *Edmonton Symptom Assessment Scale* (ESAS) [23]. This score is based on ten frequent symptoms, including nausea, pain, appetite, and depression, and is a very useful tool for detecting common symptoms and to monitor the effects of treatment by repeated measurements. Also, a number of organ-specific QoL scores are available, including the 36-item *Gastrointestinal Quality of Life Index* for gastrointestinal disorders [24].

More sophisticated QoL scores are available from the *European Organization for Research and Treatment of Cancer* (EORTC). The *EORTC QoL-C30* is one of the most frequently used tools for QoL assessment in cancer research [25], with various organ-specific modules available. The scores are validated and translated into numerous languages. Another widespread general tool for QoL assessment is the *Medical Outcomes Survey-Short Form (MOS-SF 36)* [26].

Nevertheless, quantitative outcome measures, such as survival, are of importance in palliative care as they provide information on the prognostication of a disease. Prognostic information, though limited to subgroups of patients and never to an individual patient, is helpful for counselling patients and their relatives and plays a role when the indications of palliative procedures are contemplated.

Approach to the Palliative Surgical Patient

Palliative patients suffering from an incurable disease, and regarded to be in a hopeless situation, belong to a vulnerable group of individuals. Visiting with these patients and their relatives might be a challenge for many clinicians, which relates to their own emotions, being unable to offer a cure, and the fear of taking any hope

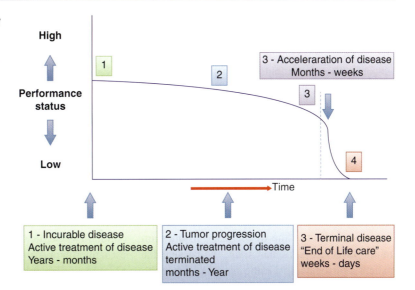

Fig. 25.1 Disease trajectory of patients with incurable malignant disease. Intensity and type of treatment has to be defined according to performance status of the patient during the disease trajectory

away from the patient. Sound principles of surgical palliative care have been described extensively by Krouse et al. [6] (Table 25.1). These principles are based on effective and empathic communication with the patient and his or her family and respect for dignity and patient autonomy. With these principles in mind, the surgeon has extended his communication tools to deal with the palliative surgical patient and his or her family more appropriately, which also includes an emphatic and human contribution to optimised end-of-life care.

Establishing Indications

The feasibility of an operation is not an indication of its performance.

The aim of palliative surgery is to improve QoL. Therefore, indications for palliative surgical procedures depend strongly on the suggested benefit for the patient and anticipated relief of symptoms after intervention. Identifying individual treatment goals for the patient is the first prerequisite in this process. Treatment goals depend on the extent of disease, predominant co-morbidity, patient age, social and psychological context, and spiritual thoughts and wishes. Furthermore,

where the patient is in the trajectory of the disease is important to take into account (Fig. 25.1). More complex procedures may be warranted in a younger and fit patient when the diagnosis of incurable cancer is established (Fig. 25.1, Phase 1) in order to achieve local tumour control and prevent the development of symptoms in the later course of the disease. This approach may not be the case for older and more fragile patients. Surgical procedures are usually not indicated in patients with rapidly deteriorating conditions who have a short life expectancy (Fig. 25.1, Phase 3 or 4).

The indications for palliative procedures may be coloured by aspects or needs other than pure medical factors. Both health-care providers and relatives may feel an urgent need that "something should be done" for a suffering patient. However, all chosen measures have to be in accordance with the patient's expectations, wishes, and individual treatment goals; otherwise, those actions are useless and outside the context of appropriate palliative care. In addition, such motivations may threaten the patient's dignity and autonomy. The dignity and autonomy of the patient are main principles of palliative care, and doctors are obliged to discourage any paternalistic interventions that may result in futile procedures with increased morbidity or mortality. The effects of any intervention are based on physical changes in the body and cannot be easily reversed. Accordingly, any complication in this context is a serious event that would most likely jeopardise the QoL and, thus, causing disastrous consequences for the remaining life of the patient: *Above all, do no harm.*

Communication

The crucial basis of good communication is a common understanding of the issue in question by the involved participants, i.e. the patient, the patient's surrogate(s), and the surgeon. Achieving a common understanding of the underlying problems for the palliative surgical patient is the cornerstone of appropriate symptom management. This approach is not specific for palliative care, but common to any field of medicine. It is widely accepted, and even regulated by the legislation in most countries, that all communication with patients be based on full disclosure. Nowadays, rather than being passive recipients of medical care, patients are active participants. However, most doctors may perceive this communication as particularly difficult when they have to break bad news on dismal prognoses. Many surgeons find themselves in such a situation rather frequently, including settings other than cancer (e.g. trauma surgery). Successful communication depends heavily on personal skills but is also a matter of education and training.

Bradley et al. [27] recently defined four areas of end-of-life issues in surgical practice:
1. The preoperative visit
2. Discussing a poor prognosis
3. Adverse outcome due to error
4. Discussing death

During the *preoperative visit*, counselling with regard to the medical facts, is only one, albeit important, aspect among others. This is an important opportunity for establishing *confidence* between the patient, family, and doctor. Confidence is obtained from information based on full disclosure with an attitude of empathy. Empathy means being open to the patient's

thoughts and emotions and should not be confused with sympathy (i.e. to share the patient's thoughts and emotions).

Exploring the patient's understanding of his or her position and the treatment goals is one of the most important objectives. Open-ended questions are considered to be the most appropriate, as well as ensuring that the patient is the focus of the conversation. One other important goal is to discuss the need for advance directives, such as the use of ICU facilities or "Do not resuscitate" orders. Doctors may be reluctant to discuss these issues, but most patients appreciate reaching a common understanding on these issues of greatest importance from an end-of-life perspective [28]. Many difficult situations can be avoided if unintended complications or events occur and these aspects have been addressed properly before any intervention.

When palliative interventions are discussed, informing the patient and family of the intention of treatment and the possible outcomes is elementary. Making sure that patients do not misinterpret a palliative intervention as an opportunity to be cured is important. The patient should also be appropriately informed about possible unfavourable aspects associated with any intervention.

Breaking bad news may be one of the greatest challenges, and every surgeon will encounter this regularly in all fields of surgery. Maguire [29] suggested guidelines and strategies for dealing with this situation. In this process, the patients will appreciate openness and honesty, which are important tools for an empathic approach. Knowing which information has been shared with the patient already, how much information the patient wishes and, finally, choosing the appropriate terms are also important. An empathic approach does not exclude information in direct terms; to the contrary, patients demand the truth and will disclose any modifications of it. Honesty and openness, together with the affirmation of a continued will to be engaged, will build up the base for new hope rather than to take hope [6].

Adverse outcomes of interventions are an inherent part of any interventional discipline.

Treatment failure may be related to insufficient preoperative investigations, wrong indications, failure to perform the procedure correctly, or other complications and circumstances beyond the surgeon's control. Most of the aspects addressed with regard to breaking bad news also apply to this situation. However, when the aim of treatment is to improve the patient's QoL, treatment failure may be perceived as being extremely disastrous for all those involved. Any preoperative efforts to establish a relationship based on mutual confidence would be of greatest importance when things go wrong. Evidence suggests that open disclosure of failures prevents, rather than stimulates, litigation, particularly when the responsible clinician takes the initiative to inform the patient [30]. Patients and surrogates expect an apology from the responsible doctor in most cases, and it is important to meet this desire [31].

Death, and talking about death, may be the point where the doctor reaches deepest into the patient's life and his or her family within the end-of-life care. Death and dying will be an important issue not only when death occurs. This topic may be taken into consideration and drawn to attention by some patients when the bad news about a serious disease or the dismal prognosis is communicated, or even before a planned operation. The circumstances and the way of sharing this message with the patient and their family are of great importance for coping with the death of a family member. This is true both at the time of death and during the following grieving process.

Clinical Scenarios

Consistent with the uniform treatment goal of curative cancer treatment, i.e. the radical removal of all cancer tissue, uniform guidelines for reaching this goal are based on accumulated evidence. However, in the palliative setting, the identification of the *individual* treatment goal has to be followed by an individualised route for each patient to reach his or her aims. In illustrative terms, the process of palliative surgical care does not follow the broad highways of guidelines for curative cancer treatment, but rather a twisting narrow

path through an unknown landscape. On this path, applying the philosophy of palliative care in clinical decision-making is the most important tool for reaching the destination safely. In other words, the identification and communication of the realistic treatment goals of the individual patient are based on maintaining the patient's autonomy, dignity, and respect. This approach is fundamental to enabling an appropriate treatment plan for achieving the highest possible QoL.

However, some clinical situations in patients with colorectal cancer, including patients with a resectable tumour in the presence of incurable metastatic disease or malignant bowel obstruction, are frequently encountered. These two scenarios are discussed in the followed sections with regard to the literature.

Treatment of Colorectal Cancer with Incurable Distant Disease: Resection or Not?

Approximately 20–25 % of all patients with colorectal cancer have distant spread at the time of diagnosis [32]. Among these patients, less than 30–50 % are amenable for liver resection with curative intent [16], and roughly 8 % will receive only symptom-related treatment [33]. According to the surgical tradition thus far, a majority of patients are recommended for resection of the primary tumour [34, 35]. Many patients may only have mild symptoms related to the tumour or be asymptomatic. Thus, the benefit of primary surgical treatment might be questionable. This approach has been brought into the discussion based on recent achievements in oncological treatment. Modern chemotherapy has increased the overall median survival from approximately 6 months with 5-fluorouracil/leucovorin alone to >24 months when treated with oxaliplatine- or irinotecan-based regimens [36, 37]. Moreover, the overall mortality and morbidity of colorectal resection is 3–5 % and 20–40 % [38], respectively, and might even be higher in patients with advanced malignancy.

Primary surgical treatment of colorectal cancer with incurable disease may aim for either the relief or prevention of symptoms, including obstruction, haemorrhage, or perforation, to mention the most serious ones. The surgical approach has been increasingly challenged by primary systemic chemotherapy, either alone or followed by surgery with curative intent. Primary chemotherapy has been advocated as the first treatment option because major surgical procedures may delay or even exclude access to chemotherapy. This scenario is well known and frequently challenges the multidisciplinary team to define the optimal treatment option for the individual patient with advanced colorectal cancer.

Tumour-related symptoms will prompt surgical treatment to achieve local control, but this may not be the case in asymptomatic patients or patients with minimal symptoms. According to recent literature on primary surgery versus chemotherapy for stage IV colorectal cancer [16, 39], the current treatment evidence is weak due to the retrospective character of most patient series and due to the lack of prospective randomised trials. Scheer et al. [16] compared the complication rates of primary surgery and primary chemotherapy, finding that patients treated with primary chemotherapy suffered from a larger tumour burden compared to patients who underwent primary resection. This difference is most likely caused by patient selection and illustrates the confounding effect of bias.

The most frequently reported complication in patients treated primarily with chemotherapy is intestinal occlusion, with a pooled frequency of 13.9 % and ranging from 5.6 % [40] to 29 % [41]. Haemorrhage and perforation occurred in 3 % and 6 % of patients treated with surgery and chemotherapy, respectively. Serious complications of chemotherapy, i.e. grade 3–4, were reported in 37 % of patients [42]. Quality of life issues were not addressed in these reviews because none of the primary publications reported the effect of primary treatment on QoL.

Primary surgery was associated with a mortality of 3 % and morbidity ranging between 18.8 and 47 %. Pooled analysis revealed the frequency of major complications, such as anastomotic leak, obstruction, or haemorrhage, in 12 % of the patients, and minor complications, such as infections of the surgical site or urinary tract, in 21 % of the patients. With regard to tumour localisation, patients with left-sided tumours (i.e. colon descendens, sigmoid, or rectum) were more likely to undergo surgical resection. However, the indication to perform surgical resection for the relief of left-sided colon obstruction is currently challenged by self-expanding metal stents (SEMS). Sebastian et al. [43] concluded in their review that SEMS treatment is highly effective with both a technical and clinical success rate of roughly 90 %, and this procedure is associated with low morbidity.

Survival appeared to be slightly longer in patients with primary resection compared to patients undergoing primary chemotherapy (14–23 months vs. 14–22 months); however, this difference is more likely due to patient selection. In multivariate analysis, the performance status of the patient, the presence of peritoneal or omental metastases, and the extent of tumour burden in the liver were significant predictors of survival, whereas the resection status was not important. In a recent study of 838 patients undergoing palliative resections for rectal cancer, perioperative mortality was 16 % in patients >80 years of age, and the median overall survival was 6 months regardless of surgical treatment [44]. Furthermore, many studies have reported on patients treated when modern, highly effective chemotherapy was not yet available. These facts underline the importance of making treatment decisions based on a comprehensive clinical evaluation of the individual patient, not only with regard to the technical feasibility of a procedure.

Malignant Bowel Obstruction

Malignant bowel obstruction (MBO) is defined as a partial or complete obstruction of the gastrointestinal (GI) tract caused by malignant tissue in the abdominal cavity. This condition may be due to either a primary cancer of the GI tract, another intra-abdominal cancer such as ovarian cancer, or intra-abdominal manifestation of an extra-abdominal primary malignancy, including breast

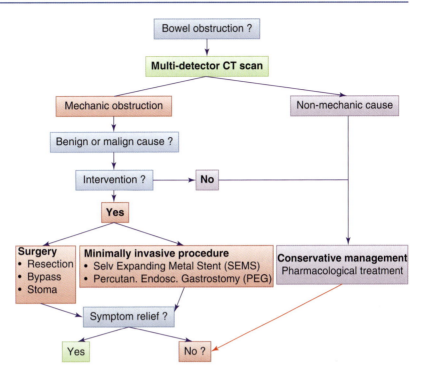

Fig. 25.2 Algorithm for evaluation and treatment of patients with suspected malignant bowel obstruction

cancer or malignant melanoma. MBO is often preceded by a long history of cancer with previous extensive multimodal treatment. Other patients may be diagnosed with colorectal cancer when they present with bowel obstruction, as roughly 20 % of all patients with colorectal cancer are diagnosed in the acute setting. However, many patients have undergone previous surgery, and about one-third of these patients may have benign causes of bowel obstruction, such as adhesions, bands, or strangulation.

MBO is a condition often seen in patients with advanced disease. Thus, this condition may have a great impact on the end stages of life. Making treatment choices that support QoL and avoiding heroic procedures and futile actions is of utmost importance. A number of treatment options are available, including conventional surgery, minimally invasive procedures, and pharmacological treatment, either in combination or alone (Table 25.2). As a general surgical principle, successful management depends on an adequate examination of the patient. Excluding other reasons for impaired bowel function is important,

including serious constipation due to opiates or other drugs, as well as identifying the patients who will benefit from any procedure to reestablish bowel function. With modern diagnostic tools, such as contrast enhanced multi-detector CT scans, assessing the nature of obstruction is possible with high diagnostic accuracy in most patients [45]. The following questions should be addressed when considering palliative surgical procedures (Fig. 25.2):

- Is the cause of obstruction mechanical?
- Is any intervention indicated?
- Which intervention is the most effective and which is least harmful?
- What are the risks associated with the procedure, and do they warrant the procedure?

Consequently, blind surgical explorations should be abandoned for the diagnosis of malignant bowel obstruction, as this may result in futile surgical procedures with detrimental effects on the patient at the end of life.

When surgical treatment for MBO is indicated, the appropriate intervention or operation should be employed under optimal conditions as in any other surgical procedure, i.e. preferably as an elective procedure performed by a competent surgical team. In contrast to other causes of intestinal obstruction, patients with malignant bowel obstruction rarely need acute surgery during the night, but a planned procedure should be aimed for based on appropriate investigations. Surgical treatment should be discouraged in the presence of ascites, peritoneal carcinomatosis, more than one level of obstruction, and high tumour burden, such as >50 % of the liver replaced by metastases, or extensive extra-abdominal spread. Previous palliative surgical procedures and other factors, such as reduced nutritional status, other comorbidities, or increased age, usually indicate that surgery is unlikely to benefit the patient. Procedures of any kind are usually contraindicated in patients with rapidly progressing disease and a limited life expectancy of ≤2 months (Fig. 25.1) [46].

The placement of SEMS should be considered in left-sided colon obstructions [47]. However, stent migration is a well-known complication that occurs more frequently in the case of external compression of the colon or in obstructions wide enough to pass with a colonoscope. Faecal impaction of the stent is another common complication and can be avoided by laxatives, such as lactulose, on a regular basis. SEMS obstruction due to tumour ingrowth may be treated by the insertion of a second stent or by argon plasma coagulation.

When surgical treatment of the malignant bowel obstruction is not indicated, other alternatives should be considered. The placement of percutaneous endoscopic gastrotomy tubes (PEG), initially designed to provide nutritional support, has been shown to provide highly effective symptom relief for intractable bowel obstruction [48]. A PEG tube may be combined with pharmacological treatment [49]. The subcutaneous injection of octreotide analogues (e.g. Sandostatin™) effectively reduces intraluminal secretion, alleviating the symptoms of bowel obstruction [50]. Other drugs, such as morphine, haloperidol, and butylscopolamine, are important supplements and may be given together as a continuous subcutaneous infusion. Corticosteroids, such as

dexamethasone, may additionally improve symptoms by reducing pain, oedema, and nausea.

The management of patients with malignant bowel obstruction is one of the most challenging clinical situations to encounter, and the balance between demands to act and resisting harmful or futile actions is important. Careful evaluation of the patient, effective and empathic communication regarding the available treatment options, and the reassurance to help even when "nothing can be done" remain the cornerstones of the successful management of malignant bowel obstruction: *Sometimes the sun can set on an unoperated bowel obstruction, especially when the sun is setting on the patient* (Krouse) [51].

References

1. Dunn GP. Principles and core competencies of surgical palliative care: an overview. Otolaryngol Clin North Am. 2009;42:1–13, vii.
2. Saunders C. The evolution of palliative care. Patient Educ Couns. 2000;41:7–13.
3. Seymour J, Clark D, Winslow M. Pain and palliative care: the emergence of new specialties. J Pain Symptom Manage. 2005;29:2–13.
4. Dunn GP, Milch RA. Introduction and historical background of palliative care: where does the surgeon fit in? J Am Coll Surg. 2001;193:325–8.
5. Statement on Principles Guiding Care at the End of Life. Bull Am Coll Surg. 1998;83.
6. Krouse RS, Jonasson O, Milch RA, Dunn GP. An evolving strategy for surgical care. J Am Coll Surg. 2004;198:149–55.
7. Dunn GP. Surgery and palliative medicine: new horizons. J Palliat Med. 1998;1:215–9.
8. Dunn GP. Patient assessment in palliative care: how to see the "big picture" and what to do when "there is no more we can do". J Am Coll Surg. 2001;193:565–73.
9. Dunn GP. Restoring palliative care as a surgical tradition. Bull Am Coll Surg. 2004;89:23–9.
10. Dunn GP. Surgical palliation in advanced disease: recent developments. Curr Oncol Rep. 2002;4:233–41.
11. Miner TJ, Jaques DP, Tavaf-Motamen H, Shriver CD. Decision making on surgical palliation based on patient outcome data. Am J Surg. 1999;177:150–4.
12. Hofmann B, Håheim LL, Søreide JA. Ethics of palliative surgery in patients with cancer. Br J Surg. 2005;92:802–9.
13. Wagman LD. Palliative surgical oncology. Surg Oncol Clin North Am. 2004;13(3):xiii–xiv.
14. Søreide JA, Grønbech JE, Mjåland O. Effects and outcomes after palliative surgical treatment of malignant dysphagia. Scand J Gastroenterol. 2006;41:376–81.

15. Lillemoe KD, Cameron JL, Kaufman HS, Yeo CJ, Pitt HA, Sauter PK. Chemical splanchnicectomy in patients with unresectable pancreatic cancer. A prospective randomized trial. Ann Surg. 1993;217:447–55; discussion 56–7.

16. Scheer MG, Sloots CE, van der Wilt GJ, Ruers TJ. Management of patients with asymptomatic colorectal cancer and synchronous irresectable metastases. Ann Oncol. 2008;19:1829–35.

17. Jeurnink SM, van Eijck CH, Steyerberg EW, Kuipers EJ, Siersema PD. Stent versus gastrojejunostomy for the palliation of gastric outlet obstruction: a systematic review. BMC Gastroenterol. 2007;7:18.

18. Easson AM, Lee KF, Brasel K, Krouse RS. Clinical research for surgeons in palliative care: challenges and opportunities. J Am Coll Surg. 2003;196:141–51.

19. Petersen MA, Larsen H, Pedersen L, Sonne N, Groenvold M. Assessing health-related quality of life in palliative care: comparing patient and physician assessments. Eur J Cancer. 2006;42:1159–66.

20. Wilson KA, Dowling AJ, Abdolell M, Tannock IF. Perception of quality of life by patients, partners and treating physicians. Qual Life Res. 2000;9:1041–52.

21. Spitzer WO, Dobson AJ, Hall J, Chesterman E, Levi J, Shepherd R, et al. Measuring the quality of life of cancer patients: a concise QL-index for use by physicians. J Chronic Dis. 1981;34:585–97.

22. ECOG Performance Status. 2010. http://ecog.dfci.harvard.edu/general/perf_stat.html.

23. Bruera E, Kuehn N, Miller MJ, Selmser P, Macmillan K. The Edmonton Symptom Assessment System (ESAS): a simple method for the assessment of palliative care patients. J Palliat Care. 1991;7:6–9.

24. Eypasch E, Williams JI, Wood-Dauphinee S, Ure BM, Schmulling C, Neugebauer E, et al. Gastrointestinal quality of life index: development, validation and application of a new instrument. Br J Surg. 1995;82:216–22.

25. Aaronson NK, Ahmedzai S, Bergman B, Bullinger M, Cull A, Duez NJ, et al. The European organization for research and treatment of cancer QLQ-C30: a quality-of-life instrument for use in international clinical trials in oncology. J Natl Cancer Inst. 1993;85:365–76.

26. Haley SM, McHorney CA, Ware Jr JE. Evaluation of the MOS SF-36 physical functioning scale (PF-10): I. Unidimensionality and reproducibility of the Rasch item scale. J Clin Epidemiol. 1994;47:671–84.

27. Bradley CT, Brasel KJ. Core competencies in palliative care for surgeons: interpersonal and communication skills. Am J Hosp Palliat Care. 2007;24:499–507.

28. Briggs LA, Kirchhoff KT, Hammes BJ, Song MK, Colvin ER. Patient-centered advance care planning in special patient populations: a pilot study. J Prof Nurs. 2004;20:47–58.

29. Maguire P. Breaking bad news. Eur J Surg Oncol. 1998;24:188–91.

30. Hebert PC, Levin AV, Robertson G. Bioethics for clinicians: 23. Disclosure of medical error. CMAJ. 2001;164:509–13.

31. Gallagher TH, Waterman AD, Ebers AG, Fraser VJ, Levinson W. Patients' and physicians' attitudes regarding the disclosure of medical errors. JAMA. 2003;289:1001–7.

32. Van Cutsem E, Verslype C, Demedts I. The treatment of advanced colorectal cancer: where are we now and where do we go? Best Pract Res Clin Gastroenterol. 2002;16:319–30.

33. Sigurdsson HK, Kørner H, Dahl O, Skarstein A, Søreide JA. Clinical characteristics and outcomes in patients with advanced rectal cancer: a national prospective cohort study. Dis Colon Rectum. 2007;50:285–91.

34. Cook AD, Single R, McCahill LE. Surgical resection of primary tumors in patients who present with stage IV colorectal cancer: an analysis of surveillance, epidemiology, and end results data, 1988 to 2000. Ann Surg Oncol. 2005;12:637–45.

35. Temple LK, Hsieh L, Wong WD, Saltz L, Schrag D. Use of surgery among elderly patients with stage IV colorectal cancer. J Clin Oncol. 2004;22:3475–84.

36. de Gramont A, Figer A, Seymour M, Homerin M, Hmissi A, Cassidy J, et al. Leucovorin and fluorouracil with or without oxaliplatin as first-line treatment in advanced colorectal cancer. J Clin Oncol. 2000;18:2938–47.

37. Douillard JY, Cunningham D, Roth AD, Navarro M, James RD, Karasek P, et al. Irinotecan combined with fluorouracil compared with fluorouracil alone as first-line treatment for metastatic colorectal cancer: a multicentre randomised trial. Lancet. 2000;355:1041–7.

38. Kørner H, Nielsen HJ, Søreide JA, Nedrebø BS, Søreide K, Knapp JC. Diagnostic accuracy of C-reactive protein for intraabdominal infections after colorectal resections. J Gastrointest Surg. 2009;13:1599–606.

39. Eisenberger A, Whelan RL, Neugut AI. Survival and symptomatic benefit from palliative primary tumor resection in patients with metastatic colorectal cancer: a review. Int J Colorectal Dis. 2008;23:559–68.

40. Muratore A, Zorzi D, Bouzari H, Amisano M, Massucco P, Sperti E, et al. Asymptomatic colorectal cancer with un-resectable liver metastases: immediate colorectal resection or up-front systemic chemotherapy? Ann Surg Oncol. 2007;14:766–70.

41. Ruo L, Gougoutas C, Paty PB, Guillem JG, Cohen AM, Wong WD. Elective bowel resection for incurable stage IV colorectal cancer: prognostic variables for asymptomatic patients. J Am Coll Surg. 2003;196:722–8.

42. Benoist S, Pautrat K, Mitry E, Rougier P, Penna C, Nordlinger B. Treatment strategy for patients with colorectal cancer and synchronous irresectable liver metastases. Br J Surg. 2005;92:1155–60.

43. Sebastian S, Johnston S, Geoghegan T, Torreggiani W, Buckley M. Pooled analysis of the efficacy and safety of self-expanding metal stenting in malignant colorectal obstruction. Am J Gastroenterol. 2004;99:2051–7.

44. Sigurdsson HK, Kørner H, Dahl O, Skarstein A, Søreide JA. Palliative surgery for rectal cancer in a national cohort. Colorectal Dis. 2008;10:336–43.

45. Hodel J, Zins M, Desmottes L, Boulay-Coletta I, Julles MC, Nakache JP, et al. Location of the transi-

tion zone in CT of small-bowel obstruction: added value of multiplanar reformations. Abdom Imaging. 2009;34:35–41.

46. Ripamonti CI, Easson AM, Gerdes H. Management of malignant bowel obstruction. Eur J Cancer. 2008;44:1105–15.

47. Finan PJ, Campbell S, Verma R, MacFie J, Gatt M, Parker MC, et al. The management of malignant large bowel obstruction: ACPGBI position statement. Colorectal Dis. 2007;9 Suppl 4:1–17.

48. Pothuri B, Montemarano M, Gerardi M, Shike M, Ben-Porat L, Sabbatini P, et al. Percutaneous endoscopic gastrostomy tube placement in patients with malignant bowel obstruction due to ovarian carcinoma. Gynecol Oncol. 2005;96:330–4.

49. Ripamonti CI. Malignant bowel obstruction: tailoring treatment to individual patients. J Support Oncol. 2008;6:114–5.

50. Ripamonti C, Panzeri C, Groff L, Galeazzi G, Boffi R. The role of somatostatin and octreotide in bowel obstruction: pre-clinical and clinical results. Tumori. 2001;87:1–9.

51. Krouse RS, McCahill LE, Easson AM, Dunn GP. When the sun can set on an unoperated bowel obstruction: management of malignant bowel obstruction. J Am Coll Surg. 2002;195:117–28.

Nausea

26

Rune Svensen

Abstract

Nausea and vomiting represent major challenges in the management of the patient with advanced cancer. An understanding of possible underlying causes as well as basic knowledge of the various receptors most commonly involved will prove useful in tailoring an effective symptomatic treatment of the individual patient. After having identified and corrected any underlying cause, a systematic use of the available antiemetics should be tried while at the same time paying attention to the environment surrounding the patient, removing as many of the emetic stimuli as possible.

Nausea is a frequent problem in palliative care, occurring in 20–30 % overall, with an increasing tendency in the terminal phase, when approximately 70 % will be affected. It is quite frequently highly distressing to the patient and at times notoriously difficult to treat. Nausea is a complex phenomenon. A number of different organs are involved, and the symptom is mediated through a large number of receptors, many of which are most likely yet to be identified [1, 2].

Nausea may be considered a central nervous problem more than a visceral one. Several key locations exist:

- The vomiting centre in the brainstem with its chemoreceptors.
- The chemoreceptor trigger zone. Interestingly this is located in an area of the brain not protected by the blood-brain barrier, thus enabling circulating chemical substances to affect the brain directly.
- The medullary area postrema and the solitary tract receiving signals from both chemo- and mechanoreceptors from distant organs, including the GI tract.
- Cerebral cortex, reacting to conscious stimuli such as anxiety, taste, smell and visual impulses.
- Meninges with its mechanoreceptors reacting to pressure changes and stretching.
- The inner ear with the vestibular system reacting to motion.
- Gastrointestinal tract with mechano- and chemoreceptors on both mucosal and serosal surfaces.

R. Svensen
Department of Gastroenterological
and Acute Surgery, Haukeland University Hospital,
NO-5021 Bergen, Norway
e-mail: rune.svensen@helse-bergen.no

G. Baatrup (ed.), *Multidisciplinary Treatment of Colorectal Cancer*,
DOI 10.1007/978-3-319-06142-9_26, © Springer International Publishing Switzerland 2015

Chemoreceptors Simplified [3]

A number of chemoreceptors involved in nausea and vomiting have been identified. Furthermore, several drugs have become available to address some of these receptors, making them useful tools in the treatment of the nauseous patient. However, the complexity of the problem and the multitude of potential culprits make the choice of the ideal drug a challenge for the physician.

- The serotonin (5-hydroxytryptamine, 5-HT) receptors in the chemoreceptor trigger zone and GI tract:
  - 5-HT$_2$
  - 5 HT$_3$
  - 5-HT$_4$
- Dopamine (D$_2$) receptors in the area postrema, solitary tract, chemoreceptor trigger zone and GI tract
- Muscarinic acetylcholine receptors in the vomiting centre and the vestibular system
- Gamma-aminobutyric acid (GABA) receptors in the cerebral cortex
- Histamine receptors in the vomiting centre

Approaching the Problem

When faced with a nauseous cancer patient, the physician will find himself far less aided by well-founded therapeutic algorithms than if the patient complained of pain. There is, for example, no parallel to the WHO pain ladder for nausea. Instead the handling of the patient will depend on the physician's ability to analyze and understand the patient's total situation, utilize knowledge of basic nausea physiopathology and act accordingly. Although the problem of nausea in the cancer patient is a challenge, a systematic approach will in most cases enable us to solve the problem, at least alleviate it.

Identify and Treat Underlying Cause, if Possible

Biochemical Disorders

1. Hypercalcaemia is not uncommon in advanced cancer cases and may be caused by the release of parathyroid hormone-related peptides (PTHrP) or through the release of calcium from skeletal metastases. Hypercalcaemia produces a nausea which is notoriously resistant to antiemetics and should be treated by reducing the levels of serum ionized calcium, for example, by rehydration, diuretics and bisphosphonates.
2. Uraemia.
3. Ketoacidosis.
4. Infection.
5. Tumour toxins.
6. Dehydration, for example, caused by fistulas and high output stomas or reduced intake.
7. Adverse drug reactions. Be especially aware of opioids, NSAIDs, digitalis and antibiotics. In cases with liver or renal deficiency, drug metabolism may be altered, and the patient might develop adverse effects even when the drug has been taken for a long period of time.
8. Treatment related (irradiation, chemotherapy, immunotherapy, hormone therapy).
9. Effects of cachexia and anorexia, which are mostly cytokine mediated [4].

Gastrointestinal Disorders and Disturbances

1. Poor oral hygiene, oral ulcerations, fungal infection or altered taste
2. Constipation, for example, caused by opioids
3. Autonomic dysfunction causing dysphagia, delayed gastric emptying and intestinal pseudo-obstruction, for example, caused by peritoneal, retroperitoneal or mesenteric metastases
4. Gastric or duodenal ulcers and gastritis
5. Mechanical bowel obstruction
6. Large intra-abdominal masses, enlarged liver and ascites

Central Nervous Disorders

1. Increased intracranial pressure, due to tumour or oedema
2. Vestibular disturbances, nausea triggered by motion
3. Meningeal distortion due to metastases or primary tumour

Conditioned Nausea

Conditioned nausea is nausea triggered by conscious sensory stimuli and mediated through receptors in the cerebral cortex. It is often underestimated as a major culprit:

1. Anxiety and despair
2. Detrimental environment around the patient with unwanted stimuli such as smell, noise, unrest, disturbing visual stimuli, bad associations, etc.
3. Nausea caused by other (untreated) symptoms such as pain, paralysis, cough, dyspnoea, hiccups, etc.

Symptomatic Management [5]

After the initial assessment of the patient, including the identification and correction of any treatable underlying cause, it is time to consider symptomatic treatment. First, however, it is important to create an environment for the patient which is not in itself an emetic. The management requires a multidisciplinary approach with good communication between its members and with the patient and the family. Concerns around meals, i.e. composition, taste, amount, presentation and fluid intake, should be addressed. The environment around the patient should be carefully assessed and modified to reduce all emetic stimuli to a minimum. Oral hygiene, especially in patients unable to drink, is particularly important.

Antiemetics

The route of administration is very important when treating nausea. To administer drugs orally to a patient suffering from heavy nausea and/or repeated vomiting will at best be a futile undertaking. The drugs should therefore initially be administered parenterally, and the conversion to oral administration should await the cessation of nausea, when the antiemetics serve a more prophylactic purpose.

The number of drugs available in most countries is substantial, and most are well documented. However, the documentation of their use in a palliative setting is far less impressive. For example, a large number of drugs have well-documented effects on chemotherapy-induced nausea and are officially approved for such use, whereas they are not approved as antiemetics in advanced cancer. The lack of an analogue to the WHO pain ladder for the treatment of nausea contributes to the confusion concerning the large number of antiemetics available. It is therefore appropriate to divide the antiemetics into groups according to the receptor involved.

Broad Spectre Antiemetic

Levomepromazine blocks $5-HT_2$-, histamine, dopamine and muscarine cholinergic receptors and is possibly the most broad-spectred antiemetic available. However, there are serious dose-dependent side effects, such as sedation, orthostatic hypotension and dryness in the mouth. The doses should probably not exceed 10–12.5 mg orally (2.5–5 mg subcutaneously), and it should be administered at bedtime.

Dopamine Blockers

Haloperidol is often the first choice in nausea caused by metabolic disturbances, including opioid-induced, uremic and hypercalcaemic nausea. The doses should not exceed 5–8 mg a day due to extrapyramidal adverse effects.

Metoclopramide is a combined prokinetic and dopamine receptor blocker. It may be advantageous in cases when there is delayed gastric emptying or autonomous dysfunction causing prolonged intestinal transit time. It should not be used in cases where there is a mechanical obstruction. The doses can be as high as 80–100 mg a day, or even higher, administered both orally and parenterally.

Domperidone is similar to metoclopramide with both antidopaminergic and prokinetic properties. It does however not cross the blood-brain barrier.

Levomepromazine, discussed under "Broad Spectre Antiemetic".

5-HT₃ Blockers

Ondansetron, granisetron, dolasetron, tropisetron and palonosetron are drugs primarily licenced to treat nausea caused by emetogenic chemotherapy. They may however prove valuable in some cases in palliative care.

Histamine Blockers

Cyclizine blocks histamine receptors in the vestibular system and the vomiting centre and is the first choice in the treatment of motion-induced nausea and in cases with meningeal distortion, in the latter case in combination with dexamethasone. It can be administered both orally and parenterally.

Cinnarizine is an alternative second-line choice.

Ranitidine, see under Antisecretory Drugs.

Muscarinic Cholinergic Blocker

Scopolamine (hyoscine hydrobromide) blocks the muscarinic cholinergic receptor in the vomiting centre and can be used for treating nausea caused by motion, similarly to the histamine blockers. It has the advantage that it can be administered transcutaneously as a patch.

GABA Blockers

Benzodiazepines may be used for treating conditioned and anxiety-induced nausea. However, anxiety should when possible be treated non-pharmacologically with reassurance, good communication and simple explanation of situations as they arise. This may require the involvement of the multidisciplinary team, including non-health professionals, such as members of the clergy, family and friends. Diazepam is strongly sedative and has a long half-life, making it a less than desirable choice for many patients with advanced cancer. In selected cases, however, the benzodiazepines may be useful.

Drugs Without Specific "Nausea" Receptor or Receptor Undefined

Dexamethasone is the first choice in cases with increased intracranial pressure, and distortion of the meninges after irradiation has been considered. An appropriate starting dose is 16 mg daily, with a gradual reduction to 2–4 mg daily reducing every 4–5 days.

Ginger or Zingiber officinale is a herb with well-documented antiemetic properties. There is however insufficient documentation for its use in palliative care. There are few side effects or drug interactions, although care should be taken if administered to patients using anticoagulants [6].

Cannabinoids (nabilone and dronabinol) are experimental drugs used to treat cancer cachexia in some countries. In addition they have antiemetic properties and are occasionally being used for chemotherapy-induced nausea. The side effects are however limiting their use (drowsiness, dizziness) [7].

Antisecretory Drugs

Proton pump inhibitors (omeprazole, lansoprazole, dexlansoprazole, esomeprazole, pantoprazole, rabeprazole) reduce gastric secretions and render it less acidic. This may be advantageous in some patients.

Ranitidine is a selective histamine 2 (H_2) blocker with a different mode of action from the other antihistamines. It is an antisecretory drug with properties comparable to the proton pump inhibitors. It reduces acid output by blocking the H_2 receptors in the parietal cells of the stomach.

Octreotide is a powerful antisecretory drug which may be used when there is mechanical obstruction of the bowel and the patient is not a candidate for surgical intervention. The doses will vary between 100 and 400 μg daily. There is a long-acting version available (LAR) where a single intramuscular injection of 10–30 mg is effective for up to 4 weeks.

Scopolamine, discussed under *"Muscarinic Cholinergic Blocker"*.

Sedation

Propolipid (propofol) may occasionally be considered in cases unresponsive to all other drugs and procedures. Propolipid is an ultrashort-acting anaesthetic with a narrow therapeutic window. It is for use in expert (anaesthesiological) hands only.

Invasive Procedures

Nasogastric tube is a useful technique for emptying a full stomach in cases of gastroparesis or bowel obstruction. It is however uncomfortable and carries a significant risk of aspiration pneumonia and should be used for short periods of time only (e.g. in preparation for surgery). If the patient requires a long-term gastric drainage, a venting gastrostomy is considered a better option [8].

Surgery. In some cases, surgery will have to be considered to re-establish a broken continuity through the GI tract. The considerations however are many and serious, and they are discussed elsewhere. Minimally or non-invasive procedures such as stenting of obstructed lower or upper GI tract will remain an option, even in those cases not eligible for major surgery.

A Proposed Algorithm for the Treatment of Nausea

1. Identify and treat the underlying cause, if possible.
2. Create an "antiemetic environment" for the patient using a multidisciplinary approach.
3. Try to identify the most probable receptor involved and choose the first antiemetic accordingly:

   (a) The first choice will often be haloperidol, levomepromazine or metoclopramide.
4. Increase the dosage until either desired effect or intolerable side effects:

   (a) If there is no response to treatment, discontinue the drug and choose an antiemetic from another receptor group. For example, substitute haloperidol (antidopaminergic) with ondansetron (anti-5-HT4) or cyclizine (antihistamine).

   (b) If there is partial response to treatment, add an antiemetic from another group.
5. Avoid polypharmacy using a multitude of different antiemetics.
6. Do not hesitate to involve other specialists, such as anaesthesiologists, specialists in palliative care, endocrinologists, surgeons, gastroenterologists, etc.

References

1. Grond S, Zech D, Diefenbach C, et al. Prevalence and pattern of symptoms in patients with cancer pain; a prospective evaluation of 1635 cancer patients referred to a pain clinic. J Pain Symptom Manage. 1994;9(6):372–82.
2. Mannix KA. Palliation of nausea and vomiting. In: Doyle D, Hanks G, Cherny N, Calman K, editors. Oxford textbook of palliative medicine. 3rd ed. Oxford/New York: Oxford University Press; 2005. p. 459–68.
3. Baines MJ. ABC of palliative care. Nausea, vomiting and intestinal obstruction. BMJ. 1997;315(7116): 1148–50.
4. Bruera E, Higginson E. Cachexia-anorexia in cancer patients. Oxford/New York: Oxford University Press; 1996.
5. Knott L. Nausea and vomiting in palliative care. UK: EMIS PatientPlus; 2009.
6. Ernst E, Pittler MH. Efficacy of ginger for nausea and vomiting: a systematic review of randomized clinical trials. Br J Anaesth. 2000;84(3):367–71.
7. Tramèr MR, Carroll D, Campbell FA, Reynolds DJM, Moore AR, McQuay HJ. Cannabinoids for control of chemotherapy induced nausea and vomiting: quantitative systematic review. BMJ. 2001;323:16–21.
8. Regnard C. Dysphagia, dyspepsia and hiccups. In: Doyle D, Hanks G, Cherny N, Calman K, editors. Oxford textbook of palliative medicine. 3rd ed. Oxford/New York: Oxford University Press; 2005. p. 473.

Part VII

Recommendations

Individualised Treatment

27

Patient-Related Factors: Patients' Preference

Birger Henning Endreseth

Abstract

As a fundamental part of the multidisciplinary treatment in colorectal cancer, treatment guidelines and decision making on treatment strategy in multidisciplinary teams have evolved. The selection of treatment strategy is primarily based on an accurate staging of the disease by means of achieving a precise cTNM stage prior to treatment. In order to be able to decide on treatment strategy in a specific patient, awareness of the impact of patient-related factors, most importantly comorbidity and physiological age, is essential. The POSSUM score, an objective model for risk prediction in surgery, and the concept of comprehensive geriatric assessment, a multidimensional assessment tool for evaluation of elderly patients, can be of help in this process. Based on this evaluation and on the patient's preference, an optimal, individualised treatment strategy for the specific patient can be achieved.

Introduction

Over the last decades, there have been an increasing number of optional treatment modalities in colorectal cancer (CRC). Traditionally, treatment of localised CRC has been major surgery with resection of the primary tumour and regional lymph nodes; lately there has been a shift from open to laparoscopic procedures [1]. Although the recommendations on oncological treatment diverge, adjuvant chemotherapy is used in selected cases, mainly in stage III colonic cancer [2], and preoperative chemoradiation is established as standard treatment in locally advanced rectal cancer [3].

There has been a considerable focus on early CRC cancer, and local treatment options, including TEM for rectal cancer and more recently submucosal endoscopic excision for colonic cancer, have been introduced [4, 5].

Furthermore, the treatment of patients with metastatic disease has undergone major advances including combinations of surgical and oncological treatment. Major surgical procedures including resections of liver, lung and peritoneum are established as a part of the optional curative treatment with acceptable postoperative morbidity and mortality rates [6]. Oncological treatment

B.H. Endreseth, MD, PhD
Department of Surgery, St. Olavs University Hospital,
Trondheim N-7006, Norway
e-mail: birger.henning.endreseth@stolav.no

with combinations of cytotoxic chemotherapy and biologic agents has improved the survival in patients with disseminated metastatic disease [7].

As a fundamental part of the multimodal treatment strategy in CRC, decision making on treatment in multidisciplinary teams has evolved. The basis for the selection of treatment strategy is an adequate staging of the disease by means of achieving a precise cTNM stage [8]. New scientific evidence is continuously implemented in national guidelines regarding the treatment of CRC patients [9]. Although specific in terms of treatment strategy in different stages of the disease, these guidelines do not differentiate between the CRC patients on an individual level.

In order to be able to decide on treatment strategy in a specific patient, knowledge of the alternative treatment options, their expected results and complications has to be evaluated in context of the patient. Awareness of the impact of patient-related factors on the treatment, most importantly comorbidity and age, is necessary in this clinical decision making. Based on this evaluation, the selected treatment strategy may deviate from the treatment guidelines, considered to be the optimal, individualised treatment in the specific case. Finally the clinician's recommendation on strategy has to be adequately presented and discussed with the patient before it is initiated.

Patient-Related Factors

Risk Prediction in CRC Surgery

Assessment of the potential risks of perioperative morbidity and mortality is important in the process of deciding on surgical treatment strategy. Traditionally this has been done by the surgeon and the anaesthesiologist, primarily based on clinical experience. Although the final decision on strategy always will have to be based on this subjective clinical evaluation, more objective models for prediction of risk could come useful in this process. Furthermore, objective preoperative information on potential risks of the treatment is essential as a part of the process of informed consent on the selected procedure.

In the context of performance evaluation of different hospital units, a comparison of crude in-hospital or 30-day mortality can be misleading due to case mix. In order to compensate for the variation in physiological condition of the patient and the severity of surgery, different risk scoring models were developed. Subsequently these multivariable regression models have proved useful in risk prediction. The number of included variables differs between the scoring systems, as does the availability of these variables and thus the possibility for effective utilisation in the clinical setting. Furthermore, the assessment of the models occurs at different points throughout the course of hospitalisation, typically in the pre-, peri- and postoperative phase. The first models introduced were devised to predict the outcome among patients undergoing surgery in general but gradually more diagnosis-related and diagnosis-specific models have been developed.

Initially meant as a tool for anaesthesiologists to improve communication and compare results of anaesthesia, the ASA classification of physical status was introduced already in 1941 [10]. Over the years this classification proved to correlate well with overall surgical mortality and developed to become an estimate of operative risk. Although vague and subjective, with a wide interobserver variability, this classification still is an important predictor of outcome after surgery in many hospitals and thus as a tool for preoperative selection among CRC patients.

At present the most widely accepted risk prediction score in gastrointestinal surgery is the POSSUM score, a Physiological and Operative Severity Score for the enUmeration of Mortality and morbidity, described by Copeland in 1991 [11]. This is a dual scoring system including assessment of both mortality and morbidity and was designed to be used in general surgery, both in the elective and emergency setting. The system consists of a 12-factor, four-grade, physiological score, in combination with a six-factor, four-grade, surgical operative severity score. Further evaluation of the POSSUM score revealed a tendency to over prediction of mortality, especially among low-risk patients, and a modification of the score, the Portsmouth POSSUM, p-POSSUM, was presented in 1998 [12]. The two systems use the same physiological and operative severity scores but different regression equations. The model for predicting morbidity is identical in the two systems. Due to limitations of applying POSSUM scoring in the oldest patients undergoing colorectal surgery, a speciality-specific model based on the POSSUM methodology have been developed, the colorectal POSSUM (CR-POSSUM) [13, 14]. In this system for prediction of mortality, the number of variables included both in the physiological and operative severity score have been reduced [15].

External validation of this model in the UK has proved it to be more accurate than the previous POSSUM models in risk prediction among CRC patients [16]. Evaluation of the applicability of all three POSSUM scores in the US has concluded with overprediction of mortality for colon cancer resections. This indicates the need for calibration when the score is applied on other health-care systems, outside the UK [17].

In general, as the different models are based on cohorts of patients from different hospitals and even from different health-care systems, an evaluation of the predictive value of the model is necessary regarding applicability in a specific hospital. Furthermore, as the quality of treatment improves and the rates of complications and mortality decrease, there has to be a continuous updating of these models in order to maintain an adequate prediction [18].

The Impact of High Age on Treatment in CRC Patients

CRC is a disease mainly affecting the elderly. In the Western world, approximately 60 % of the patients are more than 70 years at diagnosis, and, as a result of an increasing life expectancy, the incidence of CRC in older patients will continue to rise [19].

Thus, the management of elderly CRC patients represents a considerable challenge for the health-care system in the future.

The literature, primarily based on selected cohorts of elderly patients, most often supports

that surgical treatment is feasible irrespective of chronological age. In large national observational cohort series, age appears to influence on the rate of resection, both in terms of overall and curative resection rate, and on the choice of surgical procedure [20, 21].

In stage III colon cancer, adjuvant chemotherapy has been demonstrated to reduce the risk of disease recurrence and to improve survival, but the likelihood to receive chemotherapy decreases with age [22]. The same trend is seen in the use of palliative chemotherapy among older CRC patients. Furthermore, radiotherapy seems to be underutilised in the treatment of rectal cancer in the elderly [23]. To avoid a potential substandard treatment of the elderly CRC patient, knowledge regarding results of treatment in the elderly population and individual evaluation of patients in this heterogenic group is imperative.

Several series evaluating the results of elective curative major surgery in elderly CRC patients present rates of local recurrence, metastases and cancer-specific and relative survival comparable to those in younger patient cohorts [20, 22–24]. The rate of postoperative mortality and morbidity increases with age in most of these series, with a mortality of 8 % among the oldest rectal cancer patients undergoing curative major surgery [20]. The rates of postoperative morbidity range between 30 and 60 % in different series [24–26]. This illustrates the challenges of selection in older patients planned for elective CRC surgery.

During the last years, laparoscopic colorectal resection for cancer has emerged as a minimally invasive alternative. Series comparing elderly CRC patients undergoing open or laparoscopic resection have revealed a significant decrease in postoperative morbidity among those undergoing laparoscopic resection [22, 26, 27].

Furthermore, hepatic and pulmonary resections have become safer and 5-year survival rates of up to more than 50 % in selected patients have been reported [28, 29]. Major liver resections can be safely performed in elderly patients, with similar short- and long-term outcome as in their younger counterparts [28]. Although age is a prognostic factor in multivariable analysis on survival after pulmonary resection of CRC metastases, several of the presented series include elderly patients, indicating that high chronological age is not a contraindication for resection [29]. Hepatic and pulmonary resections of colorectal metastasis are feasible in selected older patients.

The rate of patients undergoing emergency surgery for CRC increases with age [21–23, 30]. Furthermore, the rate of curative resections decreases in the emergency setting and the rate of postoperative mortality increases significantly, reaching 35 % in patients aged over 80 years [30]. Colonic stenting has proved to be a safe and effective procedure and should be considered essential as a bridge to surgery or a palliative procedure in emergency treatment of CRC in elderly patients [22, 31].

Elderly rectal cancer patients treated with major rectal resection more often undergo procedures resulting in a permanent stoma than younger patients [20]. This is probably due to an assumption of increased rate of anastomotic leak and poor functional results after an anterior resection. In the literature the rate of anastomotic leak does not seem to increase with age, and although some investigators have found that increasing age has an adverse effect on postoperative functional outcome, most series find no differences between the age groups.

Moreover, the majority of elderly patients are satisfied with their functional outcome after surgery with a primary anastomosis [23, 32]. Thus, age per se does not seem to be a contraindication for primary anastomosis in major rectal resection.

The use of oncological treatment in terms of adjuvant chemotherapy in colon cancer, neoadjuvant chemoradiation in rectal cancer and in palliative treatment of metastatic disease decreases with age [20–22]. Elderly patients are usually underrepresented in clinical trials evaluating oncological treatment, and thus the information regarding the benefits and tolerability of the different treatment options among older CRC patients is limited.

As adjuvant chemotherapy in stage III colonic cancer among older patients, 5-FU-based regimens improve survival to the same extent as in younger patients. Infusional 5-FU seems to have a favourable toxicity profile compared to bolus 5-FU, and infusional 5-FU in combination with leucovorin is recommended as the treatment of choice [22]. Oral capecitabine, although proved to be as effective as 5-FU, has an increased toxicity related to renal function in older patients, while there is limited information regarding the use of the combination of oxaliplatin, 5-FU and LV (FOLFOX) in adjuvant treatment among older patients.

Oncological treatment of metastatic disease in elderly patients depends on the goal of treatment. In curative intent, a more aggressive treatment should be considered. Infusional 5-FU has the best toxic profile; the combination of 5-FU, LV and irinotecan (FOLFIRI) or oxaliplatin (FOLFOX) has similar efficacy as in younger patients and should be the standard treatment option in fit elderly patients [22, 33]. Among the biologic agents, such as vascular endothelial growth factor (VEGF) and epidermal growth factor receptor (EGFR) inhibitors, only bevacizumab has been evaluated in elderly patients. The benefit of treatment is the same as observed in younger patients, but there is an increased risk of thromboembolism in the elderly, and it should only be considered to be used in patients without cardiovascular disease [24].

Over time there have been a substantial evolvement of external radiotherapy (RT) techniques. Based on individual three-dimensional imaging reconstruction of target volume and adjacent organs, high doses can be delivered to tumour target volume with a reduced damage of normal tissue, increasing the tolerance of RT, also in elderly patients [34].

Statements on increased toxicity among elderly patients are mainly based on series presenting results after previously used RT techniques. At present it is advocated that there should be no upper age limit when including otherwise eligible patients into trails for RT treatment. Evaluation of elderly patients for RT should be done on individual basis, not according to chronological age.

Although the definitions of elderly patients diverge, the literature essentially supports similar treatment among all age categories of CRC patients. As age-related changes differ between individuals, the challenge is an adequate selection based on these individual characteristics. A major objective of cancer treatment in older patients is, in addition to survival, to prolong the patient's active life expectancy. Rather than chronological age, the concept of physiological age should be evaluated before deciding on treatment. The best estimate of a person's physiological age is achieved through a comprehensive geriatric assessment (CGA) [22, 26, 35].

In geriatric oncology, the CGA, a multidimensional assessment tool, is suggested to be used in evaluation of patients before treatment. The CGA consists of several commonly used geriatric assessment tools, evaluating comorbidity, functional status, medication use, nutrition, cognition, emotional status and social support in elderly patients. The collected information from these tests is analysed by a geriatrician, and based on this the patients can be categorised into fit, intermediate or frail. Frailty is known as a physiological state that may lead to disability, i.e. loss of a function necessary for independence, following minimal stress, indicating a decline in the functional reserve of multiple organ systems [36]. The result from the CGA is discussed by a multidisciplinary team in order to design and develop an individualised intervention plan.

The prevalence of frailty is estimated to be 10–25 % in persons aged 65 years or older [35], and in general it is recommended that patients aged 70 years or older undergo a geriatric assessment prior to treatment. As the process of CGA is considered time consuming in clinical practice, a two step procedure has been proposed [37]. The first part consists of a screening of all geriatric patients. Fit patients should receive the same oncological treatment as younger patients. Those defined as frail should undergo a complete CGA. Based on the results from the CGA, these frail patients should then receive intervention in an effort to solve the biological, clinical, or social issues limiting the applicability of standard oncological guidelines or achieve tailored treatment according to their frailty and life expectancy.

Although several trails have proved that geriatric intervention based on the concept of CGA have positive effects on different health outcomes, only a few studies have demonstrated the impact of this approach on oncological treatment in elderly patients [35, 37]. In one series CGA was described to lead to a modification of the initial treatment plan, but whether these modifications resulted in improved outcome was not evaluated [38]. In a recently published series on elderly patients undergoing elective surgery for CRC, stratification of the patients according to CGA proved to be a significant predictor of postoperative morbidity [26]. In this study neither chronological age nor ASA classification predicted postoperative complications, indicating that the concept of CGA could be of value when deciding on surgical treatment.

Patients' Preference

The decision making on treatment is primarily based on the physician's clinical evaluation prior to treatment. In this evaluation the tumour stage, the patient's comorbidity and age usually are the most important determinants of how to treat the patient. It is generally approved that the patient have the right to, and in most cases should, participate actively in decisions on their own treatment. In order to participate in this process, it is essential that the patient receives adequate information regarding the disease and the available treatment. Several series have documented that most cancer patients prefer to be involved in these decisions affecting their treatment [39].

The patient's preference is based on information regarding treatment efficacy, quality of life and proximity to end of life [40]. In most cases, the patient's decision is a trade-off between survival and quality of life. Age and previous experiences with treatment have an impact on the patient preference. The patient's social situation, having a partner or children, influence on the chosen treatment strategy, with an increased willingness to trade quality of life for a survival advantage among those living with children at home.

Among patients undergoing surgery the patient's trust in the surgeon, the surgeon's expertise and communication skills are important variables influencing on the patients preference. Furthermore, series specifically evaluating treatment of CRC have demonstrated that the avoidance of a permanent stoma was important for the patient; more than half of the patients would give up one third of their life expectancy to avoid such a surgical procedure [41].

In cases where the disease progress and the patient approach the end of life, there is an increased acceptance to higher treatment-related risk. This is typically seen in phase I trials, evaluating toxicity and appropriate dosing of experimental therapy, with a minor probability of objective benefit of treatment among the patients included. Although the patients are informed about the intent of the study, patients participate with great expectations of therapeutic benefit [39].

The process of treatment decision is complex and there is often a mismatch in treatment preferences and assumed prognosis between the physician and the patient. In the optimal process of shared decision making, these differences should merge into a mutually agreed-upon treatment plan before starting the treatment. As the disease progresses, the preferences might change both for the patient and the physician, and there should be a continuous evaluation of the individualised treatment plan.

Conclusion

The evolvement of multidisciplinary treatment in CRC has improved the results. Through individualised treatment based on adequate risk prediction before surgery and assessment of comorbidity and of the patient's preferences, an optimal treatment strategy for the specific patient can be achieved.

References

1. Reza MM, Blasco JA, Andradas E, Cantero R, Mayol J. Systematic review of laparoscopic versus open surgery for colorectal cancer. Br J Surg. 2006;93:921–8.
2. Cunningham D, Atkin W, Lenz HJ, Lynch HT, Minsky B, Nordlinger B, et al. Colorectal cancer. Lancet. 2010;375:1030–47.
3. Eriksen MT, Wibe A, Hestvik UE, Haffner J, Wiig JN. Surgical treatment of primary locally advanced rectal cancer in Norway. Eur J Surg Oncol. 2006;32: 174–80.
4. Baatrup G, Endreseth BH, Isaksen V, Kjellmo Å, Tveit KM, Nesbakken A. Preoperative staging and treatment options in T1 rectal adenocarcinoma. Acta Oncol. 2009;48:328–42.
5. Cahill RA, Leroy J, Marescaux J. Localized resection of colon cancer. Surg Oncol. 2009;18:334–42.
6. Mahmoud N, Bullard DK. Metastasectomy for stage IV colorectal cancer. Dis Colon Rectum. 2010;53: 1080–92.
7. Goldberg RM, Rothenberg ML, Van Cutsem E, Benson III AB, Blanke CD, Diasio RB, et al. The continuum of care: a paradigm for the management of metastatic colorectal cancer. Oncologist. 2007;12: 38–50.
8. UICC. TNM classification of malignant tumours. 5th ed. New York: Wiley; 1997.
9. Nasjonalt handlingsprogram med retningslinjer for diagnostikk, behandling og oppfølging av kreft i tykk og endetarm. http://ngicg.no/handlingsprogram/nasjonale_handlingsprogrammer/content_1/filelist_ee59ae57-c583-41bb-8e91-ac712e639640/1395777852047/nasjonalt_handlingsprogram_for_tykk_og_endetarmskreft.pdf.
10. Keats AS. The ASA, classification of physical status – a recapitulation. Anesthesiology. 1978;49:233–6.
11. Copeland GP, Jones D, Walters M. POSSUM: a scoring system for surgical audit. Br J Surg. 1991;78:356–60.
12. Prytherch DR, Whiteley MS, Higgins B, Weaver PC, Prout WG, Powell SJ. POSSUM and Portsmouth POSSUM for predicting mortality. Physiological and operative severity score for the enumeration of mortality and morbidity. Br J Surg. 1998;85:1217–20.
13. Tekkis PP, Kessaris N, Kocher HM, Poloniecki JD, Lyttle J, Windsor ACJ. Evaluation of POSSUM and P-POSSUM scoring systems in patients undergoing colorectal surgery. Br J Surg. 2003;90:340–5.
14. Tekkis PP, Prytherch DR, Kocher HM, Senapati A, Poloniecki JD, Stamatakis JD, et al. Development of a dedicated risk-adjustment scoring system for colorectal surgery (colorectal POSSUM). Br J Surg. 2004;91: 1174–82.
15. Risk Prediction in Surgery. http://www.riskprediction.org.uk
16. Bromage SJ, Cunliffe WJ. Validation of the CR-POSSUM risk-adjusted scoring system for major colorectal cancer surgery in a single center. Dis Colon Rectum. 2007;50:192–6.
17. Senagore AJ, Warmuth AJ, Delaney CP, Tekkis PP, Fazio VW. POSSUM, p-POSSUM, and Cr-POSSUM: Implementation issues in a United States care system for prediction of outcome for colon cancer resection. Dis Colon Rectum. 2004;47:1435–41.
18. Chandra A, Mangam S, Marzouk D. A review of risk scoring systems utilised in patients undergoing gastrointestinal surgery. J Gastrointest Surg. 2009;13: 1529–38.

19. Cancer Registry of Norway. Cancer in Norway 2005; 2006.

20. Endreseth BH, Romundstad P, Myrvold HE, Bjerkeset T, Wibe A, Norwegian Rectal Cancer Group. Rectal cancer in the elderly. Colorectal Dis. 2006;8: 471–9.

21. Van Leeuwen BL, Påhlman L, Gunnarson U, Sjovall A, Martling A. The effect of age and gender on outcome after treatment for colon carcinoma. A population-based study in the Uppsala and Stockholm region. Crit Rev Oncol Hematol. 2008;67:229–36.

22. Pallis AG, Papamichael D, Audisio R, Peeters M, Folprecht G, Lacombe D, Van Cutsem E. EORTC elderly task force experts opinion for the treatment of colon cancer in older patients. Cancer Treat Rev. 2010;36:83–90.

23. Abir F, Alva S, Longo WE. The management of rectal cancer in the elderly. Surg Oncol. 2004;13:223–4.

24. Golfinopoulus V, Pentheroudakis G, Pavlidis N. Treatment of colorectal cancer in the elderly: a review of the literature. Cancer Treat Rev. 2006;32:1–8.

25. Ugolini G, Rosati G, Montroni I, Zanotti S, Manaresi A, Giampaolo L, et al. Can elderly patients with colorectal cancer tolerate planned surgical treatment? A practical approach to a common dilemma. Colorectal Dis. 2009;11:750–5.

26. Kristjansson SR, Nesbakken A, Jordhøy MS, Skovlund E, Audisio RA, Johannesen HO, et al. Comprehensive geriatric assessment can predict complications in elderly patients after elective surgery for colorectal cancer: a prospective observational cohort study. Crit Rev Oncol Hematol. 2009. doi:10.1016/j.critrevonc.2009.11.002.

27. Tei M, Ikeda M, Haraguchi N, Takemasa I, Mizushima T, Ishii H, et al. Postoperative complications in elderly patients with colorectal cancer. Comparison of open and laparoscopic surgical procedures. Surg Laparosc Endosc Percutan Tech. 2009;19:488–92.

28. Menon KV, Al-Mukhtar A, Aldouri A, Prasad RK, Lodge PA, Toogood GJ. Outcomes after major hepatectomy in elderly patients. J Am Coll Surg. 2006;203:677–83.

29. Pfannschmidt J, Dienemann H, Hoffmann H. Surgical resection of pulmonary metastases from colorectal cancer: a systematic review of published series. Ann Torac Surg. 2007;84:324–38.

30. Iversen LH, Bulow S, Christensen IJ, Laurberg S, Harling H. on behalf of the Danish Colorectal cancer Group. Postoperative medical complications are the main cause of early death after emergency surgery for colonic cancer. Br J Surg. 2008;95:1012–9.

31. Dionigi G, Villa F, Rovera F, Boni L, Carrafiello G, Annoni M, et al. Colonic stenting for malignant disease: review of the literature. Surg Oncol. 2007;16: S153–5.

32. Eriksen MT, Wibe A, Norstein J, Haffner J, Wiig JN. on behalf of the Norwegian Rectal Cancer Group. Anastomotic leakage following routine mesorectal excision for rectal cancer in a national cohort of patients. Colorectal Dis. 2005;7:51–7.

33. Sanoff HK, Bleiberg H, Goldberg RM. Managing older patients with colorectal cancer. J Clin Oncol. 2007;25:1930–5.

34. Horiot J-C. Radiation therapy and the geriatric oncology patient. J Clin Oncol. 2007;25:1891–7.

35. Balducci L, Colloca G, Cesari M, Gambassi G. Assessment and treatment of elderly patients with cancer. Surg Oncol. 2009. doi:10.1016/j.suronc.2009. 11.008.

36. Balducci L, Extermann M. Management of cancer in the older person: a practical approach. Oncologist. 2000;5:224–37.

37. Extermann M, Aapro M, Bernabei R, Cohen HJ, Droz JP, Lichtman S, et al. Use of comprehensive geriatric assessment in older cancer patients: recommendations from the task force on CGA of the International Society of Geriatric Oncology (SIOG). Crit Rev Oncol Hematol. 2005;55:241–52.

38. Girre V, Falcou MC, Gisselbrecht M, Gridel G, Mosseri V, Bouleuc C, et al. Does a geriatric oncology consultation modify the cancer treatment plan for elderly patients? J Gerontol A Biol Sci Med Sci. 2008;63:724–30.

39. Redmond K. Assessing patient's needs and preferences in the management of advanced colorectal cancer. Br J Cancer. 1998;77 Suppl 2:5–7.

40. Zafar SY, Alexander SC, Weinfurt KP, Schulman KA, Abernethy AP. Decision making and quality of life in the treatment of cancer: a review. Support Care Cancer. 2009;17:117–27.

41. Harrison JD, Solomon MJ, Young JM, Meagher A, Butow P, Salkeld G, et al. Patient and physician preferences for surgical and adjuvant treatment options for rectal cancer. Arch Surg. 2008;143: 389–94.

Local Treatment of Rectal Cancer

28

Niels Qvist

Abstract

Local treatment with transanal tumour excision has shown to be associated with significantly decreased morbidity and mortality compared to conventional surgery (laparoscopic or open). Local treatment should be considered in select patients with early cancer or in patients with significant co-morbidity and in the very elderly patients with less oncological control as a compromise. Patient selection is important and highly dependent upon a multidisciplinary approach. The most important factors are correct preoperative staging and perioperative radiochemotherapy to minimize the risk of local recurrence. The role of local treatment in palliation of advanced disease is unknown.

Introduction

It has been shown that laparoscopic total mesorectal excision in rectal cancer may result in less blood loss, quicker return to normal diet, less pain, less narcotic use and less immune response compared to open surgery. On the other hand, it is also evident that laparoscopic surgery has no significant influence on anastomotic leakage rates and mortality compared to conventional open surgery [1]. The same applies to disease-free survival rate and local recurrence rate. No results on

functional results are reported, but there are no indications that there would be significant differences between the laparoscopic and open procedure, as the surgical procedure itself is similar. Local treatment with transanal tumour excision is associated with significant decreased risk of morbidity and mortality compared to conventional surgery [2]. Other advantages are avoidance of decreased long-term anorectal dysfunction and need for temporary or definitive colostomy in addition to short hospital stay and fast recovery. However, oncological control may be compromised in local treatment and should be restricted to highly select patients with early cancer or in patients with significant co-morbidity and in the very elderly patients with less oncological control as a compromise. Patient selection and patient information is a great challenge for the multidisciplinary group.

N. Qvist, DMSci
Surgical Department A, Odense University Hospital,
DK-5000 Odense C, Denmark
e-mail: famqvist@dadlnet.dk

G. Baatrup (ed.), *Multidisciplinary Treatment of Colorectal Cancer*,
DOI 10.1007/978-3-319-06142-9_28, © Springer International Publishing Switzerland 2015

TEM

Transanal endoscopic microsurgery (TEM) was introduced in the early 1980s as a minimally invasive procedure designed for local resection of rectal lesions that otherwise would require major abdominal or abdominoperineal resections. Compared to conventional surgery, this method results in significantly reduced morbidity and mortality rates below 1 % [3]. TEM was initially proposed for large adenomas out of reach for transanal excision and unsuitable for colonoscopic removal. Later, the indication has expanded to early rectal carcinomas [4] or for palliation in more advanced stages. However, the role of TEM in rectal cancer is still a subject of much debate. The most common controversies are:

- Preoperative tumour and lymph node staging
- Adjuvant radiochemotherapy (pre- or postoperative)
- Salvage surgery
- Palliation

Thus, the indications for TEM-surgery are highly dependent upon a multidisciplinary approach involving endoscopists, pathologists, surgeons, radiologists and oncologists.

Preoperative Staging

Malignant changes in large polyps can be very difficult to diagnose even after several biopsies. Ideally, all tumours considered for TEM should undergo meticulous endorectal ultrasonography (ERUS) with the purpose to investigate invasive growth and local lymph node involvement. Its diagnostic accuracy in the assessment of early T1 carcinomas can be up to 89 %, with a sensitivity and specificity of 92 and 50 %, respectively, in experienced hands [5], and thus superior to digital examination by colorectal specialists, computed tomography and MRI [6, 7]. Despite these results, any patient with early rectal cancer undergoing TEM is recommended to undergo a full-thickness resection, preferably including mesorectal fat allowing adequate pathological examination of the specimen.

Precise preoperative staging is imperative since the procedure does not remove any, or only a few, of the perirectal lymph nodes. This is the main reason for a higher risk of local recurrence after TEM compared to conventional surgery. The recurrence rate for T1 cancer is 0–12 %, for T2 cancer 12–28 % and for T3 cancer 36–79 % [8–10]. In past decades, TEM has usually been indicated in patients with low-risk pT1N0 adenocarcinoma. Low-risk lesions are primarily those with a small-size (<3 cm), well-differentiated histology with the absence of vascular, lymphatic or perineural invasion. When these criteria are met, survival and local recurrence rates achieved by TEM are similar to those with conventional radical surgery. Local recurrence varies between 4.2 and 9.6 % with a 5-year survival rate varying from 79 to 100 % [11–15]. In the T1 high-risk patients, the local recurrence rate was as high as 39 % [16], and in these cases, salvage surgery must be considered.

In none of the studies were the recurrence rate and long-term results significant related to invasion of the submucosal layer (sm). Lymph node involvement of 1–3 % in sm1, 8 % in sm2 and 23 % in sm3 lesion has been reported [17]. This may suggest that the indication of TEM for cure should be reserved for patients with sm1 lesion. However, larger patients' series are needed for more firm conclusions. The preoperative staging of submucosal invasion is a great challenge to the standards of the equipment. In a study using high-resolution, three-dimensional endorectal ultrasonography, the overall kappa for the concordance between ultrasonographic and histopathologic staging for the degree of submocosal invasion (slight or massive) was 0.81, and no invasive carcinomas remained undetected [18].

No preoperative investigations (ERUS, MR or CT) have revealed a sufficient sensitivity or specificity for lymph node metastasis in patients with early cancer. This has led to the development of endoscopic posterior mesorectal resection with the preservation of the anorectal function and with a low rate of morbidity [19]. In a series of 11 patients with T1 tumour, 4–20 lymph nodes (median 8) were removed in each patient and without significant complications. In two patients, lymph node metastasis was detected. Thus, combining TEM with the posterior endoscopic mesorectal excision might reduce the local recurrence rate after TEM. However, further investigations with larger prospectively evaluated patient series are needed.

Adjuvant Radiochemotherapy (RCT)

Whereas the use of preoperative neoadjuvant RCT is controversial in early T1 cancers considered for TEM, it is mandatory in T2 or larger tumours where a local recurrence rate varying from 29 to 50 % has been reported [20]. In a study with 100 patients undergoing TEM after radiotherapy (54 patients with uT2 and 46 patients with uT3 uN0), complete response or microscopic residual tumour was found in three and 15 patients, respectively [21]. Minor complications occurred in 11 patients and major complications in two patients. The cancer specific survival rate after 90 months follow-up was 89 % and the overall survival rate 72 %. Salvage abdominoperineal surgery was performed in three patients, two of whom were disease-free at 15 and 19 months. Similar results were found in another study, where the patients were randomized to either TEM or laparoscopic resections [22]. Local or distant failure was 10 % after TEM and 12 % for laparoscopic resections. The survival was 95 % for TEM and 83 % for laparoscopic resection after a median follow-up of 56 months, but the difference was not statistically significant. Other studies have shown similar results. However, in all studies, the patients were highly selected, and the treatment modality with preoperative RCT followed by TEM should be reserved for patients with a known higher risk at conventional surgery. Another and unsolved problem is the place for postoperative RCT in patients, who at histology turned out to have a higher tumour stage than T1 at the final histology examination than judged preoperatively. In general, these patients should be offered salvage surgery, as the oncological outcome after salvage is comparable to primary radical surgery [14, 15, 20, 23]. In a study which included patients with T2 lesions, that following TEM were treated with 5-FU and radiation (54 Gy), local recurrence was observed in 14 %. However, salvage was successful in less than half of the patients with local recurrence [24]. There is no available information on the results of postoperative RCT compared to salvage surgery.

Local excision may be an effective alternative treatment if patients are selected by their response to preoperative CRT [25]. Following CRT, patients with T2 or T3 tumour who achieved either partial (15 %) or complete response (85 %) no recurrences after TEM was observed within a follow-up period of at 24 months. In a similar study with TEM performed on residuals after CRT, the recurrence rate was 2.85 % with a median follow-up of 38 months [21]. Partial clinical response (pCR) rates in the region of 15–30 % have been reported following preoperative RCT. However, clinical examination is only able to identify a small proportion of patients who actually achieve a pCR [26], and only about 25–50 % of patients achieving a complete clinical response (cCR) are confirmed as having a pathologically complete response (pCR) at subsequent surgery [27]. Despite this finding, support is growing in support of the concept of 'wait and see' when a cCR is observed following neoadjuvant CRT [28].

Salvage Surgery

Salvage surgery should be considered in cases where final histological examination reveals a T2 or larger tumours or any tumour with lymphovascular invasion and has not undergone preoperative CRT. The final decision may depend on patient preference and co-morbidity. In addition, salvage surgery should be considered in younger and healthy patients with the finding of a cancerous lesion in a removed lesion that preoperatively was judged as benign. Fifty-two locally excised rectal adenocarcinomas (29 transanal excision and 23 polypectomies) were followed by radical surgery (24 abdominoperineal resection and 28 low anterior resection) within 7 (range 1–29) days [29]. Radical surgery was performed because of a cancerous polyp (*n*=42), positive margins [5], lymphovascular invasion [3] and T3-staged cancer [2]. Twelve of 52 cancers (23 %) were found to have nodal involvement and 15 of 52 (29 %) showed residual cancer in the resected specimen. Survival was comparable to the matched controls with the exception of shorter survival in T3N1 cases, but numbers were too small for a definitive conclusion. Several other studies [14, 15, 20, 23] have shown good long-term results of salvage surgery after TEM for resected lesions with a bad prognosis (T2, T3, compromised margin, invasion of lymphatic vessels or areas of poor differentiation). However, these data should be interpreted with caution since they have mainly been collected from small series and a few case reports.

Palliation

Palliation is another indication for TEM in selected cases with advanced disease and high degree of co-morbidity. It is expected that some patients in the selected population may benefit from relieving the local tumour burden with a limited procedure relating morbidity and mortality. Available data comes from only a few cases, and no study has compared TEM with any other method of palliation in rectal cancer. Finally, the effect on quality of life has not been assessed, and no recommendation on patient selection for this special indication can be given so far.

Conclusion

Significant heterogeneity and patient selection limit conclusions from the current literature. Alternate end points to local recurrence may be required in assessing the optimal surgical approach, which balances oncological control with quality of life, and the probability of dying from diseases other than rectal cancer.

TEM in low-risk tumours (uT1) have equal cancer-free survival compared to conventional surgery with highly significant lower morbidity and mortality rates. Because of selection bias in the available literature, TEM should primarily be reserved for elderly patients or patients with significant co-morbidity. Patients with inadvertent histology (T2 or larger, positive margins, lymphovascular invasion and poor differentiation) after TEM should be offered salvage surgery. Preoperative radiochemotherapy is mandatory in patients with high-risk tumours (T2–3) considered for TEM. In cases with complete response on clinical examination, a 'wait and see' strategy may be considered. In patients with no response, conventional surgery may be considered and evaluated. The role of TEM in palliation is unknown.

References

1. Breukink S, Pierie J, Wiggers T. Laparoscopic versus open total mesorectal excision for rectal cancer. Cochrane Database Syst Rev. 2006;(4):CD005200.
2. De Graaf EJ, Doornebosch PG, Tollenaar RA, Meershoek-Klein Kranenbarg E, de Boer AC, Bekkering FC, van de Velde CJ. Transanal endoscopic microsurgery versus total mesorectal excision of T1 rectal adenocarcinomas with curative intention. Eur J Surg Oncol. 2009;35(12):1280–5.
3. Middleton PF, Sutherland LM, Maddern GJ. Transanal endoscopic microscopic micoresurgery. A systematic review. Dis Colon Rectum. 2005;48:270–84.
4. Buess G. Transanal endoscopic micorsurgery (TEM). J R Coll Surg Edinb. 1993;38:239–45.
5. Kulig J, Richter P, Gurda-Duda A, et al. The role and value of endorectal ultrasonograpjy in diagnosing T1 rectal tumors. Ultrasound Med Biol. 2006;32:469–72.
6. Saclarides TJ, Bhattacharyya AK, Britton-Kuzel C, et al. Predicting lymph node metastasis in rectal cancer. Dis Colon Rectum. 1994;37:52–7.
7. Schaffzin DM, Wong WD. Endorectal ultrasound in the preoperative evaluation of rectal cancer. Clin Colorectal Cancer. 2004;4:124–32.
8. Paty PB, Nash GM, Baron P, et al. Long-term results of local excision for rectal cancer. Ann Surg. 2002;236:522–9.
9. Madoubly KM, Remzi FH, Erkek BA, et al. Recurrence after transanal excision of T1 rectal cancer. Should we be concerned? Dis Colon Rectum. 2005;48:711–9.
10. Sengupta S, Tandra JJ. Local excision of rectal cancer. What is the evidence? Dis Colon Rectum. 2001;44:1345–61.

11. Heintz A, Mörschel M, Junginger T. Comparison of results after transanal endoscopic microsurgery and radical excision for T1 carcinom of the rectum. Surg Endosc. 1998;12:1145–8.
12. Winde G, Nottberg H, Keller R, et al. Transanal endoscopic microsurgery vs. anterior resection. Dis Colon Rectum. 1996;39:969–76.
13. Stipa F, Burza A, Lucandri G, et al. Outcomes for early rectal cancer managed with transanal endoscopic microsurgery. A 5-year follow-up study. Surg Endosc. 2006;20:541–5.
14. Lee W, Lee D, Choi S, et al. Trananal endoscopic microsurgery and radical surgery for T1 and T2 rectal cancer. Surg Endosc. 2003;17:1283–7.
15. Floyd ND, Saclarides TJ. Transanal endoscopic microsurgery resection of pT1 rectal tumors. Dis Colon Rectum. 2006;49:164–8.
16. Borschitz T, Heintz A, Junginger T. The influence of histopathologic criteria on the long-term prognosis of locally excised pT1 rectal carcinomas. Results of local excision (trananal endoscopic microsurgery) and immediate reoperation. Dis Colon Rectum. 2006;49:1500–5.
17. Tytherleigh MG, Warren BF, Mortensen NJ. Management of early rectal cancer. Br J Surg. 2008;95:409–23.
18. Santoro GA, Gizzi G, Pellegrini L, et al. The value of high-resolution three-dimensional endorectal ultrasonography in the management of submucosal invasive rectal tumors. Dis Colon Rectum. 2009;52:1837–43.
19. Zerz A, Müller-Stich BP, Beck J. Endoscopic posterior mesorectal resection after transanal local excision of T1 carcinomas of the lower third of the rectum. Dis Colon Rectum. 2006;49:919–24.
20. Borschitz T, Heintz A, Junginger T. Transanal endoscopic microsurgical excision of pT2 rectal cancer. Results and possible indications. Dis Colon Rectum. 2007;50:292–301.
21. Lezoche E, Guerrieri M, Paganini AM, et al. Long-term results in patients with T2-3 N0 distal rectal cancer undergoing radiotherapy before trananal endoscopic microsurgery. Br J Surg. 2005;92:1546–52.
22. Lezoche E, Guerrieri M, Paganini AM et al. Transanal endoscopic versus total mesorectal laparoscopic resections of T2-N0 low rectal cancers after neoadjuvant treatment. A prospective randomized trial with a 3-years minimum follow-up period. Surg. Endosc. 2005;19(6):751–6.
23. Smith LE, Ko ST, Saclarides T. Transanal endoscopic microsurgery. Initial registry results. Dis Colon Rectum. 1996;39:79–84.
24. Steel Jr GD, Herndon JE, Bleday R, et al. Sphincter-sparing treatment for distal rectal adenocarcinoma. Ann Surg Oncol. 1999;6:433–41.
25. Kim JC, Yeatman TJ, Coppula D, et al. Local excision of T2 and T3 rectal cancers after downstaging chemoradiation. Ann Surg. 2001;234:352–8.
26. Guillem JG, Chessin DB, Shia J, et al. Clinical examination following preoperative chemoradiation for rectal cancer is not a reliable surrogate endpoint. J Clin Oncol. 2005;23:3475–9.
27. Tulchinsky H, Rabau M, Shacham-Shemueli E, et al. Can rectal cancers with pathological T0 after neoadjuvant chemoradiation (ypT0) be treated by transanal excision alone? Ann Surg Oncol. 2005;13:347–52.
28. Habr-Gama A, de Souza PM, Ribeiro U, et al. Low rectal cancer: impact of radiation and chemotherapy on surgical treatment. Dis Colon Rectum. 1998;41:1087–96.
29. Hahnloser D, Wolff BG, Larson DW, Ping J, et al. Immediate radical resection after local excision of rectal cancer: an oncologic compromise? Dis Colon Rectum. 2005;48:429–37.

Printing: Ten Brink, Meppel, The Netherlands
Binding: Ten Brink, Meppel, The Netherlands